About the publisher

BPP Learning Media is dedicated to supporting aspiring professionals with top quality learning material. BPP Learning Media's commitment to success is shown by our record of quality, innovation and market leadership in paper-based and e-learning materials. BPP Learning Media's study materials are written by professionally-qualified specialists who know from personal experience the importance of top quality materials for success.

About The BMJ

The BMJ (formerly the British Medical Journal) in print has a long history and has been published without interruption since 1840. The BMJ's vision is to be the world's most influential and widely read medical journal. Our mission is to lead the debate on health and to engage, inform, and stimulate doctors, researchers, and other health professionals in ways that will improve outcomes for patients. We aim to help doctors to make better decisions. BMJ, the company, advances healthcare worldwide by sharing knowledge and expertise to improve experiences, outcomes and value.

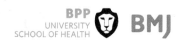

Contents

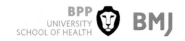

About the editors

Dr Babita Jyoti is a Radiation Oncologist with a special interest in Paediatric Proton Therapy.She graduated in Medicine in India followed by training in UK and obtained MRCP (UK) & FRCR (UK). She trained as a Clinical Oncologist at Clatterbridge Cancer Centre. She is currently working at the University of Florida Health Proton Therapy Institute in Paediatric Proton Therapy. She has been a PBL tutor and an OSCE examiner at Manchester Medical School.

Dr Ahmed Hamad is a Registrar in General Surgery with special interest in Breast Surgery at Mid Cheshire Hospitals NHS Trust. He graduated in 1992 from Cairo University School of Medicine in Egypt. Initially trained in Surgical Oncology, he received a Masters Degree in Surgery in 1997 from Cairo University. After completing his training in General Surgery, he worked as a Specialist in Surgery in different hospitals in Egypt, Saudi Arabia and Kuwait. He has become a Member of the Royal College of Surgeons of England in 2009 and in 2010, he joined the NHS, initially in General Surgery and is currently developing more experience in Breast Surgery.

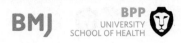

Introduction to Infectious Diseases and Public Health

"The world is changing very fast. Big will not beat small anymore. It will be the fast beating the slow." Rupert Murdoch.

The world is in the process of a major demographic transformation. Receding population growth in Western countries, especially working population, changes in age structure of most countries, open markets, new patterns and magnitudes of immigration, political and military conflicts will all lead to a completely different demographic world structure by the year 2025.

Antibiotics, one of the major breakthroughs of medicine in the 20th century, are at a crossroads. Most conventional antibiotics are gradually losing efficacy. More resistant strains of pathogens are emerging.

By looking at these major changes in demographics, one can easily see that this will inevitably be accompanied by a significant shift in the global distribution of infectious diseases. "Tropical" infections may not be tropical anymore! Historically eradicated pathogens are re-emerging. Infections previously treated with antibiotics may regain their power as life-threatening.

Taking all these factors into consideration it is apparent the focus on Infectious Diseases and Public Health needs to be on a global scale.

In this book you will find a carefully selected series of clinical reviews from The BMJ that we believe can help refresh and update knowledge on topics relevant to direct patient care in Infectious Diseases and Public Health.

Although systematic reviews and meta-analyses provide more comprehensive details, evidence and statistical analysis of certain topics, clinical reviews are of no less importance as they tend to be more applicable to the local situation than a systematic review, as it may take into account local shortages of equipment or personnel*.

In addition to relevance to day-to-day practice, we believe the fascinating diversity in this book is an advantage. From all areas in the United Kingdom to Canada to Australia, healthcare professionals from a broad range of specialties and from various grades in their careers, registrars, general practitioners, consultants and university professors have participated to deliver clinical reviews in their respective fields.

All articles are provided in a simple format and, at the same time, summarised tips and advices which can be of great value especially with the increasing work load and pressure experienced by healthcare professionals.

*Dr Norman Vetter, University of Wales College of Medicine, Cardiff, Wales, UK

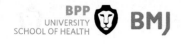

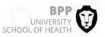

Investigating and managing pyrexia of unknown origin in adults

George M Varghese, professor[1], Paul Trowbridge, resident[2], Tom Doherty, consultant physician[3]

[1]Department of Medicine and Infectious Diseases, Christian Medical College, Vellore, India

[2]Department of Internal Medicine, Rhode Island Hospital/Brown University, Providence, USA

[3]Hospital for Tropical Diseases, London, UK

Correspondence to: G M Varghese
georgemvarghese@hotmail.com

Cite this as: BMJ 2010;341:c5470

DOI: 10.1136/bmj.c5470

http://www.bmj.com/content/341/bmj.c5470

Few clinical problems generate such a wide differential diagnosis as pyrexia (fever) of unknown origin. The initial definition proposed by Petersdorf and Beeson in 1961,[1] later revised, is "a fever of 38.3°C (101°F) or more lasting for at least three weeks for which no cause can be identified after three days of investigation in hospital or after three or more outpatient visits."[2][3][4] Essentially the term refers to a prolonged febrile illness without an obvious cause despite reasonable evaluation and diagnostic testing. A fever that is not self limiting for which no cause can be found can become a source of frustration for both patient and doctor. There is little consensus on how such patients should be investigated, although recent prospective studies have evaluated diagnostic protocols to suggest approaches to investigation.[3][5][6] We discuss evidence from epidemiological and diagnostic studies and suggest an approach to investigating and managing pyrexia of unknown origin.

Immunocompromised individuals, those with HIV infection, and patients admitted to hospital for other reasons with persistent or unexplained fever represent distinct subgroups in which the likely causes, diagnosis, and treatment of pyrexia usually differ from those in patients who are not immunocompromised. We do not discuss these subgroups in this review other than to provide definitions of pyrexia of unknown origin in different groups of patients (see box 1).

Sources and selection criteria

We searched for papers that were published between 1966 and August 2010 using appropriate MESH terms (pyrexia of unknown origin, fever of unknown origin) in the National Library of Medicine's computerised search service (PubMed and other related databases). We also consulted Cochrane database systematic reviews. We reviewed all relevant articles as well as the cited references to identify further articles.

SUMMARY POINTS

- Classic adult pyrexia of unknown origin is fever of 38.3°C or greater for at least 3 weeks with no identified cause after three days of hospital evaluation or three outpatient visits
- Common causes are infections, neoplasms, and connective tissue disorders
- A thorough history and physical examination, along with basic investigations will usually provide clues to a possible diagnosis that can guide the choice of further investigations
- If the initial evaluation provides no diagnostic clues, further investigations including imaging studies and serological tests may be indicated
- A watch and wait approach is acceptable in a clinically stable patient for whom no diagnosis can be made after extensive investigation, and the prognosis is likely to be good
- Empirical antibiotics are warranted only for individuals who are clinically unstable or neutropenic. In stable patients empirical treatment is discouraged, although NSAIDs may be used after investigations are complete. Empirical corticosteroid therapy is discouraged

How common is pyrexia of unknown origin?

The true incidence and prevalence of pyrexia of unknown origin are uncertain. A study of 153 patients reported the prevalence in hospitalised patients in the 1980s to be around 3%.[7] However, in the past two decades technological advances in diagnosis, particularly sophisticated imaging and improved culture techniques, have reduced the proportion of cases where the cause is unknown.[6]

What causes pyrexia of unknown origin?

Pyrexia of unknown origin has a wide differential diagnosis. The most frequently encountered underlying causes of the pyrexia are listed in box 2. Broadly speaking, the three most common causes are infection, neoplasia, and connective tissue disease. Many prospective and retrospective studies have shown that pyrexia of unknown origin is more often caused by an atypical presentation of a common disease than by something exotic.[5][6] Although causes of pyrexia of unknown origin vary substantially across geographical areas, a recent well conducted prospective cohort study and another retrospective evaluation from Europe reported the following proportions[8][9]—infection 15-30%, neoplasia 10-30%, connective tissue disease 33-40%, miscellaneous (such as drug fever, hyperthyroidism, and factitious fever) 5-14%, undiagnosed 20-30%.

Data from several large prospective studies suggest that infective causes are becoming less common, probably because advanced imaging techniques and improved culture methods have become more widely available.[10][11][12] For similar reasons, the proportion of cases of pyrexia of unknown origin attributed to neoplasia has steadily decreased over recent years.[5][6][13] These trends do not hold true in less developed societies where infection, often with mycobacteria, remains common and advanced diagnostic techniques are often unavailable.[14][15][16] Worth noting is that miscellaneous disorders are fairly common (see above).

How is pyrexia of unknown origin investigated?

Initial approach

History

Taking a thorough history and physical examination may often lead to a diagnosis. Repeating the history several times may elicit previously overlooked clues. Consider all symptoms as relevant since most patients with pyrexia of unknown origin present with a common disease that is atypically manifested.[5][6] Eliciting a history of comorbid conditions and previously treated diseases such as endocarditis, tuberculosis, rheumatic fever, and cancer may provide important diagnostic clues. A surgical history that

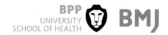

BOX 1 CLASSIFICATIONS OF PYREXIA OF UNKNOWN ORIGIN

- Classic pyrexia of unknown origin—Pyrexia for ≥3 weeks with no identified cause after evaluation in hospital for 3 days or ≥3 outpatient visits.
- Nosocomial pyrexia of unknown origin—Pyrexia in patients hospitalised for >48 hours with no infection present or incubating at admission, and in whom the diagnosis remains uncertain after ≥3 days of appropriate evaluation, which includes microbiological cultures that have been incubating for ≥2 days.
- Immunodeficient (neutropenic) pyrexia of unknown origin—Pyrexia in a patient with <500 neutrophils/μl in whom the diagnosis remains uncertain after ≥3 days of appropriate evaluation, which includes microbiological cultures that have been incubating for ≥2 days.
- HIV-associated pyrexia of unknown origin—Pyrexia in a patient with confirmed HIV infection lasting for >4 weeks as an outpatient or >3 days as an inpatient, in whom the diagnosis remains uncertain after ≥3 days of appropriate evaluation, which includes microbiological cultures that have been incubating for ≥2 days.

As classified by Durack and Street.[4]

BOX 2 COMMON CAUSES OF FEVER OF UNKNOWN ORIGIN

Infection
- Abdominal abscess
- Extrapulmonary/disseminated tuberculosis
- Infective endocarditis
- Osteoarticular infections
- Typhoid/enteric fevers
- Endemic mycosis
- Epstein-Barr virus infection
- Cytomegalovirus infection
- Brucellosis
- Leishmaniasis
- Prostatitis
- Malaria
- Rickettsial infections
- Dental abscess
- Chronic sinusitis

Neoplasm
- Lymphoma
- Hepatoma
- Hepatic metastasis
- Renal cell carcinoma
- Leukaemia
- Colon cancer
- Pancreatic cancer

Connective tissues disorder
- Systemic lupus erythematosis
- Adult onset Still's disease
- Autoimmune hepatitis
- Systemic vasculitis
- Mixed connective tissue disease
- Polymyalgia rhematica
- Inflammatory bowel disease
- Sarcoidosis
- Kikuchi's disease

Miscellaneous
- Drug fever
- Factitious fever
- Mediterranean familial fever
- Deep vein thrombosis/pulmonary embolism
- Hyperthyroidism

to endemic diseases such as malaria, histoplasmosis, or other fungal infections.

Potentially important clues may be found in aspects of the history that are not routinely discussed with patients, such as the sexual history; asking about specifics of sexual practices such as anal penetration leading to rectal abscesses may point to a possible source of infection. Ask about social habits, such as drug use, exposure to animals or pets, specifics of the patient's employment and hobbies. Enquire about unusual dietary habits, such as consumption of unpasteurised dairy products or rare meats. Check for any recent changes in medication that could have contributed to unexplained fever. A full obstetric and gynaecological history in women may provide clues to the underlying condition; for example a history of multiple miscarriages may suggest a connective tissue disease or pelvic pain may suggest tubo-ovarian pathology.

Documenting fever
A persistent fever needs to be accurately documented because the pattern of the fever and its relation with the pulse rate (particularly a temperature-pulse disparity) may point to an underlying cause. Accurate charting of the fever may require admission to hospital. Temperature-pulse disparity may have diagnostic relevance in infections with intracellular organisms such as typhoid, brucellosis, and legionellosis.

Careful physical examination
Fever could arise from pathology in any system, so a thorough physical examination is important. It should include a full neurological examination, musculoskeletal, ear-nose-throat, dermatological, lymphatic, and urogenital examinations, and fundoscopy. Box 3 lists some common symptoms and signs and the causes of pyrexia that may be associated with them. Some well known causes of pyrexia of unknown origin are associated with particular signs; for example, temporal artery tenderness in temporal arteritis, lymphadenopathy in lymphoma and disseminated tuberculosis, and a heart murmur in bacterial endocarditis. Some clinical findings, although rare, are virtually diagnostic, such as Roth's spots in infective endocarditis.

Basic investigations
The approach to investigating any patient with pyrexia of unknown origin should ideally be focused according to the patient's presentation and clinical signs. Basic laboratory and imaging studies may help to guide further evaluation. No list of tests has been widely accepted as being the minimal obligatory investigations, but basic investigations that have been suggested and used by researchers and clinicians in several studies[3 5 6 11] are listed in the first part of the diagnostic algorithm (fig 1). Additional testing for atypical presentations of diseases that are specific to certain regions, such as Lyme disease, malaria, or histoplasmosis, may also be indicated.

Further investigations
Clues gleaned from the history, physical examination, and first round of diagnostic evaluations should be the basis for subsequent investigations that are tailored to the individual patient as shown in the diagnostic algorithm (fig 1). However, in the absence of potential clues, there are some data directing what further studies are of utility. Recent prospective studies have highlighted the usefulness of early

provides information about the type of surgery performed, postoperative complications and any indwelling foreign material could also be relevant. Travel history is important because it may provide information about possible exposure

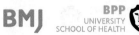

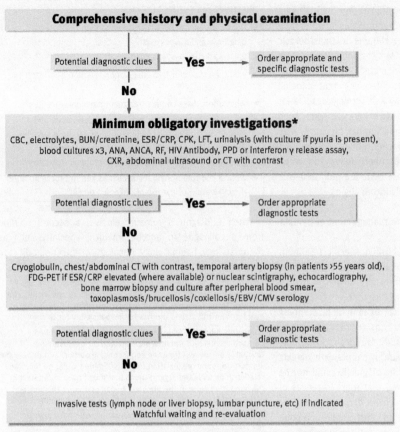

Comprehensive history and physical examination

Potential diagnostic clues — **Yes** → Order appropriate and specific diagnostic tests

No

Minimum obligatory investigations*

CBC, electrolytes, BUN/creatinine, ESR/CRP, CPK, LFT, urinalysis (with culture if pyuria is present), blood cultures x3, ANA, ANCA, RF, HIV Antibody, PPD or interferon γ release assay, CXR, abdominal ultrasound or CT with contrast

Potential diagnostic clues — **Yes** → Order appropriate diagnostic tests

No

Cryoglobulin, chest/abdominal CT with contrast, temporal artery biopsy (in patients >55 years old), FDG-PET if ESR/CRP elevated (where available) or nuclear scintigraphy, echocardiography, bone marrow biopsy and culture after peripheral blood smear, toxoplasmosis/brucellosis/coxiellosis/EBV/CMV serology

Potential diagnostic clues — **Yes** → Order appropriate diagnostic tests

No

Invasive tests (lymph node or liver biopsy, lumbar puncture, etc) if indicated
Watchful waiting and re-evaluation

*Peripheral blood smear should be done at this stage if patient has recently travelled to malaria endemic areas or if CBC suggests bone marrow involvement. CBC=complete blood count; BUN=blood urea nitrogen; ESR=erythrocyte sedimentation rate; CRP=C-reactive protein; CPK=creatine phosphokinase; LFT=liver function test; ANA=antinuclear antibody; ANCA=antineutrophilic cytoplasmic antibody; RF=rheumatoid factor; PPD=purified protein derivative; CXR=chest radiograph; CT=computed tomography; FDG-PET=fluoro-2-deoxy-D-glucose-positron emission tomography, EBV=Epstein-Barr virus, CMV=cytomegalovirus.

Algorithm for evaluation of fever of unknown origin

BOX 3 COMMON SIGNS AND SYMPTOMS AND ASSOCIATED CAUSES OF PYREXIA

- Altered mentation—tuberculous meningitis, cryptococcal meningitis, carcinomatous meningitis, brucellosis, typhoid fever, sarcoid meningitis
- Arthritis or arthralgia—systemic lupus erythematosus, infective endocarditis, Lyme disease, lymphogranuloma venereum, Whipple's disease, brucellosis, inflammatory bowel disease
- Animal contact—brucellosis, toxoplasmosis, cat scratch disease, psittacosis, leptospirosis, Q fever, rat bite fever
- Cough—tuberculosis, Q fever, typhoid fever, sarcoidosis, Legionnaires' disease
- Conjunctival suffusion—leptospirosis, relapsing fever, Rocky Mountain spotted fever
- Epistaxis—Wegener's granulomatosis, relapsing fever, psittacosis
- Epididymo-orchitis—tuberculosis, lymphoma, polyarteritis nodosa, brucellosis, leptospirosis, infectious mononucleosis
- Hepatomegaly—lymphoma, disseminated tuberculosis, metastatic carcinoma of liver, alcoholic liver disease, hepatoma, relapsing fever, granulomatous hepatitis, Q fever, typhoid fever, malaria, visceral leishmaniasis
- Lymphadenopathy—lymphoma, cat scratch disease, tuberculosis, lymphomogranuloma venereum, infectious mononucleosis, cytomegalovirus infection, toxoplasmosis, HIV infection, brucellosis, Whipple's disease, Kikuchi's disease
- Renal angle tenderness—perinephric abscess, chronic pyelonephritis
- Splenomegaly—leukaemia, lymphoma, tuberculosis, brucellosis, subacute bacterial endocarditis, cytomegalovirus infection, Epstein-Barr virus mononucleosis, rheumatoid arthritis, sarcoidosis, psittacosis, relapsing fever, alcoholic liver disease, typhoid fever, Kikuchi's disease
- Splenic abscess—subacute bacterial endocarditis, brucellosis, enteric fever, melioidosis
- Subconjunctival hemorrhage—infective endocarditis, trichinosis, leptospirosis
- Uveitis—tuberculosis, sarcoidosis, adult Still's disease, systemic lupus erythematosus, Behcet's disease

---

use of FDG-PET ([18F] fluoro-2-deoxy-D-glucose positron emission tomography), which may be useful in helping to pinpoint a source of fever.[10] [11] [17] Fluoro-2-deoxy-D-glucose is preferentially taken up by cells such as tumour and inflammatory cells, in which glucose metabolism is high. In a systematic review of eight prospective and retrospective studies including 302 patients, FDG-PET localised pathology directing further tests that led to diagnosis in over a third of patients.[18] The diagnostic yield may be increased further by simultaneously using FDG-PET with conventional computed tomography (CT). Several small retrospective studies have shown sensitivities from 56% to100%, specificities from 75% to 81%, and negative predictive values of 100%, when a combination of CT and FDG-PET scanning is used.[19] [20] [21] Notably, FDG-PET was of no diagnostic benefit unless patients had an elevated erythrocyte sedimentation rate or raised concentrations of C-reactive protein.[18]

Nuclear scintigraphy, for example with ^{67}Ga-citrate and ^{111}In labelled leukocytes, is a much cheaper and more widely available imaging technique that may perform a similar role in localising pathology, though it is more time consuming and less sensitive and specific than FDG-PET. In a retrospective study evaluating the contribution of ^{67}Ga scintigraphy in 145 cases of pyrexia of unknown origin in Belgium between 1980 and 1989, only 29% of the scans were considered helpful in diagnosis and 49% of the abnormal scans were considered noncontributory to the diagnosis.[22] The limited specificity and the generally unfavourable characteristics of ^{67}Ga scintigraphy makes it less attractive than FDG-PET. A recent retrospective study including 31 patients with pyrexia of unknown origin, ^{111}In leukocyte scintigraphy was reported to be helpful in 19% of all cases.[23] However, the probability of reaching a diagnosis was observed in 71% with a sensitivity of 75% and specificity 83%. Leukocyte scintigraphy may be helpful in diagnosing inflammatory and infectious conditions and rarely of use in neoplasm.

Several studies, including two large multicentre prospective analyses, have looked at the usefulness of other investigations in the absence of diagnostic clues. The evidence from these studies supported the use of chest CT and abdominal CT or ultrasound (if not already performed), looking specifically for: abscesses, lymph nodes, or splenomegaly; cryoglobulins (mixed cyroglobulinaemia was surprisingly common even in the absence of known risk factors); and temporal artery biopsy, particularly in patients older than 55.[6] [10] Although many previous studies supported temporal artery biopsy for patients older than 55 in the absence of clues indicating potential temporal arteritis, the authors thought this invasive procedure should be done later in the process of evaluation as temporal arteritis was a less prominent cause of pyrexia of unknown origin than previous studies had indicated.[10]

Evidence from one small but well done and recent retrospective analysis showed that bone marrow aspirate with trephine biopsy was diagnostic in nearly a fifth of patients and "helpful" for diagnosis in nearly a quarter. This was particularly, though not exclusively, true in the presence of thrombocytopenia or anaemia (haemoglobin <110 g/l). Bone marrow culture is thought to have a lower yield in immunocompetent individuals than in those who are immunocompromised, although this is probably less true in non-industrialised societies.[24] Echocardiography is a non-invasive test that may be useful even in people with negative blood culture and without an audible heart

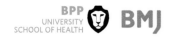

murmur. Transoesophageal echocardiography (which has a diagnostic sensitivity of 95-100%, and a specificity of 98% for endocardial vegetations) is preferable to transthoracic echocardiography (sensitivity 63%, specificity 98%).[25] Epstein-Barr virus, cytomegalovirus, toxoplasmosis, brucellosis, and coxiellosis are infections that can all present in a very non-specific way and serological tests for these infections may be useful. More invasive tests, such as lymph node or liver biopsy, and lumbar puncture, may be considered when the cause of fever remains unidentified after two step evaluation as described above and when clinical suspicion shows that these tests are indicated—see the later part of the diagnostic algorithm (fig 1).

What is a reasonable approach to management of pyrexia of unknown origin?

Once a diagnosis has been established specific treatment can be started. For patients in whom a cause for the fever is not found and who are not clinically unwell, watching and waiting is reasonable. During this time of observation re-assess the history and physical examination, stepping back to re-evaluate the data, and consider new avenues to pursue. One large prospective study found an attributable mortality of only 3.2% at five years in people with pyrexia of unknown origin where a specific diagnosis could not be reached.[26] The same study showed that most instances of pyrexia of unknown origin in which no diagnosis could be made resolved spontaneously, all of which suggests a good prognosis for people who remain without a diagnosis.[26]

In most cases where the individual is clinically stable experts consider empirical treatment to be unnecessary. Patients who are clinically unstable or neutropenic require prompt and appropriate antibiotic treatment. Empiric tuberculosis drugs may be considered where tuberculosis is prevalent and suspected but cannot be confirmed. Rifampicin may suppress fever even when not from an infectious cause. Empirical use of steroids is generally discouraged because it may mask symptoms and lead to delayed diagnosis of, for example, an underlying haematological malignancy. Several experts have recommended treatment with non-steroidal anti-inflammatory drugs for patients who have already had exhaustive investigations without finding an underlying cause. This treatment may be beneficial to patients in some situations, such as an underlying inflammatory condition. However, the theory that a patient's response to such drugs allows the doctor to differentiate neoplastic from other causes of pyrexia of unknown origin has been refuted.[27]

ADDITIONAL EDUCATIONAL RESOURCES

- Cunha B. *Fever of unknown origin*. In: Gorbach SL, Bartlett JG, Blacklow NR, eds. *Infectious diseases*, 3rd ed. 2004—well written article appropriate for helping to generate a sound differential diagnosis based on organ involvement, symptoms, or epidemiological risk factors, with a wealth of resources available within the rest of the text for specifics of infectious diseases.

- Mandell GL, Bennett JE, Dolin R. *Principles and practice of infectious disease*, 7th ed. 2009, pp 779-89—comprehensive overview of pyrexia of unknown origin. The different types of pyrexia of unknown origin with causes and approach are separately discussed.

- *Infectious Disease Clinics of North America* 2007, 21:857-1232—an entire issue of *Infectious Disease Clinics of North America* devoted to pyrexia of unknown origin, with an emphasis on the diagnostic approach.

QUESTIONS FOR FUTURE RESEARCH

- Does early use of FDG-PET combined with CT hasten diagnosis and lower costs?
- What evaluations are cost-effective?
- What is a cost-effective obligatory evaluation in a resource limited setting?
- What effect does empiric treatment have on outcomes?
- Could international standardisation of definitions and evaluation lead to the creation of large database systems through which the epidemiology and management of pyrexia of unknown origin could be properly evaluated?
- What is the role of new tests such as serum procalcitonin in the evaluation of pyrexia of unknown origin?

When a diagnosis remains elusive, a second opinion from a colleague in another medical specialty such as rheumatology, haematology, oncology, or infectious disease may be helpful.

Contributors: GMV was responsible for the initial plan; GMV and PT were responsible for data collection, interpretation, and manuscript drafting. TD was responsible for manuscript editing. GMV is the guarantor for this paper and has full responsibility for this article.

Competing interests: All authors have completed the Unified Competing Interest form at www.icmje.org/coi_disclosure.pdf (available on request from the corresponding author) and declare no support from any organisation for the submitted work: no financial relationships with any organisations that might have an interest in the submitted work in the previous 3 years: no other relationships or activities that could appear to have influenced the submitted work.

Provenance and peer review: Commissioned, externally peer reviewed.

1   Petersdorf RG, Beeson PB. Fever of unexplained origin: report on 100 cases. *Medicine (Baltimore)* 1961;40:1-30.
2   Petersdorf RG. Fever of unknown origin. An old friend revisited. *Arch Intern Med* 1992;152:21-2.
3   Knockaert DC, Vanderschueren S, Blockmans D. Fever of unknown origin in adults: 40 years on. *J Intern Med* 2003;253:263-75.
4   Durack DT, Street AC. Fever of unknown origin—reexamined and redefined. *Curr Clin Top Inf Dis* 1991;11:35-51.
5   Arnow PM, Flaherty JP. Fever of unknown origin. *Lancet* 1997;350:575-80.
6   Bleeker-Rover CP, Vos FJ, de Kleijn EM, Mudde AH, Dofferhof TS, Richter C, et al. A prospective multicenter study on fever of unknown origin: the yield of a structured diagnostic protocol. *Medicine* 2007;86:26-38.
7   Iikuni Y, Okada J, Kondo H, Kashiwazaki S. Current fever of unknown origin 1982-1992. *Intern Med* 1994;33:67-73.
8   Efstathiou SP, Pefanis AV, Tsiakou AG, Skeva II, Tsioulos DI, Achimastos AD, Mountokalakis TD. Fever of unknown origin: discrimination between infectious and non-infectious causes. *Eur J Intern Med* 2010;21:137-43.
9   Hot A, Jaisson I, Girard C, French M, Durand DV, Rousset H, et al. Yield of bone marrow examination in diagnosing the source of fever of unknown origin. *Arch Intern Med* 2009;169:2018-23.
10 De Kleijn EM, van Leir HJ, van der Meer JW. Fever of unknown origin (FUO). II. Diagnostic procedures in a prospective multicenter study of 167 patients. *Medicine* 1997;76:401-14.
11 De Kleijn EM, Vandenbroucke JP, van der Meer JW. Fever of unknown origin (FUO). I. A prospective multicenter study of 167 patients with FUO, using fixed epidemiologic entry criteria. *Medicine* 1997;76:392-400.
12 Vanderschueren S, Knockaert D, Adriaenssens T, Demey W, Durnez A, Blockmans D, et al. From prolonged febrile illness to fever of unknown origin: the challenge continues. *Arch Intern Med* 2003;163:1033-41.
13 Armstrong WS, Katz JT, Kazanjian PH. Human immunodeficiency virus-associated fever of unknown origin: a study of 70 patients in the United States and review. *Clin Infect Dis* 1999;28:341-5.
14 Saltoglu N, Tasova Y, Midikli D, Aksu HS, Sanli A, Dündar IH. Fever of unknown origin in Turkey: evaluation of 87 cases during a nine-year period of study. *J Infect* 2004;48:81-5.
15 Kejariwal D, Sarkar N, Chakraborti SK, Agarwal V, Roy S. Pyrexia of unknown origin: a prospective study of 100 cases. *J Postgrad Med* 2001;47:104-7.
16 Zheng M, Lin H, Luo S, Xu L, Zeng Y, Cheb Y. Fever of unknown origin in the elderly: nine years' experience in China. *Trop Doctor* 2008;38:221-2.
17 Bleeker-Rovers CP, Vos FJ, Mudde AH, Dofferhof As, de Geus-Oei LF, Rijnders AJ, et al. A prospective multi-centre study of the value of FDG-PET as part of a structured diagnostic protocol in patients with fever of unknown origin. *Eur J Nucl Med Mol Imaging* 2007;34:694-703.

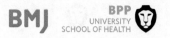

18 Bleeker-Rovers CP, van der Meer JW, Oyen WJ. Fever of unknown origin. *Semin Nucl Med* 2009;39:81-7.

19 Ferda J, Ferdova E, Zahlava J, Matejovic M, Kreuzberg B. Fever of unknown origin: a value of 18F-FDG-PET/CT with integrated full diagnostic isotropic CT imaging. *Eur J Rad* 2010;73:518-25.

20 Balink H, Collins J, Bruyn G, Gemmel F, et al. F-18 FDG PET/CT in the diagnosis of fever of unknown origin. *Clin Nucl Med* 2009;34:862-8.

21 Keider Z, Gurman-Balbir A, Gaitini D, Israel O. Fever of unknown origin: the role of 18F-FDG PET/CT. *J Nucl Med* 2008;49:1980-5.

22 Knockaert DC, Mortelmans LA, De Roo MC, Bobbaers HJ. Clinical value of gallium-67 scintigraphy in evaluation of fever of unknown origin. *Clin Infect Dis* 1994;18:601-5.

23 Kjaer A, Lebech AM. Diagnostic value of ¹¹¹In-granulocyte scintigraphy in patients with fever of unknown origin. *J Nucl Med* 2002;43:140-4.

24 Hot A, Jaisson I, Girard C, French M, Durand DV, Rousset H, et al. Yield of bone marrow examination in diagnosing the source of fever of unknown origin. *Arch Intern Med* 2009;169:2018-23.

25 Erbel R, Rohmann S, Drexler M, Mohr-Kahaly S, Gerharz CD, Iversen S, et al. Improved diagnostic value of echocardiography in patients with infective endocarditis by transoesophageal approach. A prospective study. *Eur Heart J* 1988;9:43-53.

26 Knockaert DC, Dujardin KS, Bobbaers HJ. Long-term follow-up of patients with undiagnosed fever of unknown origin. *Arch Intern Med* 1996;156:618-20.

27 Vanderschueren S, Knockaert DC, Peetermans WE, Bobbaers HJ. Lack of value of the naproxen test in the differential diagnosis of prolonged fever. *Am J Med* 2003;115:572-5.

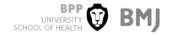

Outpatient parenteral antimicrobial therapy

Ann L N Chapman, consultant in infectious diseases

Department of Infection and Tropical Medicine, Royal Hallamshire Hospital, Sheffield Teaching Hospitals NHS Foundations Trust, Sheffield S10 2JF, UK

Correspondence to: Ann L N Chapman ann.chapman@sth.nhs.uk

Cite this as: BMJ 2013;346:f1585

DOI: 10.1136/bmj.f1585

http://www.bmj.com/content/346/bmj.f1585

Outpatient parenteral antimicrobial therapy (OPAT) allows patients to be given intravenous antibiotics in the community rather than as an inpatient. First developed in the 1970s in the US for the treatment of children with cystic fibrosis,[1] OPAT has expanded substantially and is now standard practice in many countries.[2][3] In the UK, uptake has been much slower, although OPAT is now being increasingly used in both primary and secondary care, driven by a national focus on efficiency savings in healthcare, improving patient experience, and provision of care closer to home. It is important that medical practitioners are aware both of the opportunities that OPAT presents and of the potential risks of treatment outside hospital for patients with serious and often complex infections. This article aims to describe the clinical practice of OPAT, highlight potential risks, and explore how these may be reduced.

What is OPAT?

OPAT is the administration of intravenous antimicrobial therapy to patients in an outpatient setting or in their own home. It can be used for patients with severe or deep seated infections who require parenteral treatment but are otherwise stable and well enough not to be in hospital; these patients may be discharged early to an OPAT service or may avoid hospital admission altogether.

What type of infections can be treated?

Cellulitis

OPAT is most widely used for patients with soft tissue sepsis, mainly cellulitis.[4][5] Cellulitis accounts for 1-2% of emergency hospital admissions in England and Wales, or about 80 000 admissions annually.[6] Around 30% of patients presenting to hospital with cellulitis have moderately severe infection that requires intravenous antibiotics but do not have severe systemic sepsis necessitating inpatient care.[7][8] One randomised controlled trial of twice daily intravenous cefazolin administered by a nurse at home compared with standard inpatient care showed no significant difference in duration of intravenous or subsequent oral antibiotic therapy, patient functional outcomes, or complications but reported improved patient satisfaction with home treatment.[9]

Data from several large retrospective case series show that outpatient treatment with once daily ceftriaxone is also safe and effective, with good short and long term clinical outcomes, and this is now the predominant antibiotic used for outpatient intravenous treatment of cellulitis in the UK.[4][5][10] If there is concern about possible meticillin resistant Staphylococcus aureus (MRSA) infection, teicoplanin or daptomycin are alternatives.[5] Increasingly a nurse led model of care is being used for management of cellulitis outside hospital, with treatment set out in a protocol and limited input from doctors.[11]

Bone and joint infections

Patients with bone and joint infections invariably require prolonged parenteral antibiotic courses, and several large retrospective case series have shown that outpatient treatment can be used successfully in this group.[12][13][14] Patients may receive outpatient antibiotics within a two stage revision of an infected joint or as sole therapy for septic arthritis or osteomyelitis. One UK study reported outcomes for 198 patients with a range of bone and joint infections treated by OPAT. Seventy three per cent of patients were disease free at median follow-up of 60 weeks; patients with advanced age, MRSA infection, and diabetic foot infections were more likely to have a relapse or recurrence.[12]

Infective endocarditis

US, European, and UK guidelines now recommend OPAT as part of routine clinical care for patients with infective endocarditis.[15][16][17] Although initially recommended only for uncomplicated native valve infections with low risk organisms, there is increasing evidence that OPAT is safe in more complex patients after an initial period of inpatient care, as long as the potential risks are assessed on a case by case basis and treatment is administered through a formal OPAT service with the appropriate safeguards to minimise risk.[18][19] Such safeguards include daily nurse review, once or twice weekly physician review, and the establishment of an escalation pathway for medical staff familiar with the case to be informed of potential problems.[15][16]

Other uses

Use of OPAT has been described for numerous other infections, including resistant urinary tract infections, central nervous system infections, and low risk neutropenic sepsis.[20][21][22] The availability of long acting antibiotics such as ceftriaxone, teicoplanin, and daptomycin and the diversity of models for delivering OPAT allows most stable patients requiring intravenous antimicrobials to be considered for outpatient treatment. However, there are some situations where it is less useful—for example, patients with pneumonia are best managed either with outpatient oral therapy for mild infection or intravenous antibiotics in hospital for more severe cases.[23]

Which patients are suitable?

Patients referred for outpatient treatment need to be clinically stable, both in terms of their general condition and their infection. Thus they should have stable vital signs and be at low risk of their infection progressing or developing serious complications.[2][3][24] Patients with a diagnosis of cellulitis, for example, need to be assessed by

SUMMARY POINTS

- Outpatient parenteral antimicrobial therapy (OPAT) allows patients requiring intravenous antibiotics to be treated outside hospital
- OPAT is suitable for many infections, especially cellulitis, bone and joint infections, and infective endocarditis
- Antibiotics can be administered in an outpatient unit, at home by a nurse, or at home by the patient or a carer
- Patients should be assessed by a doctor and specialist nurse to determine medical and social suitability
- Evidence suggests that OPAT is safe as long as it is administered through a formal service structure to minimise risk

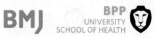

a healthcare practitioner competent to exclude other more serious conditions that could potentially be confused with cellulitis, such as septic arthritis or necrotising fasciitis. Patients with endocarditis are more likely to develop potentially life threatening complications in the first two weeks of therapy, and outpatient administration is therefore not recommended until after this period.[16] Determination of suitability will generally require a medical review, unless a protocol is in place for assessment by another trained healthcare practitioner.[11]

Other health and social issues also need to be explored. OPAT requires the patient to engage actively and reliably with therapy, and thus patients with substance misuse or serious mental health problems may not be suitable. In addition, there must be no other barrier to discharge from hospital. For example, although diabetic foot infections may be suitable for OPAT, many patients will require other care that has to be provided in hospital, including adjustment of diabetic control, vascular assessment, and surgical intervention.[25] Finally, home based care must be suitable from a social perspective—for example, an acceptable home environment, access to a telephone, adequate transport, and support from family or carers, In general the OPAT nurse, in collaboration with other professional teams, is best placed to assess these additional factors, and current OPAT guidelines recommend that patients should be assessed by both a doctor and nurse before being accepted for outpatient administration.[2 3 24]

How is OPAT delivered?

Three service models can be used to deliver OPAT, all of which have been shown to be effective: an ambulatory care centre, a nurse attending the patient's home, or self administration. The approach used varies among countries—for example, infusion centres have been the dominant model in the US whereas services in Australia tend to follow the "hospital in the home" visiting nurse model. However, it is becoming increasingly common for individual OPAT services to offer all three models, allowing treatment to be tailored to each patient's circumstances.[2] Most OPAT services described in the literature are based in acute hospitals, predominantly in specialist infectious diseases units.[4 5 13 18] Services may also be established by other inpatient specialist teams or in frontline emergency or acute medicine units[9]: in the UK, the Society of Acute Medicine has recently established a working group to promote the development of OPAT in this setting.

In the ambulatory care centre model, the patient attends a healthcare facility daily, or as required, with antibiotics administered by a healthcare practitioner. Treatment in the patient's home may be administered by community nurses, outreach nurses from the acute hospital, or nurses provided through a private healthcare company. In the third model patients (or carers) are taught to administer therapy; this has the advantages of engaging patients in their care, allowing more flexibility of dose frequency and timing, and reducing staffing costs. Despite theoretical concerns about line infections, two large retrospective studies have shown that self administration is as safe as administration by a healthcare worker in the community.[14 26]

The model of OPAT used largely determines the type of intravenous access. Options include temporary "butterfly" needles that are inserted and removed for each dose, short term peripheral cannulas or, for longer antibiotic courses, peripherally inserted central cannulas or tunnelled central lines. Bolus injections or infusions may be used, depending on the choice of antimicrobial agent(s). Infusions allow higher doses to be administered but require additional administration time and training.[27] Novel delivery devices allow patients greater freedom to continue normal daily activities. For example, portable elastomeric infusion devices can be carried in the patient's pocket or a carrying pouch and deliver continuous infusions over 24 hours.[3]

What are the benefits?

The clinical effectiveness of OPAT has been established for a wide range of infections through numerous retrospective case series, as outlined above. However, there have been few randomised controlled trials comparing OPAT with inpatient care. Furthermore, there are no published data on clinical efficacy of OPAT services based entirely in a community setting, although there are descriptions of collaborative services across primary and secondary care sectors.[9]

OPAT has been shown to be cost effective in many healthcare contexts. One retrospective study from a UK service compared the actual costs of OPAT over two years with the theoretical costs of inpatient care for the same patient cohort and found that OPAT cost 47% of equivalent inpatient national average costs.[4] However, in reality there is a wide range of funding arrangements for OPAT in operation across the UK, and in some instances OPAT may offer little cost advantage to commissioners over inpatient care. A national tariff for OPAT would allow consistency and equity and support wider use.

In addition to reducing direct costs, OPAT frees inpatient capacity, which can then be used either to admit further patients or as part of a planned reduction in bed capacity. More detailed modelling of these downstream benefits has not been undertaken but might provide added evidence of OPAT's cost effectiveness.

Finally, there is increasing evidence that OPAT is associated with a very low rate of healthcare associated infection. Despite theoretical concerns about the use of broad spectrum agents such as ceftriaxone, the risk of *Clostridium difficile* infection seems to be low: a meta-analysis of three large UK OPAT cohorts found the rate of *C difficile* infection to be 0.1%,[10] although there are no published prospective data.

What are the risks?

Despite these benefits, OPAT is associated with increased clinical risk compared with inpatient care because of the reduced level of supervision. At least 25% of patients having OPAT experience an adverse reaction of some type, ranging from mild antibiotic associated diarrhoea to severe line infections.[24] The treatment pathway—from patient selection, determination of the therapeutic regimen and intravenous access device to communication with other teams and ongoing monitoring during therapy—provides numerous opportunities for error.[28] In addition, as OPAT is used increasingly for more complex infections in patients with serious comorbidities, the likelihood of adverse events unrelated to the infection increases. A retrospective survey of US physicians involved in OPAT found that 68% had seen at least one major adverse event in their patients in the preceding year,[29] highlighting the importance of a formal governance structure. The adverse events included unexpected death, line related bacteraemia, air embolism, drug hypersensitivity, and drug induced blood dyscrasia.

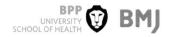

About 10% of patients will require readmission, with higher rates for patients with more complex infections.[4] [5] [14] [18] [19] In addition, many patients require further unplanned input during therapy: one study found that 12% of OPAT patients needed urgent advice or an unscheduled home visit.[30] Thus it is essential that the service has an established system for 24 hour access to clinical support and a formal (re)admission pathway to secondary care.

One further potential risk is overuse of intravenous antimicrobial therapy as an alternative to oral agents purely because an OPAT service exists. Similarly, there is also a risk that a broad spectrum once daily parenteral antimicrobial agent could be chosen in preference to a potentially more efficacious agent requiring multiple daily doses for reasons of convenience alone. OPAT should therefore operate within the context of an antibiotic stewardship programme, and it is essential that a microbiologist or infectious diseases physician is involved in both the initial design of antibiotic protocols and ongoing patient care. Several studies have found that assessment of referred patients by an infection specialist results in reduced use of intravenous therapy, improved clinical care, and substantial cost savings.[31] [32] [33]

How can the risks be reduced?

It is clear that OPAT delivered through a formal service structure is safer than when delivered through ad hoc arrangements. Several bodies have published recommendations on delivery of OPAT[2] [3] [34] and the aim of these is to ensure that the risks associated with OPAT are minimised. In the UK a consensus statement on the use of OPAT was recently published as a joint initiative between the British Society for Antimicrobial Chemotherapy and the British Infection Association.[24] It covers service structure, patient selection criteria, antimicrobial selection and delivery, frequency and type of clinical and blood test monitoring, monitoring of outcomes, and clinical governance. It recommends the core OPAT team should comprise, as a minimum, an OPAT specialist nurse, doctor, infection specialist (either an infectious diseases physician or a microbiologist), and a pharmacist. A doctor with suitable training and experience (who may also be the infection specialist, when he or she delivers hands-on clinical care) should take responsibility for management decisions for each patient, in collaboration with the team. Although patients on prolonged courses of antimicrobials can be reviewed weekly, or less frequently if stable, those receiving treatment for cellulitis should be reviewed daily to allow switching from intravenous to oral therapy as soon as clinically appropriate.

What is the future of OPAT in the UK?

OPAT offers a rare opportunity not only to improve patient choice while maintaining service quality but also to reduce healthcare costs and improve service efficiency. Use of OPAT is likely to continue to expand in the UK, as in many other countries, driven by enthusiasm for increasing care delivery in the community as well as by cost pressures and patient choice. OPAT was recently cited as one of five antimicrobial prescribing decision options in Department of Health guidance on antibiotic stewardship.[35] Services will continue to be developed both in primary and secondary care, and it is likely that integrated services across sectors will be established in order to combine primary care's capacity and expertise in home treatment with the specialist knowledge and back-up of secondary care.

SOURCES AND SELECTION CRITERIA

References were sourced through a systematic review of the literature undertaken for the UK OPAT Good Practice Recommendations in 2012. The search included all English language articles between 1998 and 2010, and was further updated with a search of PubMed, Medline, and Cochrane databases. Published OPAT guidelines from other countries and key reviews were also used, as well as the author's knowledge of the literature.

ADDITIONAL EDUCATION RESOURCES

E-OPAT (http://e-opat.com)—an online resource for setting up OPAT services from the British Society for Antimicrobial Chemotherapy

Competing interests: The author has completed the ICMJE uniform disclosure form at www.icmje.org/coi_disclosure.pdf (available on request from her) and declares: no support from any organisation for the submitted work; no financial relationships with any organisations that might have an interest in the submitted work in the previous 3 years. The author co-chaired the development of the 2012 UK OPAT good practice recommendations.

Provenance and peer review: Not commissioned; externally peer reviewed.

1 Rucker RW, Harrison GM. Outpatient intravenous medications in the management of cystic fibrosis. *Pediatrics* 1974;54:358-60.
2 Tice AD, Rehm SJ, Dalovisio JR, Bradley JS, Martinelli LP, Graham DR, et al. Practice guidelines for outpatient parenteral antibiotic therapy. IDSA guidelines. *Clin Infect Dis* 2004;38:1651-72.
3 Howden BP, Grayson ML. Hospital-in-the-home treatment of infectious diseases. *Med J Aust* 2002;176:440-5.
4 Chapman ALN, Dixon S, Andrews D, Lillie PJ, Bazaz R, Patchett JD. Clinical efficacy and cost effectiveness of outpatient parenteral antibiotic therapy (OPAT): a UK perspective. *J Antimicrob Chemother* 2009;64:1316-24.
5 Barr DA, Semple L, Seaton RA. Outpatient parenteral antimicrobial therapy (OPAT) in a teaching hospital-based practice: a retrospective cohort study describing experience and evolution over 10 years. *Int J Antimicrob Agents* 2012;39:407-13.
6 Phoenix G, Das S, Joshi M. Diagnosis and management of cellulitis. *BMJ* 2012;345:e4955.
7 CREST (Clinical Resource Efficiency Support Team). Guidelines on the management of cellulitis in adults. 2005. www.acutemed.co.uk/docs/Cellulitis%20guidelines,%20CREST,%2005.pdf.
8 Marwick C, Broomhall J, McCowan C, Phillips G, Gonzalez-McQuire S, Akhras K, et al. Severity assessment of skin and soft tissue infections: cohort study of management and outcomes for hospitalised patients. *J Antimicrob Chemother* 2011;66:387-97.
9 Corwin P, Toop L, McGeoch G, Than M, Wynn-Thomas S, Wells JE, et al. Randomised controlled trial of intravenous antibiotic treatment for cellulitis at home compared to hospital. *BMJ* 2005;330:129-32.
10 Duncan CJA, Barr DA, Seaton RA. Outpatient parenteral antimicrobial therapy with ceftriaxone, a review. *Int J Clin Pharm* 2012;34:410-7.
11 Seaton RA, Bell E, Gourlay Y, Semple L. Nurse-led management of uncomplicated cellulitis in the community: evaluation of a protocol incorporating intravenous ceftriaxone. *J Antimicrob Chemother* 2005;55:764-7.
12 Mackintosh CL, White HA, Seaton RA. Outpatient parenteral antibiotic therapy (OPAT) for bone and joint infections: experience from a UK teaching hospital-based service. *J Antimicrob Chemother* 2011;66:408-15.
13 Esposito S, Leone S, Noviello S, Ianniello F, Fiore M, Russo M, et al. Outpatient parenteral antibiotic therapy for bone and joint infections: an Italian multicenter study, *J Chemother* 2007;19:417-22.
14 Matthews PC, Conlon CP, Berendt AR, Kayley J, Jefferies L, Atkins B, et al. Outpatient parenteral antimicrobial therapy (OPAT): is it safe for selected patients to self-administer at home? A retrospective analysis of a large cohort over 13 years. *J Antimicrob Chemother* 2008;61:226-7.
15 Gould FK, Denning DW, Elliott TSJ, Foweraker J, Perry JD, Prendergast BD, et al. Guidelines for the diagnosis and antibiotic treatment of endocarditis in adults: a report of the working party of the British Society for Antimicrobial Chemotherapy. *J Antimicrob Chemother* 2012;67:269-89.
16 Habib G, Hoen B, Tornos P, Thuny F, Prendergast B, Vilacosta I, et al. Guidelines on the prevention, diagnosis, and treatment of infective endocarditis. *Eur Heart J* 2009;30:2369-413.
17 Baddour LM, Wilson WR, Bayer AS, Fowler Jr VG, Bolger AF, Levison ME, et al. Infective endocarditis: diagnosis, antimicrobial therapy, and management of complications: a statement for healthcare professionals from the Committee on Rheumatic Fever, Endocarditis, and Kawasaki Disease, Council on Cardiovascular Disease in the Young, and the Councils on Clinical Cardiology, Stroke, and Cardiovascular Surgery and Anesthesia, American Heart Association: endorsed by the Infectious Diseases Society of America. *Circulation* 2005;111:e394-434.

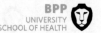

18 Amodeo MR, Clulow T, Lainchbury J, Murdoch DR, Gallagher K, Dyer A, et al. Outpatient intravenous treatment for infective endocarditis: safety, effectiveness and one-year outcomes. *J Infect* 2009;59:387-93.

19 Partridge DG, O'Brien E, Chapman ALN. Outpatient parenteral antibiotic therapy for infective endocarditis: a review of 4 years' experience at a UK centre. *Postgrad Med J* 2012;88:377-81.

20 Bazaz R, Chapman ALN, Winstanley TG. Ertapenem administered as outpatient parenteral antibiotic therapy for urinary tract infections caused by extended-spectrum- -lactamase-producing Gram-negative organisms. *J Antimicrob Chemother* 2010;65:1510-3.

21 Tice AD, Strait K, Ramey R, Hoaglund PA. Outpatient parenteral antimicrobial therapy for central nervous system infections. *Clin Infect Dis* 1999;29:1394-9.

22 Teuffel O, Ethier MC, Alibhai SM, Beyene J, Sung L. Outpatient management of cancer patients with febrile neutropenia: a systematic review and meta-analysis. *Ann Oncol* 2011;22:2358-65.

23 Ingram PR, Cerbe L, Hassell M, Wilson M, Dyer JR. Limited role for outpatient parenteral antibiotic therapy for community-acquired pneumonia. *Respirology* 2008;13:893-6.

24 Chapman ALN, Seaton RA, Cooper MA, Hedderwick S, Goodall V, Reed C, et al. Good practice recommendations for outpatient parenteral antimicrobial therapy (OPAT) in adults in the UK: a consensus statement. *J Antimicrobial Chemother* 2012;67:1053-62.

25 Lipsky BA, Berendt AR, Cornia PB, Pile JC, Peters EJG, Armstrong DG, et al. Infectious Diseases Society of America clinical practice guideline for the diagnosis and treatment of diabetic foot infections. *Clin Infect Dis* 2012;54:132-73.

26 Barr DA, Semple L, Seaton RA. Self-administration of outpatient parenteral antibiotic therapy and risk of catheter-related adverse events: a retrospective cohort study. *Eur J Clin Microbiol Infect Dis* 2012;31:2611-9.

27 Royal College of Nursing. Standards for infusion therapy. 3rd ed. 2010. www.rcn.org.uk/__data/assets/pdf_file/0005/78593/002179.pdf.

28 Gilchrist M, Franklin BD, Patel JP. An outpatient parenteral antibiotic therapy (OPAT) map to identify risks associated with an OPAT service. *J Antimicrob Chemother* 2009;64:177-83.

29 Chary A, Tice AD, Martinelli LP, Liedtke LA, Plantenga MS, Strausbaugh LJ. Experience of infectious diseases consultants with outpatient parenteral antimicrobial therapy: results of an emerging infections network survey. *Clin Infect Dis* 2006;43:1290-5.

30 Montalto M. How safe is hospital-in-the-home care? *Med J Aust* 1998;168:277-80.

31 Sharma R, Loomis W, Brown RB. Impact of mandatory inpatient infectious disease consultation on outpatient parenteral antibiotic therapy. *Am J Med Sci* 2005;330:60-4.

32 Heintz BH, Halilovic J, Christensen CL. Impact of a multidisciplinary team review of potential outpatient parenteral antimicrobial therapy prior to discharge from an academic medical centre. *Ann Pharmacother* 2011;45:1329-37.

33 Shrestha NK, Bhaskaran A, Scalera NM, Schmitt SK, Rehm SJ, Gordon SM. Contribution of infectious disease consultation toward the care of inpatients being considered for community-based parenteral anti-infective therapy. *J Hosp Med* 2012;7:365-9.

34 Nathwani D, Zambrowski JJ. Advisory group on home-based and outpatient care (AdHOC): an international consensus statement on non-inpatient parenteral therapy. *Clin Microbiol Infect* 2000;6:464-76.

35 Department of Health. Antimicrobial stewardship: start smart—then focus. DH, 2011. http://e-opat.com/wp-content/uploads/2012/07/DH-guidance-on-Antimicrobial-Stewardship-Start-Smart-then-Focus-Nov11.pdf.

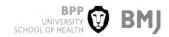

Meticillin resistant *Staphylococcus aureus* in the hospital

Jan Kluytmans, consultant microbiologist and head of infection control[1], professor of medical microbiology[2], Marc Struelens, head of the department of microbiology[3], director of Laboratoire de Référence des Staphylocoques[4], professor of medical microbiology[5]

[1]Laboratory for Microbiology and Infection Control, Amphia Hospital Breda, 4800 RK Breda, Netherlands

[2]Department of Medical Microbiology and Infection Control, VU University Medical Center Amsterdam, 1081 HV Amsterdam, Netherlands

[3]Department of Microbiology Hopital Erasme, 1070 Brussels, Belgium

[4]Laboratoire de Référence des Staphylocoques, Hopital Erasme, 1070 Brussels, Belgium

[5]Department of Microbiology and Immunology, Faculté de Médecine, Université Libre de Bruxelles, 1070 Brussels, Belgium

Correspondence to: J Kluytmans
jankluytmans@gmail.com

Cite this as: *BMJ* 2009;338:b364

DOI: 10.1136/bmj.b364

http://www.bmj.com/content/338/bmj.b364

The burden of disease from meticillin resistant *Staphylococcus aureus* (MRSA) infections is high. Around 100 000 invasive MRSA infections occurred in 2005 in the United States, and the number of associated deaths was about 19 000—more than that for HIV.[1] The epidemiology of MRSA has changed recently—infections are no longer confined to the hospital setting, but also appear in healthy people in the community with no established risk factors for acquiring MRSA. These community associated MRSA strains differ from hospital associated strains.[2] Mathematical models show that MRSA has a high potential to become endemic in the community.[3] The recent emergence of community acquired MRSA in skin and soft tissue infections calls for increased awareness among general and emergency room practitioners and a lower threshold for microbiological testing. Strategies to control hospital associated MRSA work in lower prevalence settings and may work in settings with medium to high endemic levels of hospital associated MRSA.[4]

What is MRSA and why has it become a problem?
MRSA produces penicillin binding protein 2a, which confers resistance to all β lactam antibiotics. The gene encoding this protein is carried on a mobile genetic element, the staphylococcal cassette chromosome mec (SCCmec), of which five different types have been identified.

MRSA was first reported in 1961, shortly after meticillin became available. However, it took several decades before it became a problem. For example, in the US and the United Kingdom the proportion of *S aureus* strains causing bacteraemia that were meticillin resistant started to increase around 1990, and by the start of the 21st century about half of the strains causing bacteraemia were resistant.[5] At present, hospital acquired MRSA is globally endemic except in Scandinavian countries and the Netherlands, where it is controlled by extensive measures. The worldwide emergence of MRSA is mainly the result of the extensive spread of a limited number of strains in hospitals, which are high risk settings for MRSA infection. Staphylococci spread easily between humans, either directly or indirectly by contact with healthcare workers or a contaminated environment. Because they are highly resistant to drying, staphylococci can survive for months on fomites. *Staphyloccocus aureus* is an opportunistic pathogen that mainly infects patients who have had surgery or who have invasive devices (such as intravascular catheters). Outbreaks of staphylococci are common in these patients and can be difficult to contain.

New strains
Recently, new strains of *S aureus* with diverse genetic backgrounds have acquired the meticillin resistance cassette because of the emergence of smaller and more easily acquired cassettes (types IV and V).[2] [5] These community acquired strains of MRSA successfully compete with susceptible strains outside of the hospital and can cause epidemics in closed communities and healthcare institutions.

Mortality, morbidity, and healthcare costs
A recent population based survey in Canada found a higher mortality associated with bacteraemia caused by MRSA rather than meticillin sensitive *S aureus* (MSSA) (39% v 24%) in hospital settings,[6] although others could not confirm this.[7] Observational cohort studies have consistently found that MRSA infection is associated with excess healthcare costs and prolonged hospital stay in surgical and critically ill patients, after adjusting for comorbidities and hospital events before infection.[8] In addition, in two cohort studies from Canada and the UK, MRSA did not replace MSSA but accounted for increasing rates of *S aureus* bacteraemia.[6] [7] Two surveys of all US hospitals estimated the occurrence and effects of *S aureus* infections over time.[9] [10] Infections increased from 258 000 in 1998 to 480 000 in 2005 (fig 1). In 2003, the associated incremental costs of staphylococcal disease were around $14.5bn (£10.3bn; €11bn), and nearly 60% of the infections were caused by MRSA. Therapeutic options for MRSA are limited, have more side effects, and are more costly than standard treatment with β lactam antibiotics.[11]

Who gets MRSA infection (table 1)?
Most carriers of *S aureus*, both hospital inpatients and others, are healthy asymptomatic people without evident infection.[12] In hospitals where MRSA is endemic, patients risk being colonised by spread from other patients or healthcare workers. Colonisation with *S aureus* in hospital is a risk factor for subsequent infection.[12] A recent study followed patients who carried MRSA, and during one year 23% developed at least one infection with MRSA.[13] In a population survey, groups at increased risk for invasive *S aureus* infections were those with dialysis dependence, organ transplantation, HIV infection, cancer, or diabetes.[6] In

SUMMARY POINTS

- Meticillin resistant Staphylococcus aureus (MRSA) is now a major cause of disease—in the US in 2005 more deaths were caused by MRSA than by HIV
- In addition to the well established hospital associated MRSA strains, new virulent strains have recently appeared in the general population
- Molecular technologies can rapidly detect MRSA but their cost effectiveness is unclear
- MRSA can be controlled by strict adherence to multifaceted strategies, including screening and transmission based precautions
- Clinicians must be aware of MRSA in community infections of skin and soft tissues and use a low threshold for microbiological testing
- Vancomycin is the standard treatment for serious MRSA infections. Alternative new drugs include linezolid, daptomycin, and tigecycline, which should be used with specialist advice

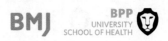

Table 1   Characteristics of hospital associated MRSA compared with community associated MRSA*

Characteristic	Hospital associated MRSA	Community associated MRSA
Patients' characteristics	Older age; underlying diseases common	Younger age; underlying diseases rare
Specific groups at risk	Patients in hospital or other healthcare facilities	Athletes, military recruits, children attending day care centres, prisoners, men who have sex with men, native Americans, native Australians, and people in contact with living pigs or veal calves
Spectrum of disease	Bacteraemia, surgical site infection, pneumonia, and urinary tract infection	Skin and soft tissue infection (such as abscesses, cellulitis, folliculitis, and impetigo); necrotising pneumonia
SCCmec types	I, II, III, and sometimes IV	IV and V
Antibiotic susceptibility	Multidrug resistant	Susceptible to most non-β lactam antibiotics
Presence of Panton-Valentine leucocidin	Rare	Common

*These characteristics were identified repeatedly when community associated MRSA first emerged. Because hospital associated MRSA is transmitted in the community and community associated MRSA spreads in hospitals the differences in characteristics are fading over time.
MRSA = meticillin resistant Staphylococcus aureus, SCCmec = staphylococcal cassette chromosome mec.

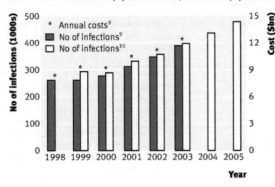

Fig 1 Trends in S aureus infections in all US hospitals from two independent surveys and associated incremental costs[9] [10]

hospital, invasive infections are most common in patients undergoing surgery or those with indwelling medical devices.[9] [10]

A new type of community acquired MRSA has recently emerged from a reservoir in animal husbandry (pigs and veal calves), and a high proportion (~30%) of people in contact with these animals become carriers.[14] The strains belong to one clonal complex (sequence type 398) and have been found in meat for sale.[15] The consequences of this reservoir in food are currently unclear.

How can we detect MRSA?
MRSA can cause the whole spectrum of staphylococcal disease (box), and no clinical feature is characteristic of MRSA infection, so its detection depends on microbiological laboratory tests. Only a minority of people in hospital who carry MRSA will be detected by testing clinical samples.[5] Asymptomatic carriers can serve as reservoirs for transmission to other patients. In countries that are still in control of MRSA, like the Netherlands and Scandinavia, screening of patients and exposed healthcare workers is part of the "search and destroy" strategy.[5] The most important carriage site for MRSA is the nose,[12] although a recent survey found that 25% of all carriers were identified only from throat swabs.[16] Adding other non-clinical sites (perineum, groin, or axilla) is probably not useful.

New rapid (around two hours of laboratory time) molecular techniques are sensitive but have a limited positive predictive value. They are therefore good screening tests, but positive results require confirmation by culture, which takes two to five days.[17]

CLINICAL SPECTRUM OF STAPHYLOCOCCAL DISEASE

Skin and soft tissue
- Impetigo, boils, carbuncles, abscesses, cellulitis, fasciitis, pyomyositis, surgical and traumatic wound infections

Foreign body associated
- Intravascular catheter, urinary catheter, surgical implant, endotracheal tubes

Intravascular
- Bacteraemia, sepsis, septic thrombophlebitis, infective endocarditis

Bone and joints
- Septic osteomyelitis, septic arthritis

Respiratory
- Pneumonia, empyema, sinusitis, otitis media

Other invasive infections
- Meningitis, surgical space infection

Toxin mediated diseases
- Staphylococcal toxic shock, food poisoning, staphylococcal scalded skin syndrome, bullous impetigo, necrotising pneumonia, necrotising osteomyelitis

How can we control MRSA?

Search and destroy
How to control MRSA in hospitals is a matter of continuing debate. At present, few countries can fully control MRSA, and they all apply the search and destroy strategy (fig 2). This strategy consists of active screening of high risk patients and exposed healthcare workers for carriage, strict implementation of transmission based precautions, and treatment of carriage using topical application of mupirocin nasal cream and washing with disinfecting agents, such as chlorhexidine. The full strategy is described in the Dutch national guidelines (www.wip.nl). Although this strategy is effective in countries with a low prevalence, it is unclear how best to adapt it for effective control of MRSA in countries where it is endemic.

Transmission based precautions
Hand hygiene remains the cornerstone for effective control of infection in hospitals. However, control of MRSA requires additional measures, like isolation. A systematic

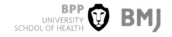

Table 2 Treatment options for meticillin resistant *Staphylococcus aureus* (MRSA) colonisation and infection

Indication and drug regimen	Adverse effects	Comments
Topical and systemic treatment to eradicate nasal carriage		
Nasal mupirocin + chlorhexidine body wash	Minor	Not effective in presence of skin breaks, extranasal colonisation, or high level of mupirocin resistance
Nasal mupirocin + chlorhexidine body wash + oral rifampicin + oral doxycycline	Hepatic toxicity and rash (related to rifampicin), photosensitivity and oesophagitis (related to doxycycline)	Contraindicated in children under 8 years
Oral treatment for mild to moderate localised skin and soft tissue infections		
Incision and drainage		May cure small abscess (<5 cm) in immunocompetent patients
Clindamycin	*Clostridium difficile* infection	Check isolate susceptibility
Co-trimoxazole	Rash and bone marrow suppression	Check isolate susceptibility; limited clinical evidence of effectiveness for treating staphylococcal infections
Doxycycline	Photosensitivity and oesophagitis	Check isolate susceptibility; contraindicated in children under 8 years; limited clinical evidence of effectiveness for treating staphylococcal infections
Linezolid	Bone marrow suppression, peripheral neuropathy, and optic neuropathy	Duration of treatment should not exceed 28 days; guidance from an infectious diseases specialist is advisable
Parenteral treatment for systemic and invasive infections		
Vancomycin	Renal toxicity with concurrent aminoglycoside use	First line treatment; monitor blood concentrations; continuous infusion preferable; check isolate susceptibility if response is poor; use adjunctive combination therapy with fluoroquinolone, rifampicin, or fusidic acid for prosthetic joint, bone, or cardiovascular infection
Teicoplanin		Monitor blood concentrations; check isolate susceptibility if response is poor
Linezolid	Bone marrow suppression, peripheral neuropathy, and optic neuropathy	Indicated in skin and soft tissue infections and pneumonia; not indicated in bacteraemia; first line treatment for glycopeptide intermediate strains; duration of treatment should not exceed 28 days (this limits treatment of bone and joint infections); guidance from an infectious diseases specialist is advisable
Daptomycin	Rhabdomyolysis, increased creatine phosphokinase concentrations	Indicated in skin and soft tissue infections and bacteraemia; not indicated in pneumonia (inactivated by surfactant); guidance from an infectious diseases specialist is advisable; check isolate susceptibility if response is poor
Tigecyclin	Nausea and vomiting	Indicated in skin and soft tissue infections but not indicated in bacteraemia or pneumonia; contraindicated in children under 8 years; guidance from an infectious diseases specialist is advisable
Necrotising pneumonia		
Linezolid + clindamycin	Bone marrow suppression, peripheral neuropathy, *Clostridium difficile* colitis	Intensive care support is needed; consider intravenous immunoglobulin if toxic is shock present; guidance from an infectious diseases specialist is advisable

See guidelines for management of MRSA.[11][23]

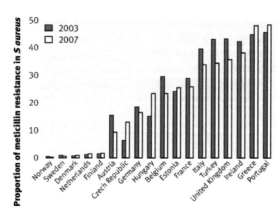

Fig 2 Trends in the proportion of meticillin resistant *S aureus* bacteraemia in Europe. Only countries reporting 500 cases or more a year were included. Reproduced from the European Antimicrobial Resistance Surveillance System database (www.rivm.nl/earss)

review found evidence that concerted efforts that included isolation could reduce the prevalence of MRSA, but the effect of isolation measures could not be assessed because of a lack of well designed studies.[4] Empirical evidence from observational cohort studies in hospitals and currently decreasing trends in several European countries after implementation of intensive national control programmes indicate that such programmes can be successful even in settings with medium to high endemic levels (fig 2). The effect of MRSA decolonisation on patients' outcomes has not been studied systematically.

Mathematical models have been developed to predict the effect of different control measures in high prevalence settings. One study using a compartmentalised model concluded that a proactive screening strategy (of high

risk patients on admission and contacts of index patients) combined with isolation could reduce the prevalence of MRSA to less than 1% within six years. To limit the need for isolation a stepwise approach combined with the use of rapid diagnostic tests was recommended.[18] Some historically controlled studies using universal screening by polymerase chain reaction showed a marked reduction in MRSA infection rates. For example, a large quasi-experimental study reported a 69.6% reduction in MRSA disease after introducing universal rapid MRSA testing and contact isolation of patients testing positive.[19] However, a well designed prospective crossover study performed in surgical patients found no significant reduction in MRSA infections.[20] Standard infection control measures, adjusted perioperative prophylaxis, and nasal decolonisation were applied in MRSA carriers. The authors commented that baseline MRSA infection rates were relatively low, limiting the power of the study, and that transmission of MRSA was ongoing in the intervention wards. Another cluster randomised crossover trial comparing polymerase chain reaction with conventional screening showed a positive effect on bed usage but no significant reduction of MRSA acquisition.[21] In this study pre-emptive isolation was used in both groups, which may not be representative for other settings. The conclusions are that the cost effectiveness of rapid screening tests remains to be established.

Restrictive use of antibiotics

Observational studies have noted the role of antibiotic use as a risk factor for nosocomial transmission of MRSA. A multicentre quasi-experimental study found an 18% reduction in the prevalence of MRSA after restricting the use of fluoroquinolones hospital wide.[22] Additional well

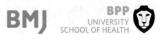

SOURCES AND SELECTION CRITERIA

We used our personal archives and also searched PubMed and the Cochrane Library (1 January 2002 to 1 July 2008) using the terms "MRSA" or "methicillin resistant *Staphylococcus aureus*", with the limits "meta-analysis and randomised controlled trial". We also reviewed the current guidelines from the US Centers for Disease Control; the Joint Working Party of the British Society for Antimicrobial Chemotherapy, Hospital Infection Society, and Infection Control Nurses Association; the Dutch Working Party on Infection Control; the Dutch Working Party on Antimicrobial Use; and the Belgian Superior Health Council. We used evidence based recommendations when available and recommendations from experts when not.

designed studies are needed to determine the effect of reducing antibiotic use in hospital on the prevalence of MRSA.

How should we treat MRSA infections (table 2)?

In the community

The worldwide rise in the prevalence of MRSA challenges the conventional approach to managing skin and soft tissue infections. Incision and drainage remain the primary treatment for boils and abscesses. Data from recent observational studies and clinical trials on the benefit of antibiotics in addition to drainage of uncomplicated infections are conflicting. Patients likely to benefit include those with large or incompletely drained abscesses, cellulitis, fever, or other signs of systemic illness. These form a minority of the patients presenting with skin and soft tissue infections, however, and antibiotics are overprescribed for this indication.

The prevalence of MRSA in community acquired infection varies widely according to region, reaching 20-50% in skin and soft tissue infections in US cities. In those areas, experts recommend changing empirical treatment of these infections from β lactams to agents with activity against MRSA (table 2). Clinical trials are ongoing to determine the most effective oral treatments. Selection of drugs for empirical regimens should be based on local susceptibility patterns. In areas with low prevalence of MRSA in the community, clinicians should still consider MRSA in the differential diagnosis of skin and soft tissue infections. They should collect specimens from purulent lesions for culture and susceptibility testing, especially in severe or recurrent infections or in the presence of risk factors for MRSA (table 1).

In the hospital

Vancomycin, a glycopeptide, is the cornerstone for treating invasive MRSA infections. An alternative agent from the same antibiotic class, teicoplanin, is available in some countries. However, these agents have limited efficacy for deep seated infections, partly because of poor diffusion into tissues—such as the lung and bone—and because of a gradual decrease in susceptibility of MRSA over recent years.[24] These glycopeptide intermediate strains have mutations that affect the synthesis of the bacterial cell wall and are not easy to detect in microbiology laboratories. In addition, genetic recombinant, high level glycopeptide resistant *S aureus* strains have been described sporadically in the US.[25] To optimise treatment with glycopeptides in these strains—although not supported by controlled studies—dose adjustment on the basis of monitoring blood concentrations and administration by continuous infusion have been advocated.

Alternative therapeutic options for parenteral treatment of invasive MRSA infection include recently licensed drugs from new antibiotic classes—linezolid, the first oxazolidinone; daptomycin, the first lipopeptide; and tigecycline, the first glycylcycline (table 2). Randomised controlled trials showed these drugs to be equivalent to vancomycin for treating skin and soft tissue infections involving MRSA.[26][27][28] Linezolid is also efficacious for treating staphylococcal pneumonia, and a trial is ongoing to test whether it is more efficacious than vancomycin in ventilator associated MRSA pneumonia, as was suggested by secondary analyses of phase III trials.

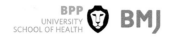

A large open label randomised controlled trial showed daptomycin to be equivalent to vancomycin for treating MRSA bacteraemia.[29] However, daptomycin resistance develops not infrequently, and daptomycin has decreased activity against glycopeptide intermediate strains, so its use should be guided by careful microbiological monitoring of activity. Other antibacterial agents active against MRSA that are in advanced clinical development include the broad spectrum cephalosporin, ceftobiprole; the lipoglycopeptides, oritavancin, dalbavancin, and telavancin; and the trimethoprim analogue, iclaprim. In severe pneumonia with signs of necrosis, respiratory failure, and haemoptysis, infection with Panton-Valentine leucocidin producing staphylococci should be suspected and a Gram stain of respiratory secretions obtained immediately to confirm this possibility. Clindamycin and linezolid repress production of the leucocidin,[30] and experts advocate treatment with high doses of these agents for necrotising staphylococcal pneumonia on the basis of experimental data and anecdotal clinical experience.[23]

Contributors: Both authors contributed to the literature search, planning, and writing of this review. JK is guarantor.

Competing interests: JK has received consulting fees from 3M, Destiny Pharma, Novabay, and Wyeth; research funds from BD, bioMérieux, and Wyeth; and speaking fees from 3M and BD. MS has received reimbursement for attending meetings from BD, bioMérieux, Pfizer; speaking fees from BD, 3M, and Pfizer; research funds from Cepheid, BD, bioMérieux, Novartis, Pfizer, Johnson & Johnson, and Wyeth; and consulting fees from 3M, Wyeth, Novartis, Eppendorf Array Technologies, and Philips Molecular Diagnostics.

Provenance and peer review: Commissioned; externally peer reviewed.

1   Klevens RM, Morrison MA, Nadle J, Petit S, Gershman K, Ray S, et al. Invasive methicillin-resistant Staphylococcus aureus infections in the United States. JAMA 2007;298:1763-71.
2   Kluytmans-VandenBergh MFQ, Kluytmans JAJW. Community-acquired methicillin-resistant Staphylococcus aureus: current perspectives. Clin Microbiol Infect 2006;12(suppl 1):9-15.
3   Cooper BS, Medley GF, Stone SP, Kibbler CC, Cookson BD, Roberts JA, et al. Methicillin-resistant Staphylococcus aureus in hospitals and the community: stealth dynamics and control catastrophes. Proc Natl Acad Sci USA 2004;101:10223-8.
4   Cooper BS, Stone SP, Kibbler CC, Cookson BD, Roberts JA, Medley GF, et al. Isolation measures in the hospital management of methicillin resistant Staphylococcus aureus (MRSA): systematic review of the literature. BMJ 2004;329:533-40.
5   Grundmann H, Aires-de-Sousa M, Boyce J, Tiemersma E. Emergence and resurgence of methicillin-resistant Staphylococcus aureus as a public-health threat. Lancet 2006;368:874-85.
6   Laupland KB, Ross T, Gregson DB. Staphylococcus aureus bloodstream infections: risk factors, outcomes, and the influence of methicillin resistance in Calgary, Canada, 2000-2006. Clin Infect Dis 2008;198:336-43.
7   Wyllie DH, Crook DW, Peto TEA. Mortality after Staphylococcus aureusbacteraemia in two acute hospitals in Oxfordshire, 1997-2003: cohort study. BMJ 2006;333:281.
8   Engemann JJ, Carmeli Y, Cosgrove SE, Fowler VG, Bronstein MZ, Trivette SL, et al. Adverse clinical and economic outcomes attributable to methicillin resistance among patients with Staphylococcus aureus surgical site infection. Clin Infect Dis 2003;36:592-8.
9   Noskin GA, Rubin RJ, Schentag JJ, Kluytmans J, Hedblom EC, Jacobson C, et al. National trends in Staphylococcus aureus infection rates: impact on economic burden and mortality over a 6-year period (1998-2003). Clin Infect Dis 2007;45:1132d0.
10   Klein E, Smith DL, Laxminarayan R. Hospitalizations and deaths caused by methicillin-resistant Staphylococcus aureus, United States, 1999-2005. Emerg Infect Dis 2007;13:1840-6.
11   Gemmel CG, Edwards DI, Fraise AP, Gould FK, Ridgway GL, Warren RE; on behalf of the Joint Working Party of the British Society for Antimicrobial Therapy, Hospital Infection Society and Infection Control Nurses Association. Guidelines for prophylaxis and treatment of methicillin-resistant Staphylococcus aureus (MRSA) infections in the UK. J Antimicrob Chemother 2006;57:589-608.
12   Kluytmans J, van Belkum A, Verbrugh H. Nasal carriage of Staphylococcus aureus: epidemiology, underlying mechanisms, and associated risks. Clin Microbiol Rev 1997;10:505-20.
13   Datta R, Huang SS. Risk of infection and death due to methicillin-resistant Staphylococcus aureus in long-term carriers. Clin Infect Dis 2008;47:176-81.
14   Van Loo I, Huijsdens X, Tiemersma E, de Neeling A, van de Sande-Bruinsma N, Beaujean D, et al. Emergence of methicillin-resistant Staphylococcus aureus of animal origin in humans. Emerg Infect Dis 2007;13:1834-9.
15   Van Loo IH, Diederen BM, Savelkoul PH, Woudenberg JH, Roosendaal R, van Belkum A, et al. Methicillin-resistant Staphylococcus aureus in meat products, the Netherlands. Emerg Infect Dis 2007;13:1753-5.
16   Mertz D, Frei R, Jaussi B, Tietz A, Stebler C, Flückiger U, et al. Throat swabs are necessary to reliably detect carriers of Staphylococcus aureus. Clin Infect Dis 2007;45:475-7.
17   De San N, Denis O, Gasasira MF, De Mendonca R, Nonhoff C, Struelens MJ. Controlled evaluation of the IDI-MRSA assay for the detection of colonization by methicillin-resistant Staphylococcus aureus in diverse mucocutaneous specimens. J Clin Microbiol 2007;45:1098-101.
18   Bootsma MC, Diekmann O, Bonten MJ. Controlling methicillin-resistant Staphylococcus aureus: quantifying the effects of interventions and rapid diagnostic testing. Proc Natl Acad Sci USA 2006;103:5620-5.
19   Robicsek A, Beaumont JL, Paule SM, Hacek DM, Thomson RB Jr, Kaul KL, et al. Universal surveillance for methicillin-resistant Staphylococcus aureus in 3 affiliated hospitals. Ann Intern Med 2008;148:409-18.
20   Harbarth S, Fankhauser C, Schrenzel J, Christenson J, Gervaz P, Bandiera-Clerc C, et al. Universal screening for methicillin-resistant Staphylococcus aureus at hospital admission and nosocomial infection in surgical patients. JAMA 2008;299:1149-57.
21   Jeyaratnam D, Whitty CJ, Phillips K, Liu D, Orezzi C, Ajoku U, et al. Impact of rapid screening tests on acquisition of methicillin resistant Staphylococcus aureus: cluster randomised crossover trial. BMJ 2008;336:927-30.
22   Charbonneau P, Parienti JJ, Thibon P, Ramakers M, Daubin C, du Cheyron D, et al. Fluoroquinolone use and methicillin-resistant Staphylococcus aureus isolation rates in hospitalized patients: a quasi experimental study. Clin Infect Dis 2006;42:778-84.
23   Nathwani D, Morgan M, Masterton RG, Dryden M, Cookson BD, French G, et al. Guidelines for UK practice for the diagnosis and management of methicillin-resistant Staphylococcus aureus (MRSA) infections presenting in the community. J Antimicrob Chemother 2008;61:976-94. Erratum in: J Antimicrob Chemother 2008;62:216.
24   Lewis JS 2nd, Ellis MW. Approaches to serious methicillin-resistant Staphylococcus aureus infections with decreased susceptibility to vancomycin: clinical significance and options for management. Curr Opin Infect Dis 2007;20:568-73.
25   Sievert DM, Rudrik JT, Patel JB, McDonald LC, Wilkins MJ, Hageman JC. Vancomycin-resistant Staphylococcus aureus in the United States, 2002-2006. Clin Infect Dis 2008;46:668-74.
26   Falagas ME, Siempos II, Vardakas KZ. Linezolid versus glycopeptide or beta-lactam for treatment of Gram-positive bacterial infections: meta-analysis of randomised controlled trials. Lancet Infect Dis 2008;8:53-66.
27   Arbeit RD, Maki D, Tally FP, Campanaro E, Eisenstein BI; Daptomycin 98-01 and 99-01 Investigators. The safety and efficacy of daptomycin for the treatment of complicated skin and skin-structure infections. Clin Infect Dis 2004;38:1673-81.
28   Florescu I, Beuran M, Dimov R, Razbadauskas A, Bochan M, Fichev G, et al; 307 Study Group. Efficacy and safety of tigecycline compared with vancomycin or linezolid for treatment of serious infections with methicillin-resistant Staphylococcus aureus or vancomycin-resistant enterococci: a phase 3, multicentre, double-blind, randomized study. J Antimicrob Chemother 2008;62(suppl 1):i17-28.
29   Fowler VG Jr, Boucher HW, Corey GR, Abrutyn E, Karchmer AW, Rupp ME, et al. Daptomycin versus standard therapy for bacteremia and endocarditis caused by Staphylococcus aureus. N Engl J Med 2006;355:653-65.
30   Dumitrescu O, Boisset S, Bes M, Benito Y, Reverdy ME, Vandenesch F, et al. Effect of antibiotics on Staphylococcus aureus producing Panton-Valentine leukocidin. Antimicrob Agents Chemother 2007;51:1515-9.

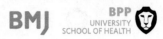

Prevention and medical management of *Clostridium difficile* infection

J Shannon-Lowe, foundation year 2 in microbiology[1], N J Matheson, specialty registrar in infectious diseases and general medicine[2], F J Cooke, specialist registrar in microbiology[1], S H Aliyu, consultant in microbiology and infectious diseases[1][2]

[1]Clinical Microbiology and Public Health Laboratory, Health Protection Agency, Addenbrooke's Hospital, Cambridge CB2 0QQ

[2]Department of Infectious Diseases, Cambridge University Hospitals NHS Foundation Trust, Addenbrooke's Hospital

Correspondence to: N J Matheson
nicholas.matheson@addenbrookes.nhs.uk

Cite this as: *BMJ* 2010;340:c1296

DOI: 10.1136/bmj.c1296

http://www.bmj.com/content/340/bmj.c1296

The incidence of *Clostridium difficile* infection in the United Kingdom has increased since the late 1990s.[1] High profile outbreaks in the United States, Canada, and northern Europe have been associated with a previously uncommon but highly virulent strain known as ribotype 027. A recent review in the *BMJ* examined the role of surgery in treating *C difficile* colitis.[2] This review focuses on the prevention and medical management of *C difficile* infection. Because few randomised controlled trials (RCTs) exist on this subject, our recommendations are based mainly on non-RCT studies and clinical governance reports.

Who becomes infected with *C difficile*?

C difficile can be cultured from the stool of 3% of healthy adults and as many as 35% of hospital inpatients.[3] Lower rates of nosocomial colonisation are seen in some studies, and may be dependent on patient population, length of hospital stay, and local infection control procedures.[w1 w2] Most colonised people remain asymptomatic. Clinical disease develops when the normal gut flora is disrupted, usually by antibiotic exposure, thereby creating conditions that favour *C difficile* proliferation within the colon. Although *C difficile* infections in England have started to decline overall, 36 097 infections in patients aged 2 years and over were reported to the UK Health Protection Agency (HPA) for the financial year ending March 2009 (www.hpa.org.uk/web/HPAwebFile/HPAweb_C/1252326222452). Elderly hospital inpatients are the main group affected, but the epidemiology of the disease is changing. Community associated infections have been increasingly recognised, as have infections in pregnant women and children, populations previously regarded as being at low risk.[4]

How does *C difficile* infection present and how is it diagnosed?

Gastrointestinal diseases associated with *C difficile* infection range from mild diarrhoea to fulminant colitis. Some "silent" infections present with abdominal pain and distension, in the absence of appreciable diarrhoea. These features may indicate severe disease, which in turn causes ileus or toxic megacolon.[w3] UK national guidelines define *C difficile* infection as one episode of unformed stool, not attributable to any other cause, occurring at the same time as a positive *C difficile* toxin assay.[1] The toxin may be detected by commercial immunoassay kits, nine of which were tested against a "gold standard" cytotoxin or toxigenic culture assay.[5] Compared with the cytotoxin assay, sensitivities ranged from 67% to 92% and specificities from 91% to 99%. Because most patients with diarrhoea do not have *C difficile* infection, these equate in practice to negative predictive values greater than 95%, but positive predictive values that may be lower than 50% (for example, in samples from the community, where prevalence is low). When *C difficile* infection is uncommon or clinically unlikely, positive test results must therefore be interpreted with care and a confirmatory test should be considered.[w4] In suspected cases of silent infection, endoscopy or abdominal computed tomography may be needed. Characteristic findings include thickening of the colonic wall, dilation, and pseudomembrane formation.[2]

How can it be prevented?

Prevention has two aspects—prevention of acquisition of *C difficile* and prevention of infection in colonised people. This requires a multifaceted approach based on the five main strategies outlined in the UK Department of Health Saving Lives campaign (www.clean-safe-care.nhs.uk)—prudent antibiotic prescribing, hand hygiene, use of personal protective equipment, environmental decontamination, and isolation or cohort nursing. In the UK, reporting of *C difficile* infections to the HPA is mandatory. Locally, surveillance of *C difficile* infections is key to identifying outbreaks and initiating control measures in a timely fashion.[6] Typing of *C difficile* isolates and molecular surveillance techniques may help investigate apparent increases in cases and improve the understanding of the transmission of epidemic strains within and between healthcare institutions.[7 w5]

How can antibiotic stewardship help prevent *C difficile* infection?

Many authors have produced "hit lists" of antibiotics with the potential to cause *C difficile* infection,[8 9] but this approach has problems.[w6] Classification into low, medium, and high risk antibiotics is practically useful (table 1), but any antibiotic, at any dose, for any length of time, will alter the colonic microbiota, potentially allowing *C difficile* to proliferate and cause disease.[w7] Prospective observational cohort studies suggest that restricting the use of the high risk agents, clindamycin and third generation cephalosporins, results in fewer cases of *C difficile* infection.[10 11 12] Although use of fluoroquinolones has been linked to the spread of the ribotype 027 strain, risk analyses have been confounded by antibiotic polypharmacy, duration of antibiotic treatment, and infection control practices.[13 14] In addition, observational data suggest that different fluoroquinolones differ in

SUMMARY POINTS

- The incidence of *Clostridium difficile* infection has increased in the past decade
- National and local surveillance of *C difficile* infection is crucial to guide implementation of control measures
- Prudent antibiotic prescribing, correct hand hygiene, use of personal protective equipment, environmental decontamination, and isolation or cohort nursing may prevent infection
- Treatment is with oral vancomycin or metronidazole, according to disease severity, with escalation of treatment in the event of non-response

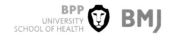

Table 1 | Antibiotics implicated in the pathogenesis of *Clostridium difficile* infection[8 9 w6]

Low risk	Medium risk	High risk
Aminoglycosides	Ampicillin and amoxicillin	Clindamycin
Vancomycin	Macrolides	Cephalosporins
Metronidazole	Tetracyclines	
Rifampicin	Fluoroquinolones	
Anti-pseudomonal penicillins	Co-trimoxazole	

propensity to cause *C difficile* infection, with gatifloxacin having the highest risk.[9]

To reduce overprescribing and inappropriate antibiotic use, the Saving Lives campaign makes the following "best practice" recommendations for antimicrobial prescribing: antibiotics should be prescribed according to local policies and guidelines for treatment and prophylaxis, avoiding broad spectrum agents; the indication for starting an antibiotic should be documented in the medical record, along with a stop or review date; intravenous antibiotics should be avoided, and the shortest treatment course likely to be effective should be prescribed; prescriptions should be reviewed daily; and single antibiotic doses should be used for surgical prophylaxis if possible. Hospital initiatives focusing on antibiotic stewardship include antibiotic ward rounds, antibiotic care bundles,[15] electronic prescribing, restricted antibiotics that require microbiology approval, and computerised decision support networks.[w8] Antibiotic pharmacists may play a major role in this regard.[w9]

What infection control measures should be instituted?
C difficile infection has been estimated to increase hospital stay by an average of 21 days,[16] although more recent studies have suggested a less pronounced effect.[w10 w11] While in hospital, infected patients may continue to excrete infective *C difficile* spores. Hand washing is paramount in preventing hospital acquired infections (www.npsa.nhs.uk/cleanyourhands). Alcohol based hand gels are highly effective against non-spore forming organisms, but they do not kill *C difficile* spores or remove them from hands. Experimental studies have shown that alcohol based hand gels are significantly less effective at reducing contamination with *C difficile* spores than washing with soap and water.[17 18] UK national guidelines recommend that healthcare workers wash their hands before and after contact with patients with suspected or confirmed *C difficile* infection, and that disposable gloves and aprons are used when handling body fluids and caring for such patients.[1]

C difficile spores can survive in the environment for months or years, and environmental contamination has been linked to the spread of *C difficile* infection in healthcare settings.[17] UK national guidelines therefore recommend various forms of environmental decontamination[1]: rooms or bed spaces of infected patients should be cleaned daily using chlorine containing cleaning agents[w12]; commodes, toilets, and bathrooms should be cleaned after each use; and after discharge of an infected patient, the room and mattress should be thoroughly cleaned using chlorine containing cleaning agents or vaporised hydrogen peroxide.[w13] Replacing electronic oral and rectal thermometers (which may be contaminated with *C difficile* spores) with disposable thermometers can significantly reduce rates of *C difficile* infection.[w14] A prospective randomised crossover study of 20 nursing units reported a significantly lower rate of nosocomial *C difficile* infection with use of disposable thermometers (0.16/1000 patient days) compared with electronic thermometers (0.37/1000 patient days; relative risk 0.44; 95% confidence interval 0.21 to 0.93),[19] and a

similar reduction was seen by an observational study that compared rates before and after the introduction of tympanic thermometers.[w15]

No RCTs or systematic reviews have assessed the value of isolation measures in preventing *C difficile* infection, but a systematic review of isolation in the hospital management of meticillin resistant *Staphylococcus aureus* (MRSA) suggested it was effective as part of a broader infection control strategy.[20] UK national guidelines recommend that patients with potentially infective diarrhoea should be moved immediately into a single room with en suite facilities,[1] but this practice has difficulties. For example, moving frail elderly patients may increase the risk of delirium.[w16] In a large outbreak, or highly endemic settings, isolating affected patients in single rooms may not be possible. The creation of *C difficile* isolation wards in hospitals with high levels of disease was successful in certain outbreaks.[6 21] Because the positive predictive value of the toxin immunoassays is suboptimal, however, transferring patients to cohort areas risks putting people without *C difficile* (false positives) at increased risk of acquiring the infection.

Are there any other ways of preventing *C difficile* infection?
The rising incidence of *C difficile* infection since the late 1990s has coincided with the widespread use of proton pump inhibitors (use increased 10-fold in the UK from 1992 to 1995), raising concerns that the two may be linked.[w17] Hospital and community studies have produced conflicting results,[8 9 22] but a meta-analysis of case-control and cohort studies including 126 999 patients suggested a significant association between proton pump inhibitors and *C difficile* infection (odds ratio 2.05; 1.47 to 2.85).[w18]

Probiotics (live micro-organisms such as *Lactobacillus* or *Bifidobacterium* taken as supplements or in yoghurt drinks to rebalance the gut flora) and prebiotics (carbohydrates such as oligofructose, inulin, and other non-digestible foodstuffs that stimulate the growth or activity of gut bacteria) have been proposed as preventive methods for *C difficile* infection.[w19] A recent double blind RCT showed that a probiotic *Lactobacillus* preparation helped prevent *C difficile* infection in a highly selected subgroup of patients receiving antibiotics,[23] but the findings may not be generalisable.[24] A previous meta-analysis failed to provide sufficient evidence for the routine clinical use of probiotics to prevent or treat *C difficile* infection.[w20] Data on prebiotics are sparse.

How is *C difficile* managed medically?
Patients with *C difficile* infection may develop electrolyte imbalance, dehydration, malnutrition, and pressure sores, so their supportive medical care must be optimised. After outbreaks at Maidstone and Tunbridge Wells NHS Trust in 2005-6, the UK Healthcare Commission criticised the general management of infected patients for inadequate monitoring and doctor review, poor fluid replacement and nutritional support, and lack of multidisciplinary assessment.[6]

In early studies, 15-23% of patients who developed *C difficile* infection became asymptomatic through stopping the offending antibiotic alone—allowing normal flora

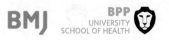

Table 2 Faecal concentrations of oral and intravenous vancomycin and metronidazole[3][25][w35]

Drug preparation	Typical faecal concentration	MIC90* (µg/ml)
Oral vancomycin (total 2 g daily)	Mean 3100 µg/g stool	0.75-2.0
Intravenous vancomycin	Clinically irrelevant	
Oral metronidazole (total 1.2 g daily)	0.4-14.9 µg/g stool†	0.2-2.0
Intravenous metronidazole (total 1.5 g daily)	5.1-24.2 µg/g stool†	

*Minimum inhibitory concentration needed to inhibit 90% of strains.
†Watery or semiformed stool.

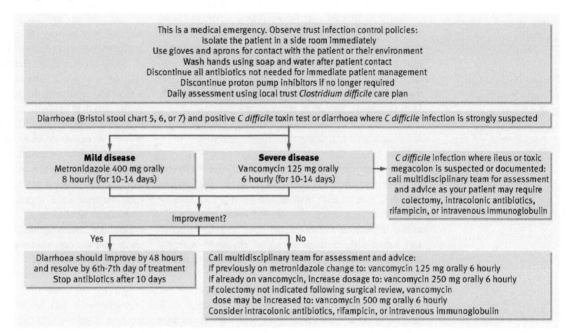

Suggested management cascade for *C difficile* infection. Severe disease: one or more of white blood cell count >15×10⁹/l, acutely rising serum creatinine (>50% above baseline), temperature >38.5°C, clinical or radiological evidence of severe colitis.[1] Multidisciplinary team may consist of microbiology, infectious diseases, gastroenterology, and surgical teams

to recolonise the colon—whereas continuing systemic antibiotics has been associated with a poor response to treatment.[3] When treatment cannot be stopped, because of concurrent infection that requires ongoing systemic antibiotics, an antibiotic with a low risk of causing *C difficile* infection may be substituted (table 1). The use of antimotility agents during active infection has been associated with toxic megacolon.[3][w7][w21]

Which antibiotics are used to treat *C difficile* infection?
Oral vancomycin was the first drug shown to be effective for *C difficile* infection, followed by oral metronidazole, and these agents remain the mainstay of treatment.[3] Whereas intravenous vancomycin is almost exclusively excreted in the urine, oral vancomycin achieves faecal concentrations many times higher than the minimum inhibitory concentrations of *C difficile* strains reported to date (table 2). After ingestion by healthy volunteers, metronidazole is completely absorbed from the gastrointestinal tract, and is undetectable in the faeces.[w22] When diarrhoea is present, however, metronidazole may achieve therapeutic values in faeces when given orally or intravenously, perhaps because of seepage across inflamed colonic mucosa.[25] UK surveillance data support the emergence of reduced susceptibility to metronidazole in some *C difficile* isolates, but the clinical importance of this is unclear.[w23]

What is the appropriate choice for initial antibiotic treatment?
In patients with severe *C difficile* infection (any of white blood cell count >15×10⁹/l, acutely rising serum creatinine (>50% above baseline), temperature over 38.5°C, or

clinical or radiographic evidence of severe colitis), UK national guidelines recommend initial treatment with oral vancomycin, on the basis of evidence from two recent RCTs that compared vancomycin and metronidazole.[1] These trials, which stratified for disease severity, showed a lower rate of treatment failure with vancomycin in patients with severe *C difficile* infection.[26][27] Only one has been fully published; it found cure rates of 76% with metronidazole versus 97% with vancomycin (P=0.002) in patients with severe disease.[26] Retrospective and prospective observational studies have also shown that response time is shorter for vancomycin than for metronidazole, which may be important in patients with severe disease.[w24][w25] In patients with mild or moderate disease, neither RCT showed that vancomycin was significantly superior.[26][27] UK national guidelines therefore still recommend oral metronidazole for initial treatment in these patient groups, because it is cheaper than oral vancomycin, and because of concern that overuse of vancomycin may result in the selection of vancomycin resistant enterococci.[1] Observational data suggest, however, that metronidazole, as well as vancomycin, may promote persistent overgrowth of vancomycin resistant enterococci.[28]

What if the patient fails to respond to initial treatment?
Treatment failure is defined as no response after one week, although most patients show signs of improvement within 48-72 hours. UK national guidelines recommend that antibiotics be reviewed daily and a plan agreed for escalating treatment in the event of non-response.[1] If diarrhoea does not improve, patients initially treated with metronidazole may be changed to vancomycin. In severe disease, aggressive treatment with escalating doses of

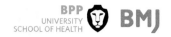

vancomycin, up to 500 mg four times daily, may be used, although no robust evidence supports this approach, and an early randomised trial comparing vancomycin 500 mg four times daily with 125 mg four times daily in 46 inpatients found no difference in outcomes.[29] In patients with adynamic ileus (which may reduce passage of oral preparations to the colon), intravenous metronidazole may be added, but the efficacy of this route of administration is unclear.[w26] Vancomycin administered as a retention enema may increase colonic antibiotic exposure, and in a recent case series examining this as adjunctive treatment, eight of nine patients completely recovered.[30] Finally, surgery may be life saving in severe disease.[2] Figure 1 shows a possible management cascade for *C difficile* infection adapted locally from UK national guidelines for use in our centre.

Are there any other treatment options for refractory disease?

Several antibiotics have been used for the treatment of refractory infection. UK national guidelines suggest considering the addition of rifampicin 300 mg twice daily for severe disease,[1] although the only RCT assessing rifampicin as an adjunct to metronidazole for *C difficile* infection was halted early because of lack of efficacy.[w27] A recent case series described the successful use of intravenous tigecycline for *C difficile* infection in four patients refractory to vancomycin and metronidazole.[w28] UK national guidelines also recommend the use of intravenous immunoglobulin (400 mg/kg) in selected severe cases,[1] although results from case reports and small series have been inconsistent and no RCTs are available to support this position.

How is recurrent *C difficile* infection diagnosed?

Recurrent *C difficile* infection (relapse of diarrhoea after initial resolution of symptoms) usually occurs within one to three weeks but has been described up two months after the initial episode.[22] The risk of recurrence after a single episode is high, with 8-50% of patients having at least a second episode after treatment with metronidazole or vancomycin.[3] Risk factors include previous relapses, age greater than 65 years, severe underlying illness, and additional antibiotic use after treatment for *C difficile* infection has been stopped.[w29 w30] Paradoxically, the antibiotics used to treat *C difficile* infection may themselves interfere with the re-establishment of the normal colonic flora, contributing to the propensity for recurrent disease.

Patients may remain positive for *C difficile* toxin despite clinical cure,[31] and UK Department of Health surveillance regards serial positive results within 28 days of the first specimen as a single episode. UK national guidelines do not recommend retesting for *C difficile* toxin within 28 days if patients remain symptomatic, but repeat testing may be appropriate at any time if symptoms relapse after resolution and recurrence needs to be confirmed.[1]

How do recommendations differ for recurrent disease?

Because recurrence may represent reinfection rather than relapse,[w31] and because evidence for clinically relevant resistance to metronidazole or vancomycin is lacking, the antibiotic that was used to treat the initial episode may be used for the first recurrence (unless this is metronidazole and the recurrence meets criteria for severe *C difficile* infection).[1] In second and subsequent recurrences, however, vancomycin is recommended. This is because stool concentrations of metronidazole wane during recovery, with much lower concentrations in formed than in watery or semiformed stools,[25] and because long term use of metronidazole may be associated with adverse effects, such as peripheral neuropathy.[32]

Observational studies have examined the use of long term, tapering, or pulsed courses of vancomycin. Slowly falling concentrations of antibiotics in the colon may suppress *C difficile* proliferation, while allowing normal colonic flora to recover, or allow *C difficile* spores to germinate, making them susceptible to subsequent intermittent doses.[32] None of the proposed regimens has been tested in an RCT, and they may all apply considerable selection pressure for vancomycin resistant enterococci. Other antimicrobial regimens, such as a short course of vancomycin and rifampicin, or rifaximin (a poorly absorbed rifamycin derivative not licensed in the UK) used as a "chaser" after vancomycin, have been reported to be successful in small numbers of patients.[w32] Low concentrations of serum antibodies against *C difficile* toxin A correlate with the risk of recurrent *C difficile* infection,[33] and a recent phase II RCT found a significant reduction in *C difficile* recurrence in patients treated with experimental monoclonal antibodies against toxins A and B.[34] Pooled intravenous immunoglobulin may also neutralise these toxins, and a small case series reported a successful clinical response to intravenous immunoglobulin in three of five patients with recurrent infection.[35] Although recommended in the UK Department of Health clinical guidelines for immunoglobulin use for selected patients with multiple recurrent *C difficile* infection in whom all other treatments have failed or are inappropriate, no RCTs support the use of intravenous immunoglobulin, and cost and availability may preclude its widespread adoption.[w33] Finally, evidence is emerging for the efficacy of faecal transplantation in patients with relapsing *C difficile* infection, mostly from small retrospective case series.[w34] Fresh stool from a healthy donor is administered by enema or nasogastric tube in an effort to reconstitute the normal colonic flora. Concerns remain about the safety of this approach, as well as its acceptability.

SOURCES AND SELECTION CRITERIA

We searched PubMed and Google Scholar for articles published from 2006 to 2009 on the treatment and prevention of *Clostridium difficile* infection and screened the reference lists of retrieved publications. We also consulted the Cochrane Library and the recent best practice guidance from the Health Protection Agency.[1]

TIPS FOR NON-SPECIALISTS

- Avoid antibiotics with a high risk of inducing *Clostridium difficile* infection, especially in patients with a history of infection
- Isolate patients with suspected *C difficile* infection, use gowns and gloves when seeing them, and remember to wash hands rather than use alcohol gel
- Pay careful attention to the supportive care (such as fluid and electrolyte replacement) of infected patients
- Stop precipitating antibiotics if possible, and if not, substitute with a lower risk agent
- Reserve metronidazole for initial treatment of patients with mild or moderate disease, then escalate treatment according to agreed local and national protocols
- Discuss patients with recurrent infection with your local microbiology department

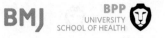

ONGOING RESEARCH

- To determine the epidemiology of community acquired *Clostridium difficile* infections in younger patients who have not received antibiotics or had contact with the healthcare system
- To determine the contribution of factors such as *C difficile* in food animals, salads and other food stuffs, pets, soil, and water
- To define diagnostic algorithms that optimise test combinations for the laboratory diagnosis of *C difficile* infection
- There is considerable interest in the development of monoclonal antibodies and toxin specific vaccines to prevent or treat *C difficile* infection, and tolevamer, a novel toxin binding polymer, is undergoing clinical trials
- Randomised controlled trials (RCTs) are urgently needed to examine treatment for fulminant, refractory, and recurrent *C difficile* infection, including new antibiotics such as tigecycline, and non-antimicrobial agents such as intravenous immunoglobulin
- An RCT examining faecal transplantation is under way in the Netherlands

Conclusions

Many cases of *C difficile* infection could be prevented by prudent antibiotic prescribing and vigorous infection control measures, which may also reduce other healthcare associated infections and limit the spread of multiresistant organisms such as MRSA and vancomycin resistant enterococci. Although evidence from RCTs supports guidance on the initial antibiotic treatment of *C difficile* infection, more data are urgently needed on the management of refractory, fulminant, and recurrent disease.

Contributors: JS-L helped in design and wrote initial drafts; NM helped in conception, merged drafts to produce the final review, and prepared the paper for submission; FJC helped in design and wrote the draft for the prevention section; SHA helped in conception, co-wrote the final version, provided critique for intellectual content, provided final approval for submission, and is guarantor.

Competing interests: None declared.

Provenance and peer review: Not commissioned; externally peer reviewed.

1 Department of Health and Health Protection Agency. Clostridium difficile infection: How to deal with the problem. 2008. www.hpa.org.uk/webw/HPAweb&HPAwebStandard/HPAweb_C/1204186173530.
2 Noblett SE, Welfare M, Seymour K. The role of surgery in Clostridium difficile colitis. BMJ 2009;338:b1563.
3 Aslam S, Hamill RJ, Musher DM. Treatment of Clostridium difficile-associated disease: old therapies and new strategies. Lancet Infect Dis 2005;5:549-57.
4 Centre for Disease Control and Prevention. Severe Clostridium difficile associated disease in populations previously at low risk. MMWR 2005;54:1201-5.
5 NHS Purchasing and Supply Agency. Evaluation report: Clostridium difficile toxin detection assays. 2009. www.pasa.nhs.uk/pasa/Doc.aspx?Path=%5bMN%5d%5bSP%5d/NHSprocurement/CEP/CEP08054.pdf.
6 Commission for Healthcare Audit and Inspection. Investigation into outbreaks of Clostridium difficile at Maidstone and Tunbridge Wells NHS Trust, October 2007.
7 Fawley WN, Freeman J, Smith C, Harmanus C, van den Berg RJ, Kuijper EJ, et al. Use of highly discriminatory fingerprinting to analyze clusters of Clostridium difficile infection cases due to epidemic ribotype 027 strains. J Clin Microbiol 2008;46:954-60.
8 Bignardi GE. Risk factors for Clostridium difficile infection. J Hosp Infect 1998;40:1-15.
9 Dial S, Kezouh A, Dascal A, Barkun A, Suissa S. Patterns of antibiotic use and risk of hospital admission because of Clostridium difficile infection. CMAJ 2008;179:767-72.
10 Climo MW, Israel DS, Wong ES, Williams D, Coudron P, Markowitz SM. Hospital-wide restriction of clindamycin: effect on the incidence of Clostridium difficile-associated diarrhea and cost. Ann Intern Med 1998;128:989-95.
11 Khan R, Cheesbrough J. Impact of changes in antibiotic policy on Clostridium difficile-associated diarrhoea (CDAD) over a five-year period in a district general hospital. J Hosp Infect 2003;54:104-8.
12 Davey P, Brown E, Fenelon L, Finch R, Gould I, Hartman G, et al. Interventions to improve antibiotic prescribing practices for hospital inpatients. Cochrane Database Syst Rev 2005;(4):CD003543.
13 Loo VG, Poirier L, Miller MA, Oughton M, Libman MD, Michaud S, et al. A predominantly clonal multi-institutional outbreak of Clostridium difficile-associated diarrhea with high morbidity and mortality. N Engl J Med 2005;353:2442-9.
14 Wilcox MH, Freeman J. Epidemic Clostridium difficile. N Engl J Med 2006;354:1201.
15 Cooke FJ, Holmes AH. The missing care bundle: antibiotic prescribing in hospitals. Int J Antimicrob Agents 2007;30:25-9.
16 Wilcox MH, Cunnliffe JG, Trundle C, Redpath C. Financial burden of hospital-acquired Clostridium difficile infection. J Hosp Infect 1996;34:23-30.
17 Gerding DN, Muto CA, Owens RC Jr. Measures to control and prevent Clostridium difficile infection. Clin Infect Dis 2008;46(suppl 1):S43-9.
18 Oughton MT, Loo VG, Dendukuri N, Fenn S, Libman MD. Hand hygiene with soap and water is superior to alcohol rub and antiseptic wipes for removal of Clostridium difficile. Infect Control Hosp Epidemiol 2009;30:939-44.
19 Jernigan JA, Siegman-Igra Y, Guerrant RC, Farr BM. A randomized crossover study of disposable thermometers for prevention of Clostridium difficile and other nosocomial infections. Infect Control Hosp Epidemiol 1998;19:494-9.
20 Cooper BS, Stone SP, Kibbler CC, Cookson BD, Roberts JA, Medley GF, et al. Systematic review of isolation policies in the hospital management of methicillin-resistant Staphylococcus aureus: a review of the literature with epidemiological and economic modelling. Health Technol Assess 2003;7:1-194.
21 Commission for Healthcare Audit and Inspection. Investigation into outbreaks of Clostridium difficile at Stoke Mandeville Hospital, Buckinghamshire Hospitals NHS Trust, July 2006.
22 Pepin J, Routhier S, Gagnon S, Brazeau I. Management and outcomes of a first recurrence of Clostridium difficile -associated disease in Quebec, Canada. Clin Infect Dis 2006;42:758-64.
23 Hickson M, D'Souza AL, Muthu N, Rogers TR, Want S, Rajkumar C, et al. Use of probiotic Lactobacillus preparation to prevent diarrhoea associated with antibiotics: randomised double blind placebo controlled trial. BMJ 2007;335:80.
24 Wilcox MH, Sandoe JA. Probiotics and diarrhea: data are not widely applicable [letter]. BMJ 2007;335:171.
25 Bolton RP, Culshaw MA. Faecal metronidazole concentrations during oral and intravenous therapy for antibiotic associated colitis due to Clostridium difficile. Gut 1986;27:1169-72.
26 Zar FA, Bakkanagari SR, Moorthi KM, Davis MB. A comparison of vancomycin and metronidazole for the treatment of Clostridium difficile-associated diarrhea, stratified by disease severity. Clin Infect Dis 2007;45:302-7.
27 Louie T, Gerson M, Grimard D, Johnson S, Poirier A, Weiss K, Louie T, Gerson M, Grimard D, et al. Results of a phase III trial comparing tolevamer, vancomycin and metronidazole in Clostridium difficile-associated diarrhea (CDAD) [abstract K-4259]. In: Program and abstracts of the 47th Interscience Conference on Antimicrobial Agents and Chemotherapy (Washington DC). ASM Press, 2007.
28 Al-Nassir WN, Sethi AK, Li Y, Pultz MJ, Riggs MM, Donskey CJ. Both oral metronidazole and oral vancomycin promote persistent overgrowth of vancomycin-resistant enterococci during treatment of Clostridium difficile-associated disease. Antimicrob Agents Chemother 2008;52:2403-6.

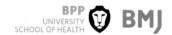

29 Fekety R, Silva J, Kauffman C, Buggy B, Deery HG. Treatment of antibiotic-associated Clostridium difficile colitis with oral vancomycin: comparison of two dosage regimens. *Am J Med* 1989;86:15-9.

30 Apisarnthanarak A, Razavi B, Mundy L. Adjunctive intracolonic vancomycin for severe Clostridium difficile colitis: case series and review of the literature. *Clin Infect Dis* 2002;35:690-6.

31 Wenisch C, Parschalk B, Hasenhündl M, Hirschl AM, Graninger W. Comparison of vancomycin, teicoplanin, metronidazole, and fusidic acid for the treatment of Clostridium difficile-associated diarrhea. *Clin Infect Dis* 1996;22:813-8.

32 Gerding DN, Muto CA, Owens RC Jr. Treatment of Clostridium difficile infection. *Clin Infect Dis* 2008;46(suppl 1):S32-42.

33 Kelly CP, LaMont JT. Clostridium difficile—more difficult than ever. *N Engl J Med* 2008;359:1932-40.

34 Lowy I, Molrine DC, Leav BA, Blair BM, Baxter R, Gerding DN, et al. Treatment with monoclonal antibodies against Clostridium difficile toxins. *N Engl J Med* 2010;362:197-205.

35 Wilcox MH. Descriptive study of intravenous immunoglobulin for the treatment of recurrent Clostridium difficile diarrhoea. *J Antimicrob Chemother* 2004;53:882-4.

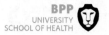

Preparing young travellers for low resource destinations

Caoimhe Nic Fhogartaigh, specialist registrar[1], Christopher Sanford, associate professor[2], Ron H Behrens, consultant physician[3]

[1]Hospital for Tropical Diseases, Mortimer Market Centre, London, UK

[2]Department of Family Medicine, University of Washington, Seattle, WA, USA

[3]Department of Clinical Research, Faculty of Infectious and Tropical Diseases, London School of Hygiene and Tropical Medicine, London WC1E 7HT

Correspondence to: R H Behrens, Travel Clinic, Hospital for Tropical Diseases, London WC1E 6JB, UK ron.behrens@lshtm.ac.uk

Cite this as: BMJ 2012;345:e7179

DOI: 10.1136/bmj.e7179

http://www.bmj.com/content/345/bmj.e7179

Increasing numbers of young adults travel to developing regions for leisure and social projects. Illness—mainly self limiting gastrointestinal or respiratory syndromes—is reported in three quarters of all such travellers.[1][2][3][4] Adverse health events occur more often in young travellers than in older ones, and these are associated with basic living conditions, longer duration of travel, and risk taking behaviours.[3][5] Road traffic crashes and injury while swimming also cause an excess number of deaths.[6]

Although extensive data are available on prevention of infectious diseases, data are lacking on accident prevention and behaviour modification to reduce health risks. Most research has focused on travellers of all ages, so extrapolation is needed to provide information on the subgroup of younger people.

Healthcare professionals are often consulted about pre-travel issues, and this review aims to provide them with published evidence and expert opinion on the major health problems that affect young people travelling to developing countries. It will also provide a framework for performing a travel health risk assessment.

What is involved in a pre-travel risk assessment?

A pre-travel risk assessment is the process of gathering information on socioeconomic, behavioural, environmental, and medical factors that are likely to affect travellers at their destination (box 1).[7] This is combined with policy recommendations and the individual's preferences to make shared decisions on the most appropriate travel health interventions. Effective communication of risk, traveller's perception of risk, attitude to preventive measures (including cost and side effects), and ability to comply with behaviour modification must all be considered.

How can infectious diseases be prevented?

What vaccinations need to be considered?
Cohorts of returning travellers have low rates of vaccine preventable diseases, with hepatitis A occurring at 1.35 per 100 000 person months and typhoid at 0.42 per 100 000 person months.[8][9] The risk may be higher in travellers on a low budget who visit developing regions. Guidelines are available on country specific vaccinations,[10][11] but individual risk assessment is needed for some vaccines.

Decisions on the need for rabies vaccination should take into account the duration of travel, whether rabies is endemic in the travel destination, age (children are at highest risk), and access to post-exposure prophylaxis with rabies immunoglobulin; however, exposure can be unpredictable. In a survey of backpackers in Bangkok (mean age 25 years), the rate of being bitten was 6.9 per 1000 person months, more than half of bites occurred within the first 10 days, and many people were poorly informed about the risk of rabies before travelling.[12] The need for immediate medical attention after a bite must be emphasised, regardless of vaccination status.

The risk of being exposed to hepatitis B during travel is low, and infection is mainly transmitted sexually in those who are visiting friends and relatives.[13] A prospective cohort study found influenza seroconversion rates of one per 100 person months after travel, making flu the most common vaccine preventable infection, and vaccination is increasingly recommended.[14] Because cost is often a problem, a discussion of risk versus benefit will enable the patient to make an informed decision on the most cost effective vaccines. Ensure that the traveller is up to date with routine vaccinations and arrange for catch-up vaccinations if necessary. In a study of people attending a pre-travel clinic in an inner city, a large proportion of whom were young travellers about to visit friends and relatives, at least a third of people needed one or more routine vaccination.[15]

How can malaria be prevented?
Plasmodium falciparum malaria occurs in 52-169 per 100 000 travellers to west Africa.[16] A cross sectional survey at two airports in Zimbabwe found that younger travellers (18-30 years) were more likely to travel to malaria risk areas, were significantly less informed about prophylaxis, and travelled for longer periods (more than four weeks), all of which were associated with lower rates of adherence to chemoprophylaxis.[17] Region specific guidance on chemoprophylaxis is available,[18][19] but malaria surveillance and travel statistics estimate risk at less than one per 100 000 travellers for many parts of South America and Southeast Asia, and it has been suggested that chemoprophylaxis is unnecessary.[20] Education through written information, instructions for chemoprophylaxis, and an outline of malaria symptoms should be provided, with advice to seek medical attention and rapid diagnostic testing should these symptoms occur, even up to six months after return. Some specialists recommend prescribed standby treatment, but a doctor should be consulted as soon as possible.[21] Data are needed on self diagnosis and treatment of malaria in young travellers.

SUMMARY POINTS

- Data on health problems encountered by young travellers are lacking and further research is needed
- Non-infectious threats are a priority in the pre-travel risk assessment
- Provide advice on injury and crime prevention, sexual health, alcohol, drug use, and prevention of infectious diseases
- Universities and volunteer organisations should emphasise pre-travel preparation, occupational health advice, and protocols to manage illness and injury overseas
- Influencing and changing behaviour is important and most difficult in this group
- Shared decision making improves understanding and compliance

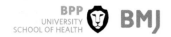

BOX 1 PERFORMING A PRE-TRAVEL RISK ASSESSMENT

The following must be ascertained to identify risks and appropriate interventions:

- Travel destination(s) including region, planned accommodation, and season of travel
- Purpose of travel: tourism, visiting friends and relatives, study, or work. Aspects to consider include planned leisure activities, nature of work or volunteering, and whether the trip is organised or self prepared
- Modes of transport, taking note of high risk travel, such as motorcycle riding
- Duration of travel
- Whether travelling alone or in a group
- Medical history: long term conditions, psychiatric illness, drugs
- Social history: alcohol use, illicit drug use, sexual history
- Previous travel experience: understanding of health risks at destination, experience of preventive strategies and barriers to uptake, particular concerns
- Behaviour: risk threshold and risk taking
- Likelihood of behaviour change

BOX 2 ADVICE ON PERSONAL SAFETY

Any threat

- Undertake pre-travel research using reputable guide books and web resources to determine threats
- Arrange insurance that is appropriate for the destination and anticipated activities
- Keep family and friends informed of your itinerary, and communicate regularly throughout the trip—for example, with a travel blog
- Register with your embassy if travelling remotely or for more than one month

Accidents and injuries

- Avoid using scooters or motorcycles and wear helmets if you do so
- Wear seatbelts in motor vehicles and on public transport if available
- Avoid travel at night and in bad weather conditions
- Avoid unsafe travel, such as a quad bike, on the back of a truck, or on the roof of a bus
- If planning sport or adventure activities, ensure safety equipment is provided and bring appropriate and well fitting clothing, footwear, and protective eye wear
- Undertake adventure sports with a companion or in a small group, with an experienced guide if your experience is limited
- Seek local advice on environmental hazards and weather conditions if planning outdoor pursuits, and carry a mobile phone if possible
- Carry a first aid kit and know how to use it
- Know the depth of water and any underwater hazards before diving; diving feet first is advised
- Pay attention to signs and surf conditions when swimming or undertaking water sports, and use flotation devices or life jackets where necessary
- Do not consume alcohol before swimming, cycling, or using a watercraft

Violence and theft

- Avoid travel to areas of conflict or political unrest
- Travel with a companion or group
- Stay in secure accommodation and use a safety deposit box
- Use only official taxi services
- Carry minimal amounts of money; a hidden money belt may be useful for holding passports and larger amounts of money
- Do not wear expensive watches or jewellery
- Dress appropriately with respect to local culture
- Avoid illicit drug use and excessive use of alcohol because of the increased risk of violent attacks and theft
- Never accept food or drink from strangers, and do not leave drinks unattended because of the risk of "spiking"
- Ensure that hired cars are roadworthy and can be locked securely
- Upload important documents onto a secure website before travel in case of theft

Environment related illness

- Seek local advice on environmental hazards, including flora, fauna, and weather conditions
- Wear protective clothing, high factor sunscreen (reapplied regularly), and insect repellent
- Carry a first aid kit
- Carry an adequate supply of water and high energy snacks
- Carry a flashlight for walking at night
- Check shoes and clothes carefully for spiders, scorpions, and so on
- Wear a stinger suit when swimming in areas with jellyfish
- Remain in vehicles when travelling through wildlife reserves
- When ascending to high altitude, adjust ascent to 300 m a day if possible; prophylactic acetazolamide may be considered but should not replace gradual ascent

---

How can diarrhoea be prevented and treated?
Travellers' diarrhoea affects 20-90% of travellers to high risk areas, including South and Southeast Asia, sub-Saharan Africa, Egypt, and South and Central America.[22] A single centre questionnaire based study that prospectively investigated illness in travellers showed that younger travellers were at greater risk of diarrhoea, and that this was associated with basic living conditions, poor hygiene, and excessive alcohol.[3]

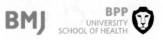

Environmental hazards to travellers[w19]	
Activity or destination	**Environmental hazards**
Summer holiday	Sunburn, heat exhaustion or heat stroke, dehydration, insect bites, animal bites, diarrhoeal disease
Urban travel	Respiratory illness due to air pollution, heat exhaustion or heat stroke, dehydration, diarrhoeal disease, insect bites
Camping or hiking	Skin blisters, hypothermia, diarrhoeal disease, insect bites, animal bites, tick borne and other zoonotic infections
Skiing	Hypothermia, frost bite, sunburn, snow blindness, avalanche risk, trauma
Mountain climbing	Skin blisters, hypothermia, frost bite, acute mountain sickness, sunburn, snow blindness, trauma
Fresh water rafting or kayaking	Drowning and cold water immersion, hypothermia, diarrhoeal disease, minor abrasions, leptospirosis, schistosomiasis in some tropical regions
Scuba diving or snorkelling	Venomous jelly fish and stingrays, abrasions, coral cuts, decompression and motion sickness

Comparable results were found in a similar study that compared young travellers (18-30 years) with older (>60 years) ones; the young travellers were also noted to have more risk taking behaviours.[5] Reviews of studies investigating diet and travellers' diarrhoea failed to show a correlation with food choice,[23] but travel destination and eating establishment were important predictors.[24] Advice should focus on self treatment and rehydration. A systematic review supported prompt antibiotic treatment (for example, ciprofloxacin) in reducing symptom duration.[25] In South and Southeast Asia, azithromycin is preferred because of fluoroquinolone resistance in *Campylobacter* spp.[26] Loperamide has a role, but it should be avoided in patients with fever or bloody diarrhoea.[27]

What should we advise young travellers about personal safety?

Advice on personal safety is often not included in the pre-travel consultation. Leggat and Klein have written a useful overview on safety.[28]

How can accidents and injuries be prevented?

Data on travel related injuries are limited, with most data focusing on mortality. Retrospective studies of deaths in US and Canadian citizens overseas showed that 25% and 18.7%, respectively, were caused by accidents,[29 30] whereas only 1% were caused by infection. The mean age was significantly younger for accidental death than for natural death (45 v 66 years).[30] The most common causes of death were motor vehicle collisions (21-27%), drowning (14-16%), and murder (9-17%).[29 31] Population based studies of road traffic crashes in resorts suggest that risk is fivefold greater for tourists than for locals.[32 33] A travel clinic based survey showed that more than 5% of tourists experience falls and recreational injuries,[3] making them a much more likely occurrence in young travellers than a serious infectious disease. Traumatic injuries may require air evacuation.[34]

In developing regions, risk of accidental injury is high. A review of the health records of tourists presenting to healthcare settings in Jamaican resorts showed that accidents were responsible for around 40% morbidity.[35] In a similar study in Mexico, accidents contributed to 50% of deaths in tourists.[w1] Indeed, accidents are associated with significantly higher proportional mortality ratios in Africa (2.7) and Southeast Asia (1.6) compared with the United States.[31] Morbidity data for developing regions are probably a gross underestimate.[w2] The World Health Organization estimates that, globally, injuries from road traffic collisions are around 20 times more common than deaths.[w3]

Various studies indicate that accidents abroad are associated with male sex,[29 35 w4 w5] younger age,[29 w6] developing countries,[34 35 w1] urban destinations,[w7] risky transport such as motorcycles and watercraft,[5 29 w4 w8] and diving into shallow water.[w9]

Proposed contributing factors include differences in safety measures at the destination compared with the traveller's home country,[w10 w11] high rates of road traffic crashes in developing countries,[w12] unfamiliar environment and activities,[35 w10 w11] poor quality equipment (including lack of safety features and seatbelts),[4 w10 w11] and alcohol and drug intake.[32 w9] Injuries in low resource settings are further complicated by limited and delayed access to healthcare and repatriation.

Strategies to prevent travel related accidents have been proposed, but no interventions have yet been evaluated. A decline in deaths overseas of Peace Corps volunteers (mostly aged 20-39 years) was attributed to a reduction in accidents after restrictions on motorcycle use were introduced.[w13] This shows that policy and legislation may have a greater impact than advice, which relies on action or a change in behaviour by the individual. Preventive strategies require collaboration between medical practitioners, the travel industry, and health officials in the host country so that measures can be implemented at multiple levels.[w8]

Recommendations for water safety and prevention of drowning have been published,[w14] and general advice on accident prevention can be found on national travel health websites.[11 12] Box 2 summarises recommendations based on expert opinion.

How can violence and attacks by criminals or terrorists be prevented?

Threats to safety and security vary between destinations, and detailed country specific information is available from government websites.[w15 w16] In surveys of young holidaymakers, 2.8-6.4% reported having been in a physical fight.[w5 w17] This type of violence was associated with male sex, alcohol, drug use, and "nightlife" destinations.[w5] In surveys of long term volunteers in developing regions, however, almost 25% reported exposure to violence, such as mugging, police violence, and political unrest.[w18] In the Peace Corps, 17% of deaths were attributable to murder; most occurred in Africa and were motivated by robbery.[w13] Again, there is no evidence on how to prevent criminal attacks. Travellers should consult the Foreign Office website before travel to identify any high risk areas or activity.

How can environment related illness be avoided?

The table outlines environmental hazards experienced by travellers.[w19] Adventure travel carries a high risk, and a questionnaire study of expedition participants (mostly aged 18-40 years) showed that 7.6% experienced health problems, ranging from insect bites and stings, to heat exhaustion and acute mountain sickness.[w20] Although acute mountain sickness is a well recognised risk in those who trek and climb mountains, it is often overlooked in non-adventure travellers to high altitude. In Cuzco (3360 m), a cross sectional airport based survey of departing travellers (mean age 32 years) reported 48.5% developed altitude sickness, as defined by the Lake Louis clinical score. Despite high rates of pre-travel advice, many of these people were unaware of this risk.[w21] Prospective collection of data on travellers and expatriates (median age 31) presenting to a Kathmandu clinic showed that male sex, tourist travel, and lack of pre-travel advice were risk factors for environment related illness.[w22] Information and preparation before travel help reduce risk. Travel health websites provide country specific information and supplementary leaflets.[11] [12] Specific advice for backpackers,[w23] a review of medically important venomous animals,[w24] and guidelines on prevention of acute mountain sickness are also available.[w25] [w26]

What should we advise on alcohol and illicit drugs?

Surveys of 18-35 year old backpackers in Australia suggest that their alcohol consumption is significantly increased while travelling.[w27] Surveys of travellers (mean age 25 years) to Southeast Asia also showed that rates of illicit drug use exceeded 50%,[w28] probably because of low cost and widespread availability. Cannabis was most popular, although ecstasy, cocaine, or lysergide (LSD) were used by 20% of those who travelled for more than 20 weeks.[w28] Large epidemiological studies on the association between alcohol and substance misuse and accidents, injuries, and psychiatric comorbidity, as well as cross sectional surveys of 16-35 year old British tourists abroad, show that these substances are associated with road traffic incidents,[32] [w29] trauma,[w9] [w30] [w31] violence,[w17] [w31] unsafe sex,[w31] and mental health problems.[w32] Substance misuse overseas carries an increased risk of dehydration, hazardous contamination, overdose, lack of social support, anxiety, and depression.[w27] [w33]

Predictors of substance misuse are male sex, smoking, previous use, lack of higher education, lone travel, and prolonged travel.[w28] The hazards of alcohol and illicit drugs should be discussed during a pre-travel consultation, with the serious penalties for possession in many countries being described.

What should we advise on sexual health?

Surveys show that young travellers have high rates of new sexual relationships (47.5%-68.9%),[w34] [w35] particularly young travellers,[w36] with 21.5-45% having multiple partners.[w35] In addition, 40% do not use condoms or use them inconsistently.[w34] [w35] [w37] Although most young people have sex with other travellers or expatriates, some have sex with local people, including sex workers.[w37] [w38] Having sex with local people increases the risk of acquiring common sexually transmitted infections and also HIV, syphilis, lymphogranuloma venereum, chancroid, and donovanosis, which are endemic in many regions.[w39]

The above studies showed that risky sexual behaviour was associated with the number of pre-travel partners,[w34] prolonged travel,[w35] high frequency of alcohol and drug use,[w34] [w35] frequent nightlife,[w35] and pre-travel expectation of sex,[w35] [w37] as well as being single,[w37] male,[w37] and homosexual or bisexual.[w37] A randomised controlled trial that compared standard pre-travel consultation, with additional provision of condoms, and a motivational brief intervention showed no effect on condom use in young travellers.[w40] Nevertheless, we should highlight sexual health risks and the role of excess alcohol and drugs, and encourage condom use. A guide to sexual health for young travellers has been published.[w41]

What extra advice should we give medical students and volunteers travelling to developing countries?

In addition to the above risks, medical students are exposed to tuberculosis and blood borne viruses. Surveys report needlestick injuries and splash exposure in 8-37% of medical students who travel to developing countries, usually when performing procedures in which they lack experience.[w42-w44] Few carry HIV postexposure prophylaxis (PEP), and reporting of exposure to blood and body fluids is poor.[w42-w44]

Stress and psychological problems due to the nature of the work, culture shock, and social isolation are also prevalent.[w45] Forty per cent of humanitarian aid workers report that their mission was more stressful than they had expected.[w46] Stress is exacerbated by the high (16-25%) rates of violence and crime experienced by aid workers.[w18] [w46] Peace Corps volunteers now undergo pre-travel screening, training in hazard avoidance, and self monitoring of physical and psychological status, and this may have contributed to the reduction in deaths from accidents and suicide in this population.[w13]

Pre-travel risk assessment and preparation—focusing on planned practical procedures and competency, access to PEP, psychological screening, adjustment to local cultural norms, personal safety, and insurance (with medical repatriation)—are essential in these groups. Ideally the consultation should be standardised for all travellers. Some organisations prohibit students undertaking invasive procedures in countries where HIV is prevalent. Simulated procedure training has been shown to reduce needlestick injuries but not exposure to splashes,[w43] so students should be provided with safety glasses. A PEP starter kit (5-7 days) should be supplied for areas of high HIV prevalence, accompanied by written instructions on immediate action and reporting if exposure occurs.[w47] Who should pay for PEP is a topic of controversy.[w42] [w44] Provision of an emergency helpline for students with health problems overseas and a post-travel consultation have been recommended.[w44] [w47]

What about people with a long term medical condition?

Chronic medical conditions, including psychiatric ones, should be reviewed as part of the risk assessment when deciding on the itinerary or deployment. Suitability and personal safety should be evaluated by both parties at the outset. Advise patients on carrying medical documentation, sufficient medication, or equipment (or a combination thereof) and provide information on how to access relevant healthcare abroad. Health insurance must cover pre-existing conditions. A written individualised self management plan is useful for some chronic conditions such as asthma. Detailed advice is available but outside the scope of this review.[w48] [w49]

How can we encourage young travellers to be more responsible for travel health problems?

Questionnaire surveys of students and backpackers suggest that many do not seek pre-travel advice. Those who do seek advice often use non-expert sources, and the information provided may not agree with that from health professionals.[w50-w52] Information evenings and written travel health advice from hostel organisations, along with web based resources and simulations, may engage and educate young people and potentially influence their perceptions and behaviour.[w52] [w53] Further research is needed into health problems in young people who travel to resource

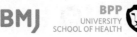

poor settings. Collaboration between the tourism and travel industry and healthcare professionals is necessary to identify the most effective methods of influencing risk taking behaviour.

SOURCES AND SELECTION CRITERIA

In this specialty, data come from population surveys, retrospective reviews, and cross sectional or cohort studies, often limited to a single centre or destination,[7] and less often from large randomised controlled trials.

We searched PubMed using combinations of words including young, youth, student, elective, volunteer, travel, traveller, health, illness, risk, advice, developing, tropical. The search was limited to the past 25 years and English language articles, and we focused on the 18-35 age group, excluding studies in children. Appropriate publications were selected from the abstracts, and additional relevant articles included from their references. We also performed searches within specific areas, such as travellers' diarrhoea. In most cases few, if any, such studies focused on young people specifically. Relevant guidelines, policies, and websites were consulted where possible for supplemental data.

ADDITIONAL EDUCATIONAL RESOURCES

Resources for healthcare professionals

- National Travel Health Network and Centre (www.nathnac. org)—Country specific guidelines for healthcare professionals on vaccination and disease prevention, as well as health and safety advice for the preparing traveller

Resources for patients

- Centres for Disease Control and Prevention (wwwnc.cdc.gov/ travel/destinations/list.htm)—Health and safety advice for the preparing traveller
- Fit for Travel (www.fitfortravel.nhs.uk/advice.aspx)—Health information for people travelling abroad from the UK, including advice for patients with asthma, diabetes, or disability, and advice on altitude and volunteer work
- Year Out Group (www.yearoutgroup.org/)—An association of independent registered organisations that provide structured programmes for young travellers planning volunteer work, expeditions, or cultural exchanges

---

Contributors: CNF conducted the searches for relevant articles. CNF and RHB reviewed the papers that informed this article. CNF wrote the first draft. All authors helped critically revise the article and form the final draft. RHB is guarantor.

Competing interests: All authors have completed the ICMJE uniform disclosure form at www.icmje.org/coi_disclosure.pdf (available on request from the corresponding author) and declare: no support from any organisation for the submitted work; RHB is supported by the UCL Hospitals Comprehensive Biomedical Research Centre Infection Theme, he is on the clinical advisory board for Sigma Tau and Norgine Pharmaceutical, and he has received support for producing an educational course from Norgine; RHB's employer has received a contract research grant from Intercell; no other relationships or activities that could appear to have influenced the submitted work.

Provenance and peer review: Commissioned; externally peer reviewed.

1   Hill DR. Health problems in a large cohort of Americans travelling to endemic countries. *J Travel Med* 2000;7:259-66.
2   Steffen R, Richenbach M, Wilhelm U, Helminger A, Schär M. Health problems after travel to developing countries. *J Infect Dis* 1987;156:84-91.
3   Rack J, Wichman O, Kamara B, Günther M, Cramer J, Schönfeld C, et al. Risk and spectrum of diseases in travellers to popular tourist destinations. *J Travel Med* 2005;12:248-53.
4   Hargarten SW, Baker TD, Guptill K. Overseas fatalities of US citizen travellers: an analysis of deaths related to international travel. *Ann Emerg Med* 1991;20:622-6.
5   Alon D, Shitrit P, Chowers M. Risk behaviours and spectrum of diseases among elderly travellers: a comparison of younger and older adults. *J Travel Med* 2010;17:250-5.
6   Steffen R. Travel medicine—prevention based on epidemiological data. *Trans R Soc Trop Med Hygiene* 1991;85:156-62.
7   Behrens RH, Stauffer WM, Barnett ED, Loutan L, Hatz CF, Matteelli A, et al. Travel case scenarios as a demonstration of risk assessment of VFR travellers: introduction to criteria and evidence-based definition and framework. *J Travel Med* 2010;17:153-62.
8   Neilsen US, Larsen CS, Howitz M, Petersen E. Hepatitis A among Danish travellers 1980-2007. *J Infect* 2009;58:47-52.
9   Ekdahl K, de Jong B, Andersson Y. Risk of travel associated typhoid and paratyphoid fevers in various regions. *J Travel Med* 2005;12:197-204.
10 National Travel Health Network and Centre. Country information. www.nathnac.org/ds/map_world.aspx.
11 Centres for Disease Control and Prevention. Travelers' health. Destinations. wwwnc.cdc.gov/travel/destinations/list.htm.
12 Piyaphanee W, Shantavasinkul P, Phumratanaprapin W, Udomchaisakul P, Wichianprasat P, Benjavongkulchai M, et al. Rabies exposure risk among foreign backpackers in Southeast Asia. *Am J Trop Med Hygiene* 2010;82:1168-71.
13 Sonder GJB, van Rijckevorsel GGC, van den Hoek A. Risk of hepatitis B for travellers: is vaccine for all travellers really necessary? *J Travel Med* 2009;16:18-22.
14 Mutsch M, Tavernini M, Marx A, Gregory V, Lin YP, Hay AJ, et al. Influenza virus infection in travellers to tropical and subtropical countries. *Clin Infect Dis* 2005;40:1282-7.
15 Hagmann S, Benavides V, Neugebauer R, Purswani M. Travel healthcare for immigrant children visiting friends and relatives abroad: retrospective analysis of a hospital-based travel health service in a US urban underserved area. *J Travel Med* 2009;16:407-12.
16 Behrens RH, Carroll B, Smith V, Alexander N. Declining incidence of malaria imported into the UK from West Africa. *Malaria J* 2008;10:235.
17 Laver SM, Wetzels J, Behrens R. Knowledge of malaria, risk perception and compliance with prophylaxis and personal and environmental protective measures in travellers exiting Zimbabwe from Harare and Victoria Falls international airport. *J Travel Med* 2001;8:298-303.
18 Chiodini P, Hill D, Lalloo D, Lea G, Walker E, Whitty C, et al. Guidelines for malaria prevention in travellers from the United Kingdom. Health Protection Agency, 2007. www.hpa.org.uk/infections/topics_az/malaria/default.htm.
19 Centres for Disease Control and Prevention. Malaria and travelers. www.cdc.gov/malaria/travelers/drugs.html.
20 Behrens RH, Carroll B, Hellgren U, Visser LG, Siikamäki H, Vestergaard LS, et al. The incidence of malaria in travellers to southeast Asia: is local malaria transmission a useful risk indicator? *Malaria J* 2010;9:266.
21 Hatz CF, Beck B, Blum J, Bourquin C, Brenneke F, Funk M, et al. Supplementum 1. Malariaschutz fur Kurzzeitaufenthalter. Swiss Federal Office of Public Health. 2006:9-10-2008.
22 Steffen R. Epidemiology of traveler's diarrhoea. *Clin Infect Dis* 2005;41:S536-40.
23 Shlim DR. Looking for evidence that personal hygiene precautions prevent traveler's diarrhoea. *Clin Infect Dis* 2005;41(suppl 8):S531-5.
24 DuPont HL, Ericsson CD, Farthing MJ, Gorbach S, Pickering LK, Rombo L, et al. Expert review of the evidence base for prevention of travelers' diarrhoea. *J Travel Med* 2009;16:149-60.
25 De Bruyn G, Hahn S, Borwick A. Antibiotic treatment for travellers' diarrhoea. *Cochrane Database Syst Rev* 2000;3:CD002242.
26 Hill DR, Beeching NJ. Travelers' diarrhea. *Current Opin Infect Dis* 2010;23:481-7.
27 Ericsson CD, DuPont HL, Okhuysen PC, Jiang ZD, DuPont MW. Loperamide plus azithromycin more effectively treats travelers' diarrhea in Mexico than azithromycin alone. *J Travel Med* 2007;14:312-9.
28 Leggat PA, Klein M. Personal safety advice for travelers abroad. *J Travel Med* 2001;8:46-51.
29 Hargarten SW, Baker TD, Guptill K. Overseas fatalities of United States citizen travellers: an analysis of deaths related to international travel. *Ann Emerg Med* 1991;20:622-6.
30 MacPherson DW, Gushulak BD, Sandhu J. Death and international travel, the Canadian experience: 1996-2004. *J Travel Med* 2007;14:77-84.
31 Guse CE, Cortés LM, Hargarten SW, Hennes HM. Fatal injuries of US citizens abroad. *J Travel Med* 2007;14:279-87.
32 Carey MJ, Aitken ME. Motorbike injuries in Bermuda: a risk for tourists. *Ann Emerg Med* 1996;28:424-9.
33 Petridou E, Askitopoulou H, Vourvahakis D, Skalkidis Y, Trichopoulos D. Epidemiology of road traffic accidents during pleasure travelling: the evidence from the island of Crete. *Accident Analys Prev* 1997;29:687-93.
34 Hargarten SW, Bouc G. Emergency air medical transport of United States citizen tourists: 1988-1990. *Air Med J* 1993;12:398-402.
35 Thompson DT, Ashley DV, Dockery-Brown CA, Binns A, Jolly CM, Jolly PE. Incidence of health crises in tourists visiting Jamaica, West Indies, 1998-2000. *J Travel Med* 2003;10:79-86.

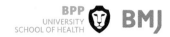

Investigation and treatment of imported malaria in non-endemic countries

Christopher J M Whitty, consultant physician and professor of international health[1][2],
Peter L Chiodini, consultant parasitologist[1], director and honorary professor[2],
David G Lalloo, professor of tropical medicine[3]

[1]Hospital for Tropical Diseases, London WC1E 6JB, UK

[2]PHE Malaria Reference Laboratory, London School of Hygiene and Tropical Medicine, London, UK

[3]Liverpool School of Tropical Medicine, Liverpool, UK

Correspondence to: C J M Whitty christopher.whitty@lshtm.ac.uk

Cite this as: BMJ 2013;346:f2900

DOI: 10.1136/bmj.f2900

http://www.bmj.com/content/346/bmj.f2900

Every year, several thousand people with malaria arrive in non-endemic countries, and about 1600 arrive in the United Kingdom alone. Case fatality in the UK, as elsewhere, is around 1% overall but varies by age and previous exposure to malaria.[1][2][3] This rate is similar to that seen in endemic countries, but the age profile of deaths is very different. In Africa mortality is highest in young children, but in imported cases it is highest in older patients, especially those over 65 years.[4][5][6] If malaria is treated early, with widely available drugs before it becomes severe, death is avoidable and a full recovery almost guaranteed. Late presentation carries a higher risk of death. The management of severe malaria is a medical emergency. This review describes how to recognise and diagnose malaria, the current treatment of uncomplicated malaria, and the management of patients with severe disease. It concentrates on adults and recent advances relevant to non-endemic high resource countries such as Europe and North America. Different challenges arise in low resource endemic settings and are not covered in this review.

What is malaria?

Malaria is a tropical parasitic disease of red blood cells transmitted by anopheles mosquitoes. Five species affect humans. The most serious, and in Europe the most common, imported form is Plasmodium falciparum malaria, which causes most deaths from imported malaria. The other common imported form is P vivax malaria. It is generally less severe but can recur several months after treatment owing to relapse from hypnozoites ("sleeping" parasites) in the liver. P ovale malaria is similar to P vivax malaria, as is P malariae malaria although it does not relapse. P knowlesi is a monkey malaria parasite that has recently been recognised to infect humans and is rare in imported cases.

Who is at risk of acquiring and dying from malaria?

Several countries that are frequented by tourists and people visiting friends and relatives have regions where the average person gets clinical malaria four or more times a year. One observational study found that around one in five travellers with a history of fever returning from sub-Saharan Africa had malaria.[7] Rates are much lower (maybe 1/100) in unwell travellers returning from malaria endemic Asia and Latin America, although the risk of malaria varies widely in these continents.[6] Failure to take effective prophylaxis is associated with acquiring malaria in several observational studies. Travellers whose families emigrated from malaria endemic countries, and who are visiting friends and relatives, are at particularly high risk of acquiring malaria, especially those of west African heritage.[2] People who travelled to visit friends and relatives account for around 65% of all malaria cases in the UK, and their reported chemoprophylaxis use is lower than for other travellers. Vivax malaria, the form of malaria most commonly imported from Asia and Latin America, had been declining over the past two decades in the UK.[8]

Observational studies of imported febrile illnesses in travellers have shown that malaria remains one of the most common potentially life threatening causes of fever in travellers.[9] Such studies also show that increasing age, delay to diagnosis,[6] and presenting in an area where malaria is seldom seen or treated increase the risk of dying from falciparum malaria once acquired (evidence from the UK only).[6] Although in Africa most deaths are in children, in non-endemic high resource settings observational studies show that older people have the greatest risk of dying from malaria if acquired, with minimal risk in children and young adults and a steadily increasing risk over the age range; case fatality in those over 65 years is 4.6% in the UK.[5][6]

How to recognise malaria in adults

The symptoms and signs of malaria are non-specific and overlap with many other common infections. Influenza is a common misdiagnosis, and case reports show that malaria has also been misdiagnosed as gastroenteritis, hepatitis, and lower respiratory tract infection.[10] The key to diagnosing malaria is to take a travel history for all patients and request a malaria test in anyone who feels unwell and has recently been to an endemic country. A history of fever will be present in most patients with malaria, but around half will have no fever at the time of presentation; absence of fever cannot exclude disease.[7] Headache, malaise, and rigors are common symptoms but not invariable. Certain symptoms and signs of severe or potentially complicated malaria—such as jaundice, seizures, or rapid breathing—can result in the misdiagnosis of malaria—for example, as hepatitis (table 1). It is therefore essential to exclude malaria with a thick and thin blood film rather than rely on clinical diagnosis based on symptoms; attempts to produce algorithms that reliably predict malaria on the basis of symptoms have been unsuccessful.[11] In patients returning from malaria endemic countries, any symptom or sign compatible with an infection should raise the possibility of malaria. Although most cases of falciparum malaria present within three months of return, case reports and Public Health England data show that some cases in travellers present up to a

SUMMARY POINTS

- Malaria is a common cause of fever in people returning from the tropics
- Falciparum malaria is potentially fatal unless treated early, and patients over 65 years are at particular risk
- In most cases, vivax malaria can be treated with chloroquine in the outpatient setting
- Resistance to antimalarial drugs used to treat falciparum malaria is widespread
- Artesunate is the drug of choice for severe malaria, but if this is not available do not delay treatment with quinine

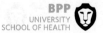

Table 1   WHO criteria for severe malaria, modified for non-endemic high resource settings (any one indicates potentially severe disease)*

Symptoms, signs, and laboratory indicators of severe disease	Adults	Children
Reduced level of consciousness	+++	+++
Seizures	+	++
Respiratory distress	++	++
Severe anaemia (haemoglobin <70 g/L)*	+	+++
Hypoglycaemia†	+	++
Renal failure	+++	+
Hyperparasitaemia (>10% red cells parasitised)	++	++
Disseminated intravascular coagulation	+	+
Shock	+	+
Warning signs of potentially complicated malaria (requires parenteral treatment):		
Jaundice	+	+
Parasite count >2%	+++	+

*+=rare; +++=uncommon; ++++=common (definition depends on age, state of immunity, and other factors).
†Common in pregnant women.

Table 2   Common licensed drugs, drug combinations, and drug doses for malaria

Drug	Dose in adults	Notes
Uncomplicated vivax, ovale, and malariae malaria		
Chloroquine	620 mg base, then 310 mg base at 6, 24, and 48 hours	
Primaquine (after chloroquine)	30 mg per day for 14 days	Test for G6PD deficiency before patients take it
Uncomplicated falciparum malaria		
Artemether-lumefantrine	4 tablets (adult) initially, followed by 5 further doses of 4 tablets at 8, 24, 36, 48, and 60 hours	
Quinine combinations	600 mg every 8 hours for 7 days or until parasites have cleared	Follow with clindamycin for 7 days, doxycycline for 7 days, or sulfadoxine-pyrimethamine once; ringing in ears a common side effect
Atovaquone-proguanil	4 tablets once a day for 3 days	Avoid if patients were on atovaquone-proguanil prophylaxis
Severe or potentially complicated malaria		
Quinine	20 mg/kg quinine intravenously, followed by 10 mg/kg 8-12 hourly until parasites have cleared	By slow infusion over 4 hours; hypoglycaemia and arrhythmias are side effects
Artesunate	2.4 mg/kg intravenously, followed by 2.4 mg/kg at 12 hours, then 2.4 mg/kg daily until parasites have cleared	As a bolus over 5 minutes

G6PD=glucose-6-phosphate dehydrogenase.

year after return, and many cases of non-falciparum malaria occur over a year later.[12]

How is malaria diagnosed?

The gold standard for malaria diagnosis in clinical practice remains microscopic examination of a blood film. Good rapid diagnostic tests for falciparum malaria with sensitivity and specificity above 97%, and fairly good ones for non-falciparum malaria,[13] are now widely available to hospitals in Europe. Most, however, are not as sensitive as an experienced microscopist and give no information about parasite density, which is important for prognosis and treatment decisions. Therefore these rapid tests should be seen as an adjunct to, rather than an alternative to, conventional microscopic diagnosis, and their sole use is not recommended. Newer polymerase chain reaction based diagnostic methods are currently used only in research settings, although they will probably become clinically useful in non-endemic settings within the next decade, especially to detect mixed infections and potentially drug resistant cases.[14]

What are the indicators of severe or complicated disease in adults?

Once malaria is diagnosed, the priority is to determine the severity of disease because this determines treatment. Table 1 shows modified World Health Organization indicators of severe disease; patients with any one of these will need parenteral treatment with antimalarial drugs. HIV positive patients have an increased risk of severe malaria and of

drug interactions.[15] Observational studies have shown that three severe syndromes predominate in adults: cerebral malaria—in practice, malaria with reduced level of consciousness, neurological signs, or seizures; renal failure; and acute lung injury (or acute respiratory distress syndrome).[16] Disseminated intravascular coagulation and shock are less common and seldom occur in isolation. In addition, jaundice (due to recent major haemolysis) or a parasite count in the blood of greater than 2%, even if the patient does not appear clinically unwell, is a sign that severe malaria is more likely to develop.

What are the indicators of severe or complicated disease in children?

Multicentre observational studies, mainly from Africa, have shown that anaemia, raised respiratory rate due to acidosis (rather than lung injury), and cerebral malaria are the most common signs of severity in young children, although this pattern varies by age, with cerebral malaria becoming more common in older children.[17]

What about malaria in pregnancy?

Treat pregnant women as having potentially complicated malaria, although not all will need parenteral treatment. The risks associated with severe disease are greater than in non-pregnant women, and there are serious risks to the pregnancy, including miscarriage, in otherwise non-severe disease.[18] The management of malaria in pregnancy has particular challenges,[19] because of the risks the disease poses to the pregnancy and because the theoretical risks

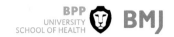

of teratogenicity of antimalarial drugs need to be balanced with the substantial risks of undertreating; specialist advice is strongly recommended. Data from animals suggest that artemisinin drugs are teratogenic in early pregnancy, but human data are reassuring, with no current evidence of increased risk.[20] Hypoglycaemia is a problem in pregnant women with malaria,[21] and any pregnant woman with a reduced level of consciousness should be given glucose while awaiting blood glucose measurements.

How is uncomplicated non-falciparum malaria managed?

Several case reports indicate that vivax malaria, and possibly ovale and malariae malaria, cause severe disease more often than was once thought,[22] and their label as "benign" malaria is misleading. However, patients with non-falciparum malaria need to be admitted only if they have indicators of severe disease (table 1) or cannot take oral drugs. Provided the laboratory making the diagnosis is experienced and unlikely to have mistaken falciparum or rare mixed species infection (<1%), chloroquine remains the drug of choice to treat vivax, ovale, and malariae malaria. There is limited but growing chloroquine resistance in vivax in eastern Asia and the Pacific.[23] Evidence from clinical trials and a systematic review shows that most patients with vivax malaria, even those from South Asia or East Asia, respond to chloroquine within three days (see table 2 for dosing).[24] Good evidence from clinical trials shows that artemisinin combination treatment (ACT) or quinine both work against vivax malaria at the same doses as those used for falciparum malaria (see below) if there is uncertainty about species or in patients with mixed infections.[25]

The biggest difficulty in managing patients with vivax or ovale malaria is that they can relapse several times after an initial episode, often more than a year after initial infection. Chloroquine and ACT treat the initial infection but do not kill the hypnozoites in the liver, which cause recurrent malaria. Primaquine is the only drug currently licensed to kill these hypnozoites and prevent or reduce the risk of relapse.[26] Apart from the need for a two week course, primaquine has two disadvantages. Firstly, resistance is gradually spreading, particularly in Oceania and eastern Asia, so that higher doses are now needed.[27] In the United States and UK, the current recommended dose for vivax malaria in adults is 30 mg a day for 14 days (15 mg a day for ovale). In addition, case reports and observational studies have found that treatment with primaquine in patients with phenotypic glucose-6-phosphate dehydrogenase (G6PD) deficiency can lead to haemolysis, which can be life threatening. G6DP deficiency therefore needs to be excluded before the drug is taken.[28] G6PD deficiency can affect more than 10% of the population in malaria endemic countries, although its prevalence is lower in people with malaria.[29] [30] Patients should not take primaquine until their G6PD status is known, but treatment with chloroquine must not be delayed. Unfortunately, the only new anti-hypnozoite drug likely to be licensed in the next few years, tafenoquine, has similar risks with G6PD deficiency.

How should uncomplicated falciparum malaria be managed?

The severity of uncomplicated falciparum malaria is difficult to assess at presentation owing to the complex life cycle of the parasites, so all patients presenting with falciparum malaria in non-endemic countries should be admitted. Patients can seem well initially and then deteriorate despite treatment, and in around 20% of patients the parasite count rises in the first 24 hours despite adequate treatment.[7] Do not assume that patients who once lived in endemic countries but now are settled in non-endemic countries retain immunity. Clinical studies show that although being born in endemic Africa reduces the risk of dying from malaria, admission to intensive care and death can still occur.[6] [31]

Provided oral treatments can be tolerated, parenteral treatment is not needed if there are no clinical or laboratory signs of severity (table 1). Because of a lack of evidence, guidelines vary about the threshold parasite count above which to give parenteral treatment in patients without symptoms or signs of severity: UK guidelines (designed for non-endemic countries) suggest parasite counts over 2%, whereas WHO suggests over 5%. Chloroquine resistance is near universal, so this drug should not be used. A variety of drug combinations are effective against uncomplicated falciparum malaria (table 2). Falciparum malaria should always be treated with a combination of at least two drugs. Commonly used options include ACTs, quinine combined with another drug, and atovaquone-proguanil. Most non-endemic countries have evidence based expert recommendations that are periodically updated on the basis of trends in epidemiology of imported malaria, emerging drug resistance, and local availability of drugs.[32] [33]

There is good evidence from large trials and systematic reviews that ACT or quinine based combinations will be effective in malaria from Africa, most of Asia, and Latin America; ACT drugs are generally better tolerated and reduce parasite counts more rapidly.[34] Two ACTs, artemether-lumefantrine and dihydroartemisinin-piperaquine, are currently licensed in Europe and may become available in the US.

Is malaria resistance increasing?

P falciparum has developed resistance to several older antimalarials, and resistance continues to evolve. Several clinical studies show clear evidence of early emerging artemisinin resistance in South East Asia (Cambodia, Thailand, and parts of Burma), although ACTs still work clinically.[35] Clinical trials have also noted partial quinine resistance in the same area. Several recent trials have found no evidence that quinine or artesunate resistance is a serious clinical problem outside these areas. Resistance to some older companion drugs (such as sulfadoxine-pyrimethamine) is widespread, but well conducted trials (in endemic countries) and observational data (in imported cases) show that the combinations in table 2 are effective for most (>95%) cases of imported malaria. Atovaquone-proguanil has been associated with occasional treatment failure in some case reports, so many centres do not use it as first line treatment[36]; it should not be used in people who have been taking it prophylactically. Atovaquone-proguanil may be appropriate second line treatment for the rare cases of treatment failure with effective first line combinations, particularly those from South East Asia. Falciparum malaria does not relapse and patients can be reassured that they are unlikely to have recurrent malaria if they complete a full course of treatment. Any further attacks (generally within six weeks) usually represent treatment failure. Warn travellers about the growing problem of poor quality and counterfeit antimalarial drugs in many endemic countries.[37]

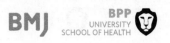

How should severe and potentially complicated malaria be managed?

Severe malaria is a medical emergency, and the main priority is for patients to receive adequate doses of effective drugs as soon as possible. Quinine (quinidine in the US, which is broadly equivalent) or artesunate are the two drugs used for parenteral treatment of severe malaria. Clear evidence from large randomised trials now shows that although quinine remains effective, artesunate is associated with a survival advantage (relative risk reduction of 22-34%) in adults and children in Asia and Africa.[38] [39] Previously, the poor quality and limited availability of parenteral artesunate has been a problem in many non-endemic countries. However, although not licensed in Europe or the US, parenteral artesunate of reliable quality can now be sourced (including through the Centers for Disease Control and Prevention in the US). Patients should always be started on parenteral quinine while trying to obtain artesunate if it is not initially available to avoid delay in effective treatment. In adults, artesunate confers the greatest survival benefit in those with very high parasite counts (>10%).[22] Parenteral quinine and quinidine are associated with hypoglycaemia and arrhythmia so should be used with caution in patients with cardiac problems.

Other than antimalarials, good management of patients with severe malaria largely depends on supportive care, including dialysis or haemofiltration in those with renal failure and respiratory support for those with acute lung injury. Various adjunctive treatments have been tried in cerebral malaria—including steroids, mannitol, and anti-tumour necrosis factor—none of which has shown a survival advantage.

For many years, there has been controversy over the use of exchange transfusion or automated red blood cell exchange to reduce parasite counts in patients with hyperparasitaemia (generally >10%).[40] The advent of treatment with artesunate, when available, renders this debate irrelevant. Unlike quinine, artesunate kills parasites of all stages and rapidly reduces parasite counts. Exchange transfusion is now rarely indicated and should be used only after discussion with a specialist centre.

The optimum management of fluids in adults and children has, in the absence of good data, been highly controversial. A recent trial in African children showed convincingly that aggressive fluid management was associated with increased mortality.[41] Good data on the optimal management of fluids in adults or children in high resource settings are limited. In adults, particularly those with renal failure, the risks of undertreating acidosis and any pre-renal component if fluids are withheld must be balanced against provoking pulmonary oedema if excess fluids are used. Most doctors used to treating severe malaria are wary about the overuse of fluids once pre-renal failure has been ruled out by short, small fluid challenges; unlike in bacterial sepsis, shock is rare in adults with malaria.

Clinical observational studies have shown a clear association between severe malaria and Gram negative sepsis in children, and reductions in the incidence of malaria in populations have been associated with reductions in Gram negative bacteria.[42] [43] Broad spectrum antibiotics should therefore be considered in all children with severe malaria. Data from adults are limited, but the association seems to be less pronounced, so routine antibiotics are not needed.[44] Case reports suggest that broad spectrum antibiotics should be given to the rare adult patients who have shock with malaria.

Acute respiratory distress syndrome is the most feared late complication of malaria in adults. In severe malaria, this can occur several days after treatment has started, including when parasites have cleared from the blood. As with other causes of the syndrome, it is important to maintain oxygenation with respiratory support in intensive care and treat the underlying infection. No adjunctive treatments have been shown to improve outcomes in patients with this complication. Respiratory distress is also a poor prognostic sign in African children,[11] but less so in Asia (perhaps because of greater availability of blood transfusions)[45]; it is almost always caused by acidosis rather than lung injury.[11]

What is the prognosis after malaria?

The outlook for adults who survive an initial episode of malaria is good, even for those with severe malaria. Serious neurological sequelae occur in less than 5% of adults with severe malaria, although few series have been large enough to provide confident estimates. Many of the estimates in the literature are based on expert opinion rather than data.[46] [47] Renal failure and lung injury almost invariably resolve if patients survive. Neurological deficits in children who have had cerebral malaria are now recognised to be more common, up to 30% in some series,[48] but these are often more subtle than for other serious neurological infections, such as meningitis.[49]

SOURCES AND SELECTION CRITERIA

We searched the Cochrane Library and PubMed for recent relevant trials and observational studies on imported malaria. The search was supplemented where relevant by data from the UK Malaria Reference Laboratory and expert opinion from the PHE Advisory Committee on Malaria Prevention in UK Travellers (ACMP) and World Health Organization expert guidelines. Good epidemiological data are available on imported malaria in Europe and North America and on diagnostic tests. There are high quality trials of malaria treatment in endemic countries but few large well conducted trials of treatment in travellers, so data on treatment have to be extrapolated from endemic settings.

ADDITIONAL EDUCATIONAL RESOURCES

Resources for healthcare professionals

- WHO World Malaria Report 2012. www.who.int/malaria/publications/world_malaria_report_2012/en/. Describes the current state of malaria in the world
- WHO management of severe malaria: a practical handbook. 2013. www.who.int/malaria/publications/atoz/9789241548526/en/index.html. Explains the management of severe malaria

Resources for patients

- National Travel Health Network and Centre. www.nathnac.org/travel/factsheets/malaria_chemoprophylaxis.htm. Information leaflet for travellers on chemoprophylaxis
- Advisory Committee on Prevention of Malaria in UK. www.hpa.org.uk/infections/topics_az/malaria/guidelines.htm. Travellers' handbook

PLC is supported by the UCL Hospitals Comprehensive Biomedical Research Centre Infection Theme.

Contributions: All authors contributed to the writing of this paper. CW is guarantor.

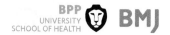
Competing interests: We have read and understood the BMJ Group policy on declaration of interests and declare the following interests: None.

Provenance and peer review: Commissioned; externally peer reviewed.

1 Mali S, Kachur SP, Arguin PM; Division of Parasitic Diseases and Malaria, Center for Global Health; Centers for Disease Control and Prevention (CDC). Malaria surveillance—United States, 2010. *MMWR Surveill Summ* 2012;61:1-17.

2 Smith AD, Bradley DJ, Smith V, Blaze M, Behrens RH, Chiodini PL, et al. Imported malaria and high risk groups: observational study using UK surveillance data 1987-2006. *BMJ* 2008;337:a120.

3 Seringe E, Thellier M, Fontanet A, Legros F, Bouchaud O, Ancelle T, et al. Severe imported Plasmodium falciparum malaria, France, 1996-2003. *Emerg Infect Dis* 2011;17:807-13.

4 WHO. World malaria report 2012. 2012. www.who.int/malaria/publications/world_malaria_report_2012/en/.

5 Ladhani S, Garbash M, Whitty CJM, Chiodini PL, Aibara RJ, Riordan FA, et al. Prospective, national clinical and epidemiologic study on imported childhood malaria in the United Kingdom and the Republic of Ireland. *Pediatr Infect Dis J* 2010;29:434-8.

6 Checkley AM, Smith A, Smith V, Blaze M, Bradley D, Chiodini PL, et al. Risk factors for mortality from imported falciparum malaria in the United Kingdom over 20 years: an observational study. *BMJ* 2012;344:e2116.

7 Nic Fhogartaigh C, Hughes H, Armstrong M, Herbert S, McGregor A, Ustianowski A, et al. Falciparum malaria as a cause of fever in adult travellers returning to the United Kingdom: observational study of risk by geographical area. *QJM* 2008;101:649-56.

8 Public Health England. Malaria 2011. www.malaria-reference.co.uk/.

9 Odolini S, Parola P, Gkrania-Klotsas E, Caumes E, Schlagenhauf P, López-Vélez, et al. Travel-related imported infections in Europe, EuroTravNet 2009. *Clin Microbiol Infect* 2012;18:468-74.

10 Kyriacou DN, Spira AM, Talan DA, Mabey DC. Emergency department presentation and misdiagnosis of imported falciparum malaria. *Ann Emerg Med* 1996;27:696-9.

11 Chandramohan D, Jaffar S, Greenwood BM. Use of clinical algorithms for diagnosing malaria. *Trop Med Int Health* 2002;7:45-52.

12 Bottieau E, Clerinx J, Van Den Enden E, Van Esbroeck M, Colebunders R, Van Gompel A, et al. Imported non-Plasmodium falciparum malaria: a five-year prospective study in a European referral center. *Am J Trop Med Hyg* 2006;75:133-8.

13 Abba K, Deeks JJ, Olliaro P, Naing CM, Jackson SM, Takwoingi Y, et al. Rapid diagnostic tests for diagnosing uncomplicated P. falciparum malaria in endemic countries. *Cochrane Database Syst Rev* 2011;7:CD008122.

14 Robinson T, Campino SG, Auburn S, Assefa SA, Polley SD, Manske M, et al. Drug-resistant genotypes and multi-clonality in Plasmodium falciparum analysed by direct genome sequencing from peripheral blood of malaria patients. *PLoS One* 2011;6:e23204.

15 Kamya MR, Byakika-Kibwika P, Gasasira AF, Havlir D, Rosenthal PJ, Dorsey G, et al. The effect of HIV on malaria in the context of the current standard of care for HIV-infected populations in Africa. *Future Virol* 2012;7:699-708.

16 WHO. Management of severe malaria: a practical handbook. 2nd ed. 2000. www.rbm.who.int/docs/hbsm.pdf.

17 Marsh K, Forster D, Waruiru C, Mwangi I, Winstanley M, Marsh V, et al. Indicators of life-threatening malaria in African children. *N Engl J Med* 1995;332:1399-404.

18 Desai M, ter Kuile FO, Nosten F, McGready R, Asamoa K, Brabin B, et al. Epidemiology and burden of malaria in pregnancy. *Lancet Infect Dis* 2007;7:93-104.

19 Whitty CJM, Edmonds S, Mutabingwa TK. Malaria in pregnancy. *BJOG* 2005;112:1189-95.

20 Manyando C, Kayentao K, D'Alessandro U, Okafor HU, Juma E, Hamed K. A systematic review of the safety and efficacy of artemether-lumefantrine against uncomplicated Plasmodium falciparum malaria during pregnancy. *Malar J* 2012;11:141.

21 Ali AA, Elhassan EM, Magzoub MM, Elbashir MI, Adam I. Hypoglycaemia and severe Plasmodium falciparum malaria among pregnant Sudanese women in an area characterized by unstable malaria transmission. *Parasit Vectors* 2011;4:88.

22 Kochar DK, Das A, Kochar SK, Saxena V, Sirohi P, Garg S, et al. Severe Plasmodium vivax malaria: a report on serial cases from Bikaner in northwestern India. *Am J Trop Med Hyg* 2009;80:194-8.

23 Baird JK. Resistance to chloroquine unhinges vivax malaria therapeutics. *Antimicrob Agents Chemother* 2011;55:1827-30.

24 Naing C, Aung K, Win DK, Wah MJ. Efficacy and safety of chloroquine for treatment in patients with uncomplicated Plasmodium vivax infections in endemic countries. *Trans R Soc Trop Med Hyg* 2010;104:695-705.

25 Douglas NM, Anstey NM, Angus BJ, Nosten F, Price RN. Artemisinin combination therapy for vivax malaria. *Lancet Infect Dis* 2010;10:405-16.

26 Baird JK, Hoffman SL. Primaquine therapy for malaria. *Clin Infect Dis* 2004;39:1336e45.

27 Fernando D, Rodrigo C, Rajapakse S. Primaquine in vivax malaria: an update and review on management issues. *Malar J* 2011;10:351.

28 Clyde DF. Clinical problems associated with the use of primaquine as a tissue schizontocidal and gametocytocidal drug. *Bull World Health Organ* 1981;59:391-5.

29 Leslie T, Briceño M, Mayan I, Mohammed N, Klinkenberg E, Sibley CH, et al. The impact of phenotypic and genotypic G6PD deficiency on risk of plasmodium vivax infection: a case-control study amongst Afghan refugees in Pakistan. *PLoS Med* 2010;7:e1000283.

30 Howes RE, Piel FB, Patil AP, Nyangiri OA, Gething PW, Dewi M, et al. G6PD deficiency prevalence and estimates of affected populations in malaria endemic countries: a geostatistical model-based map. *PLoS Med* 2012;9:e1001339.

31 Bunn A, Escombe R, Armstrong M, Whitty CJM, Doherty JF. Falciparum malaria in malaria-naive travellers and African visitors. *QJM* 2004;97:645-9.

32 Public Health England. Malaria reference laboratory (malaria RL). www.hpa.org.uk/ProductsServices/MicrobiologyPathology/LaboratoriesAndReferenceFacilities/MalariaReferenceLaboratory/.

33 Centers for Disease Control and Prevention. Malaria. www.cdc.gov/MALARIA/.

34 Sinclair D, Zani B, Donegan S, Olliaro P, Garner P. Artemisinin-based combination therapy for treating uncomplicated malaria. *Cochrane Database Syst Rev* 2009;3:CD007483.

35 Phyo AP, Nkhoma S, Stepniewska K, Ashley EA, Nair S, McGready R, et al. Emergence of artemisinin-resistant malaria on the western border of Thailand: a longitudinal study. *Lancet* 2012;379:1960-6.

36 Sutherland CJ, Laundy M, Price N, Burke M, Fivelman QL, Pasvol G, et al. Mutations in the Plasmodium falciparum cytochrome b gene are associated with delayed parasite recrudescence in malaria patients treated with atovaquone-proguanil. *Malar J* 2008;7:240.

37 Nayyar GM, Breman JG, Newton PN, Herrington J. Poor-quality antimalarial drugs in southeast Asia and sub-Saharan Africa. *Lancet Infect Dis* 2012;12:488-96.

38 Dondorp A, Nosten F, Stepniewska K, Day N, White N; South East Asian Quinine Artesunate Malaria Trial (SEAQUAMAT) group. Artesunate versus quinine for treatment of severe falciparum malaria: a randomised trial. *Lancet* 2005;366:717-25.

39 Dondorp AM, Fanello CI, Hendriksen IC, Gomes E, Seni A, Chhaganlal KD, et al. Artesunate versus quinine in the treatment of severe falciparum malaria in African children (AQUAMAT): an open-label, randomised trial. *Lancet* 2010;376:1647-57.

40 Griffith KS, Lewis LS, Mali S, Parise ME. Treatment of malaria in the United States: a systematic review. *JAMA* 2007;297:2264-77.

41 Maitland K, Kiguli S, Opoka RO, Engoru C, Olupot-Olupot P, Akech SO, et al. Mortality after fluid bolus in African children with severe infection. *N Engl J Med* 2011;364:2483-95.

42 Scott JA, Berkley JA, Mwangi I, Ochola L, Uyoga S, Macharia A, et al. Relation between falciparum malaria and bacteraemia in Kenyan children: a population-based, case-control study and a longitudinal study. *Lancet* 2011;378:1316-23.

43 Nadjm B, Amos B, Mtove G, Ostermann J, Chonya S, Wangai H, et al. WHO guidelines for antimicrobial treatment in children admitted to hospital in an area of intense Plasmodium falciparum transmission: prospective study. *BMJ* 2010;340:c1350.

44 Marks ME, Armstrong M, Suvari MM, Batson S, Whitty CJM, Chiodini PL, et al. Severe imported falciparum malaria among adults requiring intensive care: a retrospective study at the hospital for tropical diseases, London. *BMC Infect Dis* 2013;13:118.

45 Al-Taiar A, Jaffar S, Assabri A, Al-Habori M, Azazy A, Al-Mahdi N, et al. Severe malaria in children in Yemen: two site observational study. *BMJ* 2006;333:827.

46 Lubell Y, Staedke SG, Greenwood BM, Kamya MR, Molyneux M, Newton PN, et al. Likely health outcomes for untreated acute febrile illness in the tropics in decision and economic models; a Delphi survey. *PLoS One* 2011;6:e17439.

47 Nguyen TH, Day NP, Ly VC, Waller D, Mai NT, Bethell DB, et al. Post-malaria neurological syndrome. *Lancet* 1996;348:917-21.

48 Birbeck GL, Molyneux ME, Kaplan PW, Seydel KB, Chimalizeni YF, Kawaza K, et al. Blantyre Malaria Project Epilepsy Study (BMPES) of neurological outcomes in retinopathy-positive paediatric cerebral malaria survivors: a prospective cohort study. *Lancet Neurol* 2010;9:1173-81.

49 Idro R, Ndiritu M, Ogutu B, Mithwani S, Maitland K, Berkley J, et al. Burden, features, and outcome of neurological involvement in acute falciparum malaria in Kenyan children. *JAMA* 2007;297:2232-40.

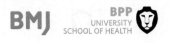

Dengue fever

Senanayake A M Kularatne, senior professor of medicine

Department of Medicine, Faculty of Medicine, University of Peradeniya, Peradeniya, Sri Lanka

Correspondence to: Senanayake A M Kularatne samkul@sltnet.lk

Cite this as: BMJ 2015;351:h4661

DOI: 10.1136/bmj.h4661

http://www.bmj.com/content/351/bmj.h4661

ABSTRACT

This clinical review has been developed for The BMJ in collaboration with BMJ Best Practice, based on a regularly updated web/mobile topic that supports evidence based decision making at the point of care. To view the complete and current version, please refer to the dengue fever (http://bestpractice.bmj.com/best-practice/monograph/1197.html) topic on the BMJ Best Practice website.

Dengue fever is a globally important arboviral infection transmitted by mosquitoes of the Aedes genus (primarily Aedes aegypti, but also A albopictus), an insect found in tropical and subtropical regions.[1] Dengue infection causes a range of severe and non-severe clinical manifestations.[2] The incubation period is 3-14 days (average 7 days).

Who gets dengue fever?

Around two fifths of the world's population (those in tropical and subtropical countries), or up to 2.5 billion people, are at risk of dengue infection.[1] An estimated 50 million infections occur annually worldwide, with 0.5 million of these cases being admitted to hospital for dengue haemorrhagic fever. Approximately 90% of these cases are in children aged less than 5 years.[1] The epidemiology is, however, changing both regionally and globally. Classic dengue fever is more common in adults than in children.[3]

The infection is now endemic in more than 100 countries, particularly the South East Asia region, western Pacific region, and the Americas.[1][4][5][6] Severe manifestations such as dengue haemorrhagic fever and dengue shock syndrome, as well as other unusual manifestations, are increasingly being reported in previously unaffected regions.[5][6] Multiple epidemics of dengue fever occurred in the United States in the 18th to early 20th centuries. After an absence of 56 years, dengue fever has re-emerged in US states such as Texas and Hawaii, and 796 cases were reported in the US from 2001 to 2007.[2] Dengue haemorrhagic fever has been reported in many tropical US territories, and the DENV-2 virus has been implicated in some of these cases.[7]

All cases of dengue fever in the United Kingdom have been acquired as a result of travel to endemic areas. The Health Protection Agency reported 406 cases of dengue fever in England, Wales, and Northern Ireland in 2010, compared with 166 in 2009.

What causes dengue fever?

Dengue fever is caused by four antigenically distinct dengue virus serotypes: DENV-1, DENV-2, DENV-3, and DENV-4. All four have the capacity to cause severe disease. They are RNA viruses that belong to the Flavivirus genus/Flaviviridae family, which also includes the yellow fever virus, West Nile virus, Japanese encephalitis virus, and the St Louis encephalitis virus.[1]

The primary vector for spread of infection is A aegypti, a highly domesticated, day biting mosquito, with A albopictus also responsible for transmission. Although the mosquitoes are of Asian origin, they now occur in Africa, Europe, and the US. International travel and transportation of goods has helped the spread of both vector and virus. A considerable genetic variation occurs within each viral serotype, thereby forming phylogenetically distinct genotypes. The virion consists of three structural proteins plus a lipoprotein envelope and seven non-structural proteins, of which non-structural protein 1 (NS1) has diagnostic and pathological importance. Infection with any one serotype confers lifelong immunity to that specific serotype; cross protection to other serotypes, however, lasts only a few months.[1][2][8] Some studies have shown that infection with the DENV-1 or DENV-2 serotype may result in more severe infection.[9][10]

Pathogenesis is linked to the host immune response, which is triggered by infection with the virus.[11] Primary infection is usually benign. Secondary infection with a different serotype or multiple infections with different serotypes may, however, cause severe infection that can be classified as either dengue haemorrhagic fever or dengue shock syndrome, depending on the clinical signs.

Antigen-presenting dendritic cells, the humoral immune response, and the cell mediated immune response are involved in the pathogenesis. Proliferation of memory T cells and the production of pro-inflammatory cytokines lead to vascular endothelial cell dysfunction, which results in plasma leakage. The concentration of cytokines such as interferon-γ, tumour necrosis factor-α, and interleukin 10 is higher, and the levels of nitric oxide and some complement factors are reduced. NS1 is a modulator of the complement pathway and plays a role in low levels of complement factors.[12][13] After infection, specific cross reactive antibodies, as well as CD4 and CD8 T cells, remain in the body for years.[2]

Infants can develop severe dengue fever during a primary infection (which is usually benign) owing to transplacental transfer of antibodies from an immune mother. This subsequently amplifies the infant's immune response to the primary infection.[12]

Can dengue fever be prevented?

Primary prevention
The World Health Organization recommends strategies for the prevention and control of dengue infection,[1][2] and authorities in dengue endemic regions may also produce their own prevention programmes and initiatives. The key

---

THE BOTTOM LINE

- Dengue fever is a globally important arboviral infection transmitted by the Aedes genus of mosquito (primarily A aegypti, but also A albopictus), found in tropical and subtropical regions
- The infection is endemic in more than 100 countries, particularly the South East Asia region, western Pacific region, and the Americas
- The incubation period is 3-14 days (average 7 days)
- Clinical features include fever, headache, myalgia/arthralgia, and skin flushing/rash, together with leucopenia, thrombocytopenia, and increased liver function
- Severe thrombocytopenia, haemorrhage, and plasma leakage are the key diagnostic features of the more severe forms of infection
- Confirmatory tests include detection of viral antigen or nucleic acid and serology
- Fluid therapy and the identification of the critical phase are the most important aspects of management

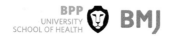

Table 1   Confirmatory laboratory tests for dengue fever

Tests	How it works	Advantages	Disadvantages
Viral antigen detection	Detection of non-structural protein 1 using enzyme linked immunosorbent assay (ELISA) or rapid kits is useful in early diagnosis and can be ordered from days 1-5 of illness.[20] A serum specimen should be used. A positive result confirms diagnosis	Easy to perform; rapid tests can be used in the field and provide results in a few hours; early diagnosis is possible, which may affect management[2]	May be as sensitive as viral nucleic acid detection; however, does not identify serotype[2]
Viral nucleic acid detection	Reverse transcriptase-polymerase chain reaction is method of choice and can be ordered in the first 5 days of fever onset. Tissue, whole blood, serum, or plasma specimen can be used. A positive result confirms diagnosis	Most sensitive and specific test available, especially in early infection; early diagnosis is possible, which may affect management; can identify serotype[2]	Expensive, requires laboratory facilities and expertise, not rapid (takes 24-48 hours), cannot differentiate between primary and secondary infection, potential for false positive results owing to contamination[2]
Serology	Serology results may be negative in first 5 days of illness; therefore, IgM ELISA and IgG ELISA are tests of choice after first 5 days of illness (polymerase chain reaction is more sensitive in first 5 days). Presence of IgG in first few days of infection strongly suggests secondary infection. Positive IgM and IgG in single serum sample is highly suggestive of dengue infection, whereas IgM or IgG seroconversion in paired serum samples or a fourfold IgG titre increase in paired serum samples confirms the diagnosis.[2] Whole blood, serum, or plasma specimen can be used. IgM rapid tests are commercially available and easy to use; however, their accuracy is poor as cross reaction with other infectious agents and in autoimmune disorders can occur. Haemagglutination inhibition test is useful for diagnosing secondary dengue infection (that is, titre ≥1:1280)	Inexpensive, easy to perform, more readily available in dengue endemic areas, can distinguish between primary and secondary infection (that is, IgM to IgG ratio <1.2 suggests secondary infection)[2]	Disadvantages: lower specificity than other tests; requires two serum samples; delays confirmation of diagnosis[2]

BOX 1 MEASURES TO PREVENT THE SPREAD OF DENGUE FEVER[1]

- Regular removal of all sources of stagnant water to prevent mosquito breeding grounds
- Appropriate clothing to cover exposed skin, especially during the day, and the use of insecticides, mosquito repellents, mosquito coils, and mosquito nets
- Mosquito nets and coils placed around sick patients to prevent transmission

---

to all prevention programmes is disease surveillance to detect epidemics (box 1). Communities in dengue endemic regions should be educated to recognise symptoms and prevent transmission.

Various worldwide initiatives are in the process of testing genetically modified mosquitoes to help stop the spread of dengue fever.[14] A tetravalent vaccine is being developed and may be available in the future.[1 6 15]

Screening
Screening is not applicable as dengue fever is a communicable disease. However, populations may be screened for epidemiological purposes or to check for previous exposure to dengue virus.

Secondary prevention
Recurrence is possible, with different serotypes leading to a secondary infection. The usual primary prevention measures should therefore be followed after recovery from an initial infection.

How is dengue fever diagnosed?
Dengue fever should be considered in any patient presenting with fever, generalised skin flushing, leucopenia, and thrombocytopenia. A correct diagnosis early in the course of infection is important to prevent complications.

History
Dengue fever should be suspected in any patients residing in countries where the infection is endemic and in those who travelled in such areas within the past two weeks.

The onset of symptoms after the incubation period is usually abrupt. Fever is characteristic of infection and is often abrupt in onset with high spikes of 39.4-40.5°C. It may also be biphasic and have a remittent pattern or be low grade, and generally lasts for five to seven days. In young children fever may cause febrile seizures or delirium. Patients with rapid defervescence may be about to enter the critical phase of infection.[2 6]

Aches and pains, particularly backache, arthralgia, myalgia, and bone pain, are common. Headache is also typical of infection and is generally constant and towards the front of the head. It usually improves within a few days. Severe retro-orbital pain on eye movement or with a little pressure applied to the eyeball is also usual.

Gastrointestinal symptoms (for example, anorexia, nausea or vomiting, epigastric discomfort or pain), lethargy or restlessness, collapse, or dizziness may also be present. Patients often report a lack of appetite or changes to taste sensation. Gastrointestinal symptoms, weakness, and dizziness may be more noticeable in dengue haemorrhagic fever. Upper respiratory tract symptoms (for example, cough, sore throat) are usually absent, although they may atypically occur in mild infection.

Physical examination
Diffuse skin flushing of the face, neck, and chest develop early with infection. This evolves into a maculopapular or rubelliform rash of the whole body, usually on day 3 or 4 of the fever. Blanching may occur when the skin is pressed.[16] The rash fades with time, and during the convalescent phase appears as pallid areas.

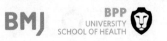

Table 2 World Health Organization guide to severity of infection[2]

Patient groups	Features	Setting for patient management
A	No warning signs (particularly when fever subsides); able to tolerate adequate volume of oral fluids and pass urine at least once every 6 hours; near normal blood counts and haematocrit	Home
B	Developing warning signs; co-existing risk factors for serious infection (for example, pregnancy, extremes of age, obesity, diabetes, renal impairment, haemolytic diseases); poor family or social support (for example, patients who live alone or live far from medical facilities and do not have reliable transport); increasing haematocrit or a rapidly decreasing platelet count	Hospital
C	Established warning signs; in critical phase of infection, with severe plasma leakage (with or without shock), severe haemorrhage, or severe organ impairment (for example, hepatic or renal impairment, cardiomyopathy, encephalopathy, or encephalitis)	Emergency medical intervention with access to intensive care facilities and blood transfusion

---

BOX 2 WARNING SIGNS OF IMPENDING CRITICAL PHASE OF INFECTION[6]

- Abdominal pain or tenderness
- Persistent vomiting
- Accumulation of clinical fluid (for example, ascites, pleural effusion)
- Mucosal bleeding
- Lethargy or restlessness
- Liver enlargement >2 cm
- Increase in haematocrit with rapid decrease in platelet count

---

BOX 3 LABORATORY CRITERIA FOR DIAGNOSIS OF DENGUE HAEMORRHAGIC FEVER OR DENGUE SHOCK SYNDROME[1][2]

- Rapidly developing, severe thrombocytopenia
- Decreased total white cell count and neutrophils and changing neutrophil to lymphocyte ratio
- Increased haematocrit (20% increase from baseline is objective evidence of plasma leakage)
- Hypoalbuminaemia (serum albumin <35 g/L suggests plasma leakage)
- Increased liver function test results (aspartate aminotransferase:alanine aminotransferase >2)

Haemorrhagic signs include petechiae, purpura, or a positive tourniquet test (blood pressure cuff inflated to a point midway between systolic and diastolic blood pressures for five minutes; the test is positive if ≥10 petechiae per square inch appear on the forearm). More major haemorrhage can manifest as epistaxis, gingival bleeding, haematemesis, melaena, vaginal bleeding (in women of childbearing age), or bleeding from a venepuncture site. These signs can occur with either dengue fever or dengue haemorrhagic fever.[1][2]

Hepatomegaly may be present. Plasma leakage is a sign of dengue haemorrhagic fever, and clinical evidence of this includes the presence of ascites, postural dizziness, or pleural effusion.[1][2]

Circulatory collapse (that is, cold clammy skin, rapid and weak pulse with narrowing of pulse pressure <20 mm Hg with decreased diastolic pressure, postural drop of blood pressure >20 mm Hg, capillary refill time greater than three seconds, reduced urine output) indicates the presence of shock and supports a diagnosis of dengue shock syndrome.[1][2]

Phases of infection
Dengue infection has three distinct phases[2]: febrile, critical, and convalescent. The febrile phase is characterised by a sudden high grade fever and dehydration that can last two to seven days.[2] The critical phase (box 2) is characterised by plasma leakage, bleeding, shock, and organ impairment and lasts for about 24 to 48 hours. It usually starts around the time of defervescence (this does not always occur), typically days 3 to 7 of the infection.

Patients with dengue haemorrhagic fever or dengue shock syndrome go through all three stages. The critical phase is bypassed in patients with dengue fever.[1][2][17]

Laboratory investigations

Initial laboratory investigations
A full blood count should be ordered initially in all patients with symptoms. Typically, leucopenia and thrombocytopenia occur as early as the second day of fever.[1] Leucopenia, in combination with a positive tourniquet test, in a dengue endemic area has a positive predictive value of 70-80%.[18][19] Leucopenia (with neutropenia) persists throughout the febrile period. In classic dengue fever (box 3), thrombocytopenia is usually mild, although it may also be severe.[1]

The haematocrit may also rise about 10% in patients with dengue fever owing to dehydration.[1] The results of liver function tests are usually increased, particularly for alanine and aspartate aminotransferases.[1] Clotting studies are not required for diagnosis but may play a useful role in the management of the infection in patients with haemorrhagic signs.

Confirmatory laboratory investigations
Confirmatory tests should be carried out if possible.[1][2] This is important because dengue fever can be confused with many non-dengue illnesses. Four types of diagnostic test are available for confirmation of dengue virus infection (table 1).

The choice of test depends on numerous factors, including local availability, cost, time of sample collection, available facilities, and technical expertise. Although direct methods such as viral nucleic acid or viral antigen detection are more specific, they are more costly and labour intensive. Indirect methods (that is, serology) are less specific but are more accessible, faster, and less costly.[2] The identification of viral nucleic acid or viral antigen, plus the detection of an antibody response (serology), is preferable to either approach alone.[2] Detection of viral nucleic acid or viral antigen is primarily done in the first five days of illness, and serological tests after the fifth day. Some tests differentiate between viral serotypes, although this is not useful clinically.

Virus isolation is possible during the initial viraemic phase. This test is accessible only in some locations and is generally not recommended as results are usually not available in a clinically meaningful time frame.

Imaging
Imaging studies are required only if dengue haemorrhagic fever or dengue shock syndrome is suspected. A lateral decubitus chest radiograph of the right side of the chest can be ordered to detect clinically undetectable pleural effusion in the early phase of plasma leakage. Ultrasonography of the abdomen is useful to detect the presence of ascites and plasma leak or other disease related changes in abdominal

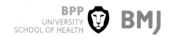

organs, including the liver, gallbladder (oedema may precede plasma leakage), and kidneys.[1][2]

How is dengue fever managed?

Treatment approach

Treatment is supportive, as no specific antiviral therapy is available for dengue infection, and is based on guidance produced by WHO and other region specific authorities.[1][2][6][17][21][22] The only recognised treatment in dengue fever is maintaining adequate hydration, and in dengue haemorrhagic fever and dengue shock syndrome treatment is fluid replacement therapy. In dengue endemic regions, the triage of patients with suspected dengue infection should be done in a specifically designated area of the hospital.

Early diagnosis and optimal clinical management reduce the associated morbidity and mortality. Delays in diagnosis, incorrect diagnosis, use of improper treatments (for example, non-steroidal anti-inflammatory drugs), and surgical interventions are all considered harmful. Educating the public about the signs and symptoms of dengue infection and when to seek medical advice is the key to optimal diagnosis and treatment.

Severity of infection

The most commonly used and practical treatment plan is produced by WHO and is based on the severity of infection.[2] This classification separates patients into one of three groups (table 2), depending on the clinical presentation.

Group A

Patients classified as being in group A have the following features and can be managed at home:

- No warning signs (particularly when fever subsides)
- Able to tolerate an adequate volume of oral fluids and pass urine at least once every six hours
- Near normal blood counts and haematocrit.

Group B

Patients classified as being in group B have the following features and require hospital admission:

- Developing warning signs
- Co-existing risk factors for serious infection (for example, pregnancy, extremes of age, obesity, diabetes, renal impairment, haemolytic diseases)
- Poor family or social support (for example, patients live alone or far from medical facilities and without reliable transport)
- Increasing haematocrit or a rapidly decreasing platelet count.

Group C

Patients classified as being in group C have the following features and require emergency medical intervention:

- Established warning signs
- In the critical phase of infection, with severe plasma leakage (with or without shock), severe haemorrhage, or severe organ impairment (for example, hepatic or renal impairment, cardiomyopathy, encephalopathy, or encephalitis).

Management of group C patients

These patients require emergency medical intervention. At presentation, patients may be in compensated or decompensated shock. Access to intensive care facilities and blood transfusion should be available. Intravenous crystalloids and colloids administered rapidly are recommended, according to algorithms produced by WHO.[1][2] An attempt should be made to work out how long patients have been in the critical phase and their previous fluid balance.

The total fluid quota for 48 hours should be calculated based on the formula[1][17]:

maintenance (M)+5% fluid deficit

where M=100 mL/kg for the first 10 kg of body weight, 50 mL/kg for the second 10 kg of body weight, and 20 mL/kg for every kilogram over 20 kg of body weight up to 50 kg; and 5% fluid deficit is calculated as 50 mL/kg of body weight up to 50 kg

For example, for an adult who weighs 50 kg, the total fluid quota for 48 hours would be 4600 mL.

The formula may be used for children and adults, although the rate of administering treatment differs between these patient groups, and local protocols should be followed. Ideal body weight should be used in the formula for children.

Other formulas for fluid replacement therapy have been reported, so local protocols should be consulted and followed. The infusion rate should be adjusted according to the usual monitoring variables, and therapy is usually required for only 24-48 hours, with a gradual reduction once the rate of plasma leakage decreases towards the end of the critical phase.[2]

Giving colloids (for example, dextran 70% or 6% starch) over crystalloids (for example, 0.9% normal saline, Ringer's lactate) has no clinical advantage.[23][24][25] (B evidence.) WHO guidelines clearly indicate when colloids should be used (for example, intractable shock, resistance to crystalloid resuscitation).[1][2]

Patients should be monitored closely throughout, including vital signs, peripheral perfusion, pulse pressure, capillary refill time, fluid balance, haematocrit, platelet count, urine output, temperature, blood glucose, liver function tests, renal profile, coagulation profile, and other organ function tests as indicated.

Usually the patient's condition will become stable within a few hours of fluid therapy. If patients remain unstable, other contributory causes such as metabolic acidosis, electrolyte imbalances (for example, hypocalcaemia, hypoglycaemia), myocarditis, or hepatic necrosis should be investigated and managed appropriately. If patients do not improve and the haematocrit falls, internal bleeding should be suspected and a blood transfusion carried out immediately; caution is, however, advised owing to the risk of fluid overload. Consensus is now for early use of colloids and blood transfusion in refractory unstable patients.

Over-enthusiastic treatment and too rapid hydration can lead to fluid overload, causing pulmonary oedema, facial congestion, raised jugular venous pressure, pleural effusion, or ascites. These complications should be treated with restriction of intravenous fluid therapy and bolus doses of intravenous furosemide (frusemide) until patients are stable. Although less common, the disease may take a different course as a result of the complications listed in table 3.

Management of group B patients

These patients require hospital admission. The severity of infection should be assessed. If patients are not in the early critical phase (that is, with plasma leakage) they should be encouraged to take fluids orally (for example, approximately

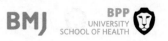

Table 3   Complications of dengue fever

Complications	Clinical features and management
Fluid overload	Overenthusiastic treatment and too rapid hydration can lead to fluid overload, causing pulmonary oedema, facial congestion, raised jugular venous pressure, pleural effusion, or ascites. These complications should be treated with restriction of intravenous fluid therapy and bolus doses of intravenous furosemide (frusemide) until the patient is stable
Acalculous cholecystitis	Should be considered in patients with prominent right upper quadrant pain and tenderness, and persistent nausea and vomiting. Ultrasonography is recommended for diagnosis. Intravenous broad spectrum antibiotics and conservative management are recommended[1]
Acute respiratory distress syndrome	Should be considered in patients with dyspnoea and hypoxia. Chest radiograph shows diffuse shadows. Management includes assisted ventilation and oxygen therapy
Rhabdomyolysis	A rare complication owing to the infection causing myonecrosis. Should be considered in patients with muscle pain. Diagnostic tests include serum creatine kinase level, electrolytes, and myoglobin levels (blood and urine).[1] Treatment includes hydration, urine alkalinisation, and diuretic therapy
Postviral fatigue syndrome	Some patients may experience postviral fatigue syndrome for a variable duration after infection[1]
Myocarditis	Should be considered in patients with excessive or unusual tiredness, chest discomfort, hypoxia, tachycardia or bradycardia, and electrocardiographic changes, including T wave inversion or bundle branch blocks. Troponin T or I estimation and echocardiography should be ordered to assess severity. Management is supportive. Bed rest is recommended, as well as oxygen therapy. Fluid should be administered carefully to prevent fluid overload, which may cause heart failure or pulmonary oedema.[28] One or two doses of intravenous hydrocortisone may be beneficial (personal experience)
Hepatitis	Invariably, patients with dengue infection have increased liver enzymes suggestive of anicteric hepatitis. In some patients, these levels may increase substantially and the liver may become enlarged and tender. Liver function tests and coagulation profile should be monitored regularly. Patients need rest and supportive treatment. These patients are at higher risk of developing dengue haemorrhagic fever. They are also at a high risk of developing severe hepatic necrosis and hepatic encephalopathy.[1][40] May lead to acute liver failure
Hepatic encephalopathy	Should be considered in patients presenting with altered level of consciousness, jaundice, and asterixis (liver flap or flapping tremor). Those with pre-existing liver disease are at a higher risk. If liver enzymes increase >10-fold or continue to increase, the risk of developing this complication is high.[1] Standard management is recommended, including fluid restriction. Corticosteroids may be considered to reduce cerebral oedema. Plasmapheresis and haemodialysis may be considered if there is clinical deterioration. Meticulous fluid management to prevent shock and avoidance of hepatotoxic drugs help to prevent this complication.[1] Patients may go on to develop hypoglycaemia, bleeding, respiratory distress, electrolyte imbalances, and sepsis
Encephalitis	Should be considered in patients with an altered level of consciousness and convulsions. Electroencephalography is useful to support the diagnosis and monitor progression. Supportive treatments, including anticonvulsants, are indicated[1]
Acute pancreatitis	Should be considered in patients with prominent gastrointestinal manifestations, including central abdominal pain and vomiting. Serum amylase level is high, and ultrasound examination supports the diagnosis.[1] Management is conservative
Acute appendicitis	Should be considered in patients with fever and pain and tenderness in the right iliac fossa. Often, patients are admitted to a surgical ward for appendectomy; this, however, may be detrimental to the patient owing to the high risk of perioperative bleeding. Patients should be managed conservatively[1]
Acute renal failure	A rare complication due to multiple organ impairment or myoglobinuria. Diagnosed by acutely increasing urea and creatinine levels. Renal replacement therapy may be required[1]
Haemophagocytic syndrome	Should be considered in patients who develop pancytopenia (usually anaemia)[1]

2500 mL/24 hours for adults, or age appropriate maintenance fluid requirement for children). If this is not possible, or patients enter the critical phase (indicated by rising haematocrit, hypoalbuminaemia, progressive leucopenia, thrombocytopenia, third space fluid loss, and narrowing of pulse pressure with postural drop), intravenous fluid replacement therapy with 0.9% saline (or Ringer's lactate) should be started using the maintenance (M)+5% fluid deficit formula.[1][17] Patients should be monitored closely throughout, including vital signs, peripheral perfusion, fluid balance, haematocrit, platelet count, urine output, temperature, blood glucose, liver function tests, renal profile, and coagulation profile.

Management of group A patients

These patients can be managed at home and should be encouraged to take oral fluids (for example, approximately 2500 mL/24 hours for adults, or age appropriate maintenance fluid requirement for children). Oral rehydration products, fruit juices, and clear soups are better than water. Red or brown fluids should be avoided, as these may lead to confusion about haematemesis.

Patients should be advised to rest. Tepid sponging may be used for fever and paracetamol in usual doses for pain or fever. Non-steroidal anti-inflammatory drugs should be avoided as they increase bleeding tendency.

Patients should be given an instruction leaflet outlining the warning signs and be advised to return to hospital immediately if any develop. Blood counts should be performed daily.

Pregnancy

Pregnancy is a risk factor for higher maternal mortality and poor antenatal outcomes. The incidence of caesarean sections, pre-eclampsia, preterm deliveries, reduced birth weight, and vertical transmission of the infection is higher.[26] Close observation and meticulous management is therefore important in this patient group. Fluid intake is the same as for non-pregnant women; prepregnancy body weight should be used in the formula.[1][27]

As pregnancy is associated with various physiological changes such as high pulse rate, low blood pressure, wider pulse pressure, decreased haemoglobin and haematocrit values, and decreased platelet count, baseline variables should be noted on the first day of infection and subsequent results interpreted with caution. It should be remembered that other pregnancy related conditions, such as pre-eclampsia and HELLP (haemolysis, elevated liver enzyme levels, and low platelet levels) syndrome, may also alter laboratory variables.[1][27]

Detection of plasma leakage (for example, ascites, pleural effusion) is difficult in pregnant women, and so early ultrasonography is recommended.[1][27]

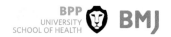

Children

As the tendency for children to develop dengue haemorrhagic fever or dengue shock syndrome is increased, laboratory variables such as haematocrit, platelet count, and urine output should be monitored regularly.

Assessment of the severity of symptoms in infants aged less than 1 year is difficult compared with that in older children and adults. Infants have less respiratory reserve and are more susceptible to electrolyte imbalances and hepatic impairment. The plasma leakage that occurs in children may be shorter and respond faster to fluid resuscitation.[1]

Convalescence and discharge

Convalescence can be recognised by the improvement in clinical variables as well as the patient's appetite and wellbeing. Patients may develop a diuresis, and hypokalaemia may follow. If hypokalaemia occurs, intravenous fluids should be replaced by potassium rich fluid. During recovery patients may also develop a rash or generalised pruritus. Once wellbeing is achieved and patients remain afebrile for 48 hours with an increasing platelet count and stable haematocrit, they can be discharged.[2]

Adjunctive therapies

Prophylactic platelet transfusions are rarely required (even with very low platelet counts) and are not recommended except in the presence of active bleeding. The clinical value of fresh frozen plasma, corticosteroids, intravenous immunoglobulin, and antibiotics is controversial and more evidence is required before they can be recommended.[1 28]

Disease notification

In dengue endemic regions, suspected, probable, and confirmed cases of dengue fever should be reported to the relevant authorities as soon as possible so that measures can be instituted to prevent transmission.[2]

What are the complications of dengue fever?

Prognosis

The mortality rate for severe dengue fever is 0.8-2.5%.[1] Children are at an increased risk of severe infection and death, although severe infection in adults is increasingly being reported.[1 4 5 6] The risk of children aged 1-5 years dying from dengue fever is fourfold higher than in children aged 11-15 years.[20] Even though dengue haemorrhagic fever and dengue shock syndrome are uncommon in adults, a higher morbidity and mortality rate has been reported, especially in older people, which is related to an increased risk of organ impairment.[1 6 29 30 31]

Long term sequelae

Once patients have recovered, no long term sequelae are associated with dengue fever; some patients may, however, experience postviral fatigue syndrome. Platelet count gradually increases during convalescence, although some patients may develop temporary thrombocytosis during recovery. Complete normalisation of liver function test results may take up to four weeks.

Recurrence

Recurrence is possible with a different dengue virus serotype, leading to secondary dengue infection. Third and fourth recurrences of clinical infection can also occur, but the clinical impact is not clear. Once immunity has developed to all four serotypes, lifelong immunity to each occurs.

Monitoring

Patients do not require monitoring and regular follow-up beyond the acute infectious period. It is advisable to review blood counts and liver function for up to four weeks after discharge.

Patient instructions

Patients should be reassured that there are no long term sequelae associated with dengue fever after recovery, and that they may resume normal activities once physically capable. Based on empirical evidence, patients should be advised to avoid alcohol and strenuous activities during convalescence, as liver function may take up to three weeks to return to normal.

Are there any emerging treatments?

Corticosteroids

Although some studies report that corticosteroids are effective in dengue fever, more evidence is required before they are recommended.[28 32] (C evidence.) In one randomised controlled trial use of oral prednisolone during the early acute phase of dengue fever was not associated with prolongation of viraemia or other adverse effects. The study was not powered to assess efficacy, but it found no reduction in the development of shock or other recognised complications of dengue fever.[33]

Antiviral drugs

The development of a safe and effective antiviral drug that is active against the dengue virus is a priority. Although this has been attempted, no successful outcomes have been achieved.[34] Balapiravir is a prodrug of a nucleoside analogue (R1479) and an inhibitor of hepatitis C virus replication in vivo. It was found to be ineffective as a candidate drug in a randomised, double blind placebo controlled trial of balapiravir in adults with dengue fever.[35]

Vaccines

A tetravalent vaccine is currently being developed and may be available in the future.[1 6] Trial results have shown promise.[36 37 38 39 40]

Competing interests: I have read and understood the BMJ Policy on competing interests and declare the following: none.

Provenance and peer review: Commissioned; externally peer reviewed.

This clinical review series has been developed for The BMJ in collaboration with BMJ Best Practice (http://bestpractice.bmj. com), an independent product produced by BMJ Publishing Group Limited. BMJ Best Practice comprises web/mobile topics that support evidence-based decision making at the point of care. Peer review of the content in this clinical review was carried out exclusively according to BMJ Best Practice's own, independent process (http://bestpractice.bmj.com/best-practice/marketing/how-is-best-practice-produced.html). This adaptation of a BMJ Best Practice topic for a clinical review in The BMJ uses only a portion of content from the latest available web version of BMJ Best Practice. BMJ Best Practice is updated on an ongoing basis, and the content of any BMJ Best Practice topic is expected to change periodically including subsequent to its publication as a clinical review in The BMJ. To view

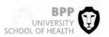
ADDITIONAL EDUCATIONAL RESOURCES

Resources for healthcare professionals

- Guidelines on management of dengue fever and dengue haemorrhagic fever in adults (www. epid.gov.lk/web/images/pdf/Publication/guidelines_for_the_management_of_df_and_dhf_in_ adults.pdf)—guidelines developed by a team of experienced doctors and specific to adults
- Comprehensive guideline for prevention and control of dengue and dengue haemorrhagic fever (www.searo.who.int/entity/vector_borne_tropical_diseases/documents/SEAROTPS60/en)— outlines recommendations for management of dengue fever/dengue haemorrhagic fever and focuses on topics of relevance to member states of the South East Asia region
- Dengue guidelines for diagnosis, treatment, prevention and control: new edition (http:// whqlibdoc.who.int/publications/2009/9789241547871_eng.pdf?ua=1)—outlines clinical management of dengue fever for all phases of infection and includes a stepwise approach to management, differentiating between patient groups

Resource for patients

- Centers for Disease Control and Prevention (CDC): dengue—prevention (www.cdc.gov/Dengue/ prevention/)—discusses ways to reduce the risk of dengue infection

the complete and current versions of all BMJ Best Practice topics, please refer to the BMJ Best Practice website (http://bestpractice.bmj. com).

Content from BMJ Best Practice is intended to support, aid and supplement the expertise, discretion and judgement of licensed medical health professionals who remain solely responsible for decisions regarding diagnosis and treatment of their patients. Content from BMJ Best Practice is not intended to function as a substitute for a licensed medical health professional's judgement. BMJ Best Practice reflects evidence available to its authors and licensors prior to publication. BMJ relies on its authors to confirm the accuracy of the information presented to reflect generally accepted practices. While BMJ seeks to ensure BMJ Best Practice is up to date and accurate, it does not warrant that is the case. Content from BMJ Best Practice is supplied on an "as is" basis and any statements made to the contrary are void. BMJ Best Practice does not endorse drugs, diagnose patients, or recommend therapy. The full disclaimer applicable to BMJ Best Practice can be found at http://bestpractice. bmj.com/best-practice/marketing/disclaimer.html.

1   World Health Organization, Regional Office for South-East Asia. Comprehensive guidelines for prevention and control of dengue and dengue haemorrhagic fever—revised and expanded edition. 2011. www.searo.who.int/entity/vector_borne_tropical_diseases/documents/ SEAROTPS60/en/.

2   World Health Organization, Special Programme for Research and Training in Tropical Diseases (TDR). Dengue guidelines for diagnosis, treatment, prevention and control: new edition. 2009. http:// whqlibdoc.who.int/publications/2009/9789241547871_eng.pdf?ua=1.

3   Kalayanarooj S, Vaughn DW, Nimmannitya S, et al. Early clinical and laboratory indicators of acute dengue illness. J Infect Dis1997;176:313-21.

4   Halstead SB. Dengue. Lancet2007;370:1644-52.

5   Guzman MG, Kouri G. Dengue and dengue haemorrhagic fever in America: lessons and challenges. J Clin Virol2007;27:1-13.

6   Teixeira MG, Barreto M. Diagnosis and management of dengue: clinical review. BMJ2009;339:1189-93.

7   Wilder-Smith A, Gubler DJ. Geographic expansion of dengue: the impact of international travel. Med Clin North Am2008;92:1377-90.

8   Webster DP, Farrar J, Rowland-Jones S. Progress towards dengue vaccine. Lancet Infect Dis2009;9:678-87.

9   Pichainarong N, Mongkalangoon N, Kalyanarooj S, et al. Relationship between body size and severity of dengue haemorrhagic fever among children aged 0-14 years. South East J Trop Med Public Health2006;37:283-8.

10   Guzman MG, Kouri GP, Bravo J, et al. Dengue haemorrhagic fever in Cuba 1981, retrospective seroepidemiological study. Am J Trop Med Hyg1990;42:179-84.

11   Stephenson JR. Understanding dengue pathogenesis: implication for vaccine design. Bull World Health Organ2005;83:308-14.

12   Whitehorn J, Simmons CP. The pathogenesis of dengue. Vaccine2011;29:7221-8.

13   Libraty DH, Young PR, Pickering D, et al. High circulating levels of the dengue virus nonstructural protein NS1 early in dengue illness correlate with development of dengue haemorrhagic fever. J Infect Dis2002;186:1165-8.

14   Baldacchino F, Caputo B, Chandre F, et al. Control methods against invasive Aedes mosquitoes in Europe: a review. Pest Manag Sci2015, published online 21 May.

15   Villar L, Dayan GH, Arredondo-García JL, et al; CYD15 Study Group. Efficacy of a tetravalent dengue vaccine in children in Latin America. N Engl J Med2015;372:113-23.

16   Premaratne R, Pathmeswaran A, Amarasekara ND, et al. A clinical guide for early detection of dengue fever and timing of investigations to detect patients likely to develop complications. Trans R Soc Trop Med Hyg2009;103:127-31.

SOURCES AND SELECTION CRITERIA

I searched Medline and PubMed from 1980 to date, limited to publications in English. My search strategy used a combination of key words, including "dengue", "DHF", "US", "Africa", "Europe", "Asia", "WHO", and "Complications". I supplemented these sources with selected systematic reviews. Additional information cited includes evidence based national guidelines, published consensus statements, and WHO publications.

17   Ministry of Health, Sri Lanka. Guidelines on management of dengue fever and dengue haemorrhagic fever in children and adolescents: revised and expanded edition. Nov 2012. www.epid.gov.lk/web/ images/pdf/Publication/gmdfca12.pdf.

18   Kalayanarooj S, Nimmanitya S, Suntayakorn S, et al. Can doctors make an accurate diagnosis of dengue infection at an early stage? Dengue Bull1999;23:1-9.

19   Sawasdivorn S, Vibulvattanakit S, Sasavatpakdee M, et al. Efficacy of clinical diagnosis of dengue fever in paediatric age groups as determined by WHO case definition 1997 in Thailand. Dengue Bull2001;25:56-64.

20   Lima Mda R, Nogueira RM, Schatzmayr HG, et al. Comparison of three commercially available dengue NS1 antigen capture assays for acute diagnosis of dengue in Brazil. PLoS Negl Trop Dis2010;4:e738.

21   Centers for Disease Control and Prevention. Clinical guidance: dengue virus. Jun 2014. www.cdc.gov/dengue/clinicalLab/clinical.html.

22   Ashley EA. Dengue fever. Trends Anaesth Crit Care2011;1:39-41.

23   Dung NM, Day NP, Tam DT, et al. Fluid replacement in dengue shock syndrome: randomized, double-blind comparison of four intravenous fluid regimens. Clin Infect Dis1999;29:787-94.

24   Ngo NT, Cao XT, Kneen R, et al. Acute management of dengue shock syndrome: randomized double-blind comparison of 4 intravenous fluid regimens in the first hour. Clin Infect Dis2001;32:204-13.

25   Wills BA, Nguyen MD, Ha TL, et al. Comparison of three fluid solutions for resuscitation in dengue shock syndrome. N Engl J Med2005;353:877-89.

26   Pouliot SH, Xiong X, Harille RM, et al. Maternal dengue and pregnancy outcomes: a systemic review. Obstet Gynecol Surv2010;65:107-18.

27   Ministry of Health, Sri Lanka. Guidelines on management of dengue fever and dengue haemorrhagic fever in adults: revised and expanded edition. Nov 2012. www.epid.gov.lk/web/images/pdf/ Publication/guidelines_for_the_management_of_df_and_dhf_in_ adults.pdf.

28   Rajapakse S. Corticosteroids in the treatment of dengue illness. Trans R Soc Trop Med Hyg2009;103:122-6.

29   Kularatne SA, Patirage MM, Pathirage PV, et al. Cardiac complication of a dengue fever outbreak of Sri Lanka, 2005. Trans R Soc Trop Med Hyg2007;101:804-8.

30   Kularatne SA, Pathirage MM, Gunasena S. A case series of dengue fever with altered consciousness and electroencephalogram changes in Sri Lanka. Trans R Soc Trop Med Hyg2008;102:1053-4.

31   Gulati S, Maheshwari A. Atypical manifestations of dengue. Trop Med Int Health2007;12:1087-95.

32   Zhang F, Kramer CV. Corticosteroids for dengue infection. Cochrane Database Syst Rev2014;7:CD003488.

33   Tam DT, Ngoc TV, Tien NT, et al. Effects of short-course oral corticosteroid therapy in early dengue infection in Vietnamese patients: a randomized, placebo-controlled trial. Clin Infect Dis2012;55:1216-24.

34   Noble CG, Chen YL, Dong H, et al. Strategies for development of dengue virus inhibitors. Antiviral Res2010;85:450-62.

35   Nguyen NM, Tran CN, Phung LK, et al. A randomized, double-blind placebo controlled trial of balapiravir, a polymerase inhibitor, in adult dengue patients. J Infect Dis2013;207:1442-50.

36   Sabchareon A, Wallace D, Sirivichayakul C, et al. Protective efficacy of the recombinant, live-attenuated, CYD tetravalent dengue vaccine in Thai schoolchildren: a randomised, controlled phase 2b trial. Lancet2012;380:1559-67.

37   Lanata CF, Andrade T, Gil AI, et al. Immunogenicity and safety of tetravalent dengue vaccine in 2-11 year-olds previously vaccinated against yellow fever: randomized, controlled, phase II study in Piura, Peru. Vaccine2012;30:5935-41.

38   Leo YS, Wilder-Smith A, Archuleta S, et al. Immunogenicity and safety of recombinant tetravalent dengue vaccine (CYD-TDV) in individuals aged 2-45 years: phase II randomized controlled trial in Singapore. Hum Vaccin Immunother2012;8:1259-71.

39   Durbin AP, Kirkpatrick BD, Pierce KK, et al. A single dose of any of four different live attenuated tetravalent dengue vaccines is safe and immunogenic in flavivirus-naive adults: a randomized, double-blind clinical trial. J Infect Dis2013;207:957-65.

40   Capeding MR, Tran NH, Hadinegoro SR, et al; CYD14 Study Group. Clinical efficacy and safety of a novel tetravalent dengue vaccine in healthy children in Asia: a phase 3, randomised, observer-masked, placebo-controlled trial. Lancet2014;384:1358-65.

41   Kularatne SA, Imbulpitiya IV, Abeysekera RA, et al. Extensive haemorrhagic necrosis of liver is an unpredictable fatal complication in dengue infection: a postmortem study. BMC Infect Dis2014;14:141.

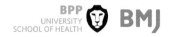

Diagnosis and management of cellulitis

Gokulan Phoenix, core surgical trainee year 1 (London Deanery)[1], Saroj Das, consultant vascular surgeon[2], Meera Joshi, core surgical trainee year 1 (Oxford Deanery)[3]

[1]Department of General Surgery, Chelsea and Westminster Hospital, London SW10 9NH

[2]Department of General Surgery, the Hillingdon Hospitals, London

[3]Department of General Surgery, Wexham Park Hospital, Oxford

Correspondence to: G Phoenix
gokulan.phoenix@nhs.net

Cite this as: BMJ 2012;345:e4955

DOI: 10.1136/bmj.e4955

http://www.bmj.com/content/345/bmj.e4955

Cellulitis is an acute, spreading, pyogenic inflammation of the lower dermis and associated subcutaneous tissue. It is a skin and soft tissue infection that results in high morbidity and severe financial costs to healthcare providers worldwide. Cellulitis is managed by several clinical specialists including primary care physicians, surgeons, general medics, and dermatologists. We assess the most recent evidence in the diagnosis and management of cellulitis.

What is the extent of the problem?

In 2008-9 there were 82113 hospital admissions in England and Wales lasting a mean length of 7.2 days[1]; an estimated £133m (€170m; $209m) was spent on bed stay alone.[2] Cellulitis accounted for 1.6% of emergency hospital admissions during 2008-9.[3]

In Australia, hospital admissions for cellulitis have risen to 11.5 people per 10000 (2001-2) with the average admission lasting 5.9 days.[4] In the US more than 600000 hospitalisations were recorded in 2010,[5] representing 3.7% of all emergency admissions.[6] In all, 14.2 million Americans visited primary care physicians, hospital outpatient departments, and emergency services with skin and soft tissue infections in 2005, an increase from 321 to 481 visits per 100000 (50% increase; P=0.003) since 1997. Over 95% of this change was attributed to abscesses and cellulitis. Hospital visits for abscesses and cellulitis have increased from 173 to 325 per 1000 population (88% increase; P<0.001).[7]

What causes cellulitis?

Cellulitis is caused by a wide range of organisms (see table 1). The majority of cases are caused by *Streptococcus pyogenes* or *Staphylococcus aureus*. A review of prospective and retrospective laboratory studies found that *S aureus* accounted for 51% of all aspiration and punch biopsy cultures positive for cellulitis, and *Streptococcus* accounted for 27%.[8]

A prospective study demonstrated that the majority of *S aureus* infections in the US are now meticillin resistant; among 389 blood culture isolates of *S aureus*, 63% (244) were CA-MRSA.[14]

A multicentre study of 11 US hospitals reported a prevalence of MRSA ranging from 15% to 74% (59% overall).[15]

A recent review reports an increase in CA-MRSA rates in Europe.[16]

Who is at risk of cellulitis?

No link with age or gender has been established. However, a recent prospective case controlled study comprising 150 patients with cellulitis and 300 controls found white people to be at higher risk.[17] Alcohol intake and smoking have been disproved as risk factors in case-control studies.[18]

Commonly identified risk factors are listed in box 1. General systemic risk factors include venous insufficiency, regarded to be the most frequent[19]; lymphoedema, both a predisposing factor and a complication of cellulitis[20]; peripheral vascular disease; diabetes mellitus; and obesity.[9] Local factors include tinea pedis, ulcers, trauma, and insect bites.[9]

Can cellulitis be prevented in those at risk?

Besides the management of lymphoedema, there is no evidence to support the active management of other risk factors including diabetes mellitus, peripheral vascular disease, and tinea pedis.

In lymphoedema, decongestive lymphatic therapy, consisting of manipulation of the lymphatic system through massage, has been associated with reduced recurrence of cellulitis. In a prospective study of 299 people who underwent decongestive lymphatic therapy the incidence of cellulitis infections decreased from 1.10 to 0.65 infections per person per year.[21]

How is the diagnosis of cellulitis made?

Clinical diagnosis

Cellulitis most commonly affects the lower extremities, and often presents as an acute, tender, erythematous, and swollen area of skin. In severe cases blisters, ulcers, oedema, associated lymphangitis, and lymphadenopathy may be present. Constitutional features include fever and malaise. In the late stages widespread features of sepsis including hypotension and tachycardia may also be present.

Other conditions can masquerade as cellulitis. Several differential diagnoses (see table 2), especially in the lower limbs, can present with similar signs and symptoms. In a recent prospective study of 145 patients, 28% of patients were incorrectly diagnosed with lower limb cellulitis. The diagnosis most commonly mistaken as cellulitis was (venous) stasis dermatitis (37%).[22]

In view of the potential for misdiagnosis on clinical observation alone, investigations are sometimes recommended to help confirm or refute the diagnosis.

Blood investigations

In a prospective study of 150 people admitted to the emergency department that examined the feasibility of using C reactive protein level and white cell count as indicators of bacterial infections including cellulitis, white cell counts had a specificity of 84.5% and a sensitivity of 43.0% and

SUMMARY POINTS

- Cellulitis episodes in the United States, the United Kingdom, and Australia have risen over the past decade, with an increase in community acquired meticillin resistant *Staphylococcus aureus* (CA-MRSA) cases of cellulitis in the US, and to a lesser extent the UK and Australia. Antibiotic resistant strains of CA-MRSA are already emerging

- Diagnosis is based on clinical findings with investigations lending weight to confirm or refute diagnosis

- Existing guidelines need revision, taking into consideration CA-MRSA and other emerging strains as well as using new clinical classification systems such as the Dundee criteria

- Use outpatient parenteral antibiotic therapy if available

- More randomised control trials assessing the management of predisposing factors and long term therapy for recurrent cellulitis are required

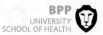

Table 1 Treatment recommendations for cellulitis based on organisms[9 10 11 12 13]

Clinical presentation	Organism	Antibiotic
Typical cellulitis	Streptococcus pyogenes	Amoxicillin or flucloxacillin
Typical cellulitis—pus forming	Staphylococcus aureus	Flucloxacillin
Typical cellulitis in the US—pus forming	CA-MRSA, HA-MRSA	Doxycycline or minocycline or clindamycin or vancomycin
Penicillin allergy	NA	Erythromycin or clarithromycin or clindamycin
Cat or dog bite	Pasteurella multocida	Co-amoxiclav; if allergic to penicillin: doxycycline and metronidazole
Freshwater exposure	Aeromonas hydrophila	Ciprofloxacin
Saltwater exposure	Vibrio vulnificus	Doxycycline
Necrotising fasciitis	Polymicrobial; with common causes including group A streptococci, *Staphylococcus aureus*, and anaerobes	Benzylpenicillin, ciprofloxacin, and clindamycin
Butchers and fish handlers	Erysipelothrix	Penicillin; if allergic to penicillin: ciprofloxacin

Table 2 Common differential diagnoses for cellulitis with defining characteristics[10]

Differential	Defining characteristics
Stasis dermatitis	Absence of pain or fever; circumferential; bilateral
Acute arthritis	Involvement of joint; pain on movement
Pyoderma gangrenosum	Ulcerations on the legs; history of inflammatory bowel disease
Hypersensitivity/drug reaction	Exposure to allergen or drug; pruritus; absence of fever; absence of fever or pain
Deep vein thrombosis	Absence of skin changes or fever
Necrotising fasciitis	Severe pain, swelling and fever; rapid progression; pain out of proportion; systemic toxicity; skin crepitus; necrosis; ecchymosis

---

BOX 1 PREDISPOSING RISK FACTORS FOR LOWER LIMB CELLULITIS[9 17]

General

- Non-modifiable—pregnant; white race
- Modifiable—venous insufficiency; lymphoedema; peripheral arterial disease; immunosuppression; diabetes

Local

- Non-modifiable—trauma; animal and insect bites; tattoos
- Modifiable—ulcers; eczema; athlete's foot (tinea pedis); burns

---

C reactive protein had a sensitivity of 67.1%, specificity of 94.8% (positive predictive value 94.6% and negative predictive value 67.9%).[23] An elevated level of C reactive protein is a better indicator of bacterial infection than an elevated white cell count but a normal level of C reactive protein cannot rule out an infection. Blood investigations do not appear to be clinically useful for diagnosis.

Microbiology

Prospective studies have shown true positive rates from blood cultures in those with suspected cellulitis are between 2-4%.[24 25] In a retrospective study of 757 people admitted to a medical centre with cellulitis, blood cultures were performed for 553 people (73%)—only 11 (2%) were positive. Eight of 11 patients with positive blood cultures were changed from empirical treatment with cefazolin to penicillin. Furthermore, all those in the study, including those with systemic toxicity, recovered, whether a blood culture was taken or not. The cost of negative blood cultures was $34 950 (£22 255; €28 560) and the cost for the 11 positive cultures was $1100, amounting to an excess cost of $36 050. The authors concluded blood cultures were neither clinically effective or cost effective.[20] National guidelines, including the Northern Ireland Clinical Resource Efficiency Support Team (CREST) 2005 guidelines on the management of cellulitis in adults, recommend taking blood cultures only in patients that have significant systemic upset including pyrexia (>38°C).[10]

In a prospective study of 50 patients with cellulitis, cultures from skin biopsies and aspirations that showed true positives were found to be 20% and 10% respectively.[25]

CREST guidelines suggest the use of skin biopsies and aspirations in only selected patients, where the diagnosis of cellulitis is in doubt.[10]

In regard to wound swabs, a multicentre prospective study from France that analysed wound swab samples from 214 patients with lower limb cellulitis identified 183 (85.5%) positive cultures; *S aureus* and *Streptococcus* being the most frequently isolated micro-organisms (56% and 21% respectively). Sensitivities from the swabs showed resistance to the empirical antibiotics that had initially been used, prompting a change in antibiotics.[26] CREST guidelines suggest the use of swabs on open cellulitis wounds.[10]

Imaging

Imaging techniques are useful when there is a suspicion of an underlying abscess associated with cellulitis, necrotising fasciitis, or when the diagnosis of cellulitis is uncertain. In a retrospective study of 542 emergency department patients for whom the clinical diagnosis of cellulitis was in doubt, 109 (17%) were found to have a deep vein thrombosis on Doppler ultrasound.[27]

In a prospective observational study of 216 adult emergency department patients with a clinical diagnosis of lower limb cellulitis, an ultrasonography scan changed the management in 71 patients (56%) in regard to the need for drainage of underlying abscesses. In the pre-test group that were believed not to need drainage of any underlying abscess, ultrasonography resulted in a change in management in 32 of 44 patients (73%), including 16 in whom drainage was eliminated. In the pre-test group that was believed to not need further drainage, ultrasonography changed the management in 39 of 82 (48%), with 33 receiving drainage and six receiving further diagnostic imaging. Ultrasound may therefore guide management of cellulitis by detection of occult abscess, prevention of invasive procedures, and providing guidance for further imaging or consultation.[28]

Other imaging studies, such as MRI (magnetic resonance imaging) may be useful in those with an equivocal diagnosis of cellulitis or with suspicion of necrotising fasciitis. According to CREST guidelines, the physician should be alert to the possibility of necrotising fasciitis upon presentation

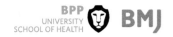

Table 3 Eron clinical classification system³⁴

Class	Systemic toxicity	Comorbidities	Oral v intravenous antibiotics	Outpatient v hospital admission
I	No sign	None	Oral	Outpatient
II	May or may not have systemic illness	Peripheral vascular disease, obesity, venous insufficiency	Intravenous	Hospital admission for 48 hours then outpatient parenteral antibiotic therapy
III	Significant systemic toxicity—confusion, tachycardia, tachypnoea, hypotension	Unstable	Intravenous	Hospital
IV	Sepsis syndrome/necrotising fasciitis	Unstable	Intravenous with or without surgical debridement	Hospital

Table 4 Eron classification v Dundee classification¹⁵ ³³

Parameter	Eron (2003)	Dundee (2010)
Strength of evidence	Expert opinion	Retrospective study of 205 consecutive patients
Incorporated into guidelines?	CREST and NHS acute trusts	NA
Validated?	Yes	Yes
Criteria	Comorbidities including obesity and peripheral vascular disease	The importance of comorbidities
	Systemic toxicity: pyrexia (>38°c), hypotension, tachypnoea, and tachycardia	Obesity and peripheral vascular disease not counted towards hospital admission
		Up to date definition of systemic inflammatory response syndrome (SIRS)
		Standardised and validated early warning scores

of tense oedema, skin necrosis, crepitus, paraesthesia with an elevated white cell count greater than 14×10⁹/L, and in the haemodynamically stable patient an MRI scan is warranted.¹⁰ In a prospective study of 36 patients with a clinical diagnosis of acute infectious cellulitis, MRI demonstrated necrotising fasciitis in 16 people, all of whom underwent surgical debridement. Distinct MRI features were found in people with necrotising soft tissue infections, including hyper-attenuating signals on T2 weighted images at the deep fasciae and poorly defined areas of hyper-intense signal on T2 weighted images within muscles. In cellulitis, signal intensity abnormalities are only within the subcutaneous fat.²⁹

What is the treatment of cellulitis?
General measures include rest, elevation of any affected limbs, and analgesia. The area of cellulitis should be clearly marked and reviewed daily for progression or regression to assess the efficacy of the antibiotic regimen.¹⁰

However, there is still uncertainty regarding the optimal antibiotic choice, duration, and route of antibiotic therapy, and the use of corticosteroids. A recent Cochrane review could not draw any definitive conclusions on the optimal antibiotics, duration, or route of administration from an analysis of 25 randomised controlled trials, as no two trials had compared the same antibiotics.³⁰ A summary of the main antibiotics that are currently recommended in US and UK national guidelines, as well as in large prospective studies, are provided in table 1.

CREST guidelines still recommend flucloxacillin for the majority of cases of cellulitis caused by S aureus, Streptococcus, or when the organism has not been identified,¹⁰ but clinicians should take into account the rise in CA-MRSA rates. The 2011 Infectious Diseases Society of America national guidelines have now recommended patients with pus forming cellulitis to be treated with antibiotics that target CA-MRSA.¹¹

The efficacy of other agents that target CA-MRSA has been studied. One retrospective cohort study has shown doxycycline or minocycline to be effective in 95% of patients (n=276) with CA-MRSA.¹² Clindamycin is also therapeutic, with susceptibility in isolates as high as 93%. However,

the development of resistance is not uncommon and as it associated with cases of *Clostridium difficile*, it should be discontinued on the development of diarrhoea.³¹ In those with severe cellulitis requiring admission to hospital, linezolid and vancomycin were found to have good efficacy.³²

When should a person be admitted to hospital for intravenous antibiotics?
The Cochrane review from 2010 also states the need for further evaluation of oral versus intravenous antibiotics as well as the efficacy of outpatient parenteral antibiotic therapy (OPAT).³⁰

In a prospective study of 205 consecutive adults admitted to a Scottish hospital for cellulitis, 43% were found to be overtreated based on CREST guidelines. The study suggests they possibly could have been managed as outpatients on oral antibiotics.³³ The CREST guidelines determine route of administration based on the Eron clinical classification system, taking into consideration the presence of systemic toxicity and comorbidities.

Eron classification v Dundee classification
The Eron classification is based on expert opinions, and is among the most widely used classification systems for diagnosis and treatment of cellulitis.³⁴ The Eron classification is summarised in table 3.

However, new criteria such as the 2011 Dundee classification are also available³³—a comparison between the two is provided in table 4. Seventy per cent of people that, based on Eron recommendations, would be treated with inpatient stay and intravenous antibiotics meet the criteria for outpatient management based on the Dundee criteria.³³ Further validation of the Dundee criteria is required.

Outpatient parenteral antibiotic therapy (OPAT)
A prospective study on 344 episodes of treatment administered by a UK OPAT service showed that 87% of patients were cured, readmission rate was 6.3%, and patient satisfaction was high. OPAT costs 41% of inpatient costs when calculated using conservative cost measurements. The authors of the study concluded that clinicians should use OPAT where available³⁵; this is supported by CREST guidelines.¹⁰

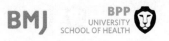

SOURCES AND SELECTION CRITERIA

We searched PubMed and the Cochrane library for recent and clinically relevant cohort studies and randomised controlled trials on cellulitis, using the search terms "cellulitis", "erysipelas", "diagnosis", "investigation", "recurrence", "complications" and "management". For position statements and guidelines we consulted the British Lymphology Society (BLS), National Health Service Clinical Knowledge Summaries (CKS), Clinical Resource Efficiency Support Team (CREST), and Infectious Disease Society of America (IDSA).

ONGOING RESEARCH

- UK Dermatology Clinical Trials Network. Prophylactic antibiotics for the treatment of cellulitis at home (PATCH) I study—a multicentre randomised control trial in the UK assessing the efficacy of a one year course of penicillin V prophylaxis versus placebo in patients with recurrent cellulitis

ADDITIONAL EDUCATIONAL RESOURCES

Resources for healthcare professionals
- Kilburn SA, Featherstone P, Higgins B, Brindle R. Interventions for cellulitis and erysipelas. *Cochrane Database Syst Rev* 2010;6:CD004299—the most recent review of randomised controlled trials on various antimicrobial options for cellulitis, with evidence for the most commonly used antibiotics
- Thomas K, Crook A, Foster K, Mason J, Chalmers J, et al; for the UK Dermatology Clinical Trials Network's PATCH Trial Team. Prophylactic antibiotics for the prevention of cellulitis (erysipelas) of the leg: results of the UK Dermatology Clinical Trials Network's PATCH II trial. *Br J Dermatol* 2012;166:169-78—a recent randomised controlled trial that assessed the efficacy of long term prophylactic penicillin V for recurrent cellulitis. No statistical significance was seen in the reduction in rates of recurrence with penicillin V
- Chronic oedema and lymphoedema *BMJ* learning module. http://learning.bmj.com/learning/module-intro/lymphoedema-.html?moduleId=10029385—*BMJ* module on the diagnosis, investigation, and treatment of lymphoedema associated with cellulitis

Information resources for patients
- Cellulitis Support Group. www.mdjunction.com/cellulitis—forums for cellulitis sufferers to discuss various treatment options (free registration required)

When should a switch to oral antibiotics be made?

CREST guidelines suggest indications for a switch to oral therapy are apyrexia (<37.8°C) for 48 hours, regression of cellulitis from a clearly marked area (on daily review), and a falling C reactive protein level.[10]

When to seek further advice?

CREST and NHS Clinical Knowledge Summaries guidelines suggest that if there is doubt in the diagnosis, atypical presentations, or no improvement in clinical symptoms and signs after 48 hours, then advice from a dermatologist or microbiologist or both should be sought.[29]

Can recurrence be prevented?

Several prospective and retrospective studies suggest a high proportion of cellulitis sufferers develop recurrent episodes, especially in those with untreated predisposing factors.[9] [20] One retrospective study reported 47% recurrence in a cohort of 171 people who had suffered one prior episode.[20]

Antibiotic prophylaxis

The Dermatology Clinical Trials Networks PATCH II trial (prophylactic antibiotics for the treatment of cellulitis at home II) was a large, multicentre, randomised trial in the UK that assessed the efficacy of 6 months of penicillin V prophylaxis in reducing recurrence. A total of 123 participants were randomised into those treated with penicillin (n=60) versus placebo (n=63); recurrence rates were 20% and 33% respectively (hazard ratio 0.53, 95% confidence interval 0.26 to 1.07, P=0.08) with no difference in the number of adverse effects between both groups.[13] The authors of this study conclude that there is no statistical significance seen in the reduction of cellulitis rates for penicillin V for prophylaxis, but there are promising results and longer term prophylaxis (for one year) may be required. The PATCH I trial, which assesses one year penicillin V prophylaxis, is under way.[13] CREST guidelines advise antibiotic prophylaxis with penicillin V or erythromycin for 1 to 2 years in patients with two or more previous episodes of cellulitis.[10]

Contributors: SD planned and initiated the manuscript. GP planned and contributed to the manuscript and provided figures. MJ contributed to the manuscript and provided figures. SD critically revised drafts of the article and approved the content of the final version to be published. SD is guarantor.

Competing interests: All authors have completed the ICMJE uniform disclosure form at www.icmje.org/coi_disclosure.pdf (available on request from the corresponding author) and declare: no support from any organisation for the submitted work; no financial relationships with any organisations that might have an interest in the submitted work in the previous three years; no other relationships or activities that could appear to have influenced the submitted work.

Provenance and peer review: Not commissioned; externally peer reviewed.

1. Department of Health. Hospital episode statistics. Primary diagnosis 2008-2009. NHS Information Centre, 2010. www.hesonline.nhs.uk.
2. NHS. Institute for innovation and improvement. Quality and service improvement tools. 2008. www.institute.nhs.uk/quality_and_service_improvement_tools/quality_and_service_improvement_tools/length_of_stay.html.
3. Blunt I, Bardsley M, Dixon J. Trends in emergency admissions in England 2004-9. The Nuffield Trust, 2010. www.nuffieldtrust.org.uk/sites/files/nuffield/Trends_in_emergency_admissions_REPORT.pdf.
4. Australian Institute of Health and Welfare. Australian hospital statistics 2001-02. 2003. www.aihw.gov.au/publication-detail/?id=6442467479.
5. Agency for Healthcare Research and Quality. HCUP Databases. Healthcare Cost and Utilization Project (HCUP). Overview of the Nationwide Inpatient Sample (NIS). June 2012. www.hcup-us.ahrq.gov/nisoverview.jsp.
6. National Hospital Ambulatory Medical Care Survey: 2008 Emergency Department Summary. www.cdc.gov/nchs/fastats/ervisits.htm.
7. Hersh AL, Chambers HF, Maselli JH, Gonzales R. National trends in ambulatory visits and antibiotic prescribing for skin and soft-tissue infections. *Arch Intern Med* 2008;168:1585-91.
8. Chira S, Miller LG. Staphylococcus aureus is the most common identified cause of cellulitis: a systematic review. *Epidemiol Infect* 2010;138:313-7.
9. Cox NH, Colver GB, Paterson WD. Management and morbidity of cellulitis of the leg. *J R Soc Med* 1998;91:634-7.
10. Clinical Resource Efficiency Support Team (2005) Guidelines on the management of cellulitis in adults. Crest, Belfast. http://www.acutemed.co.uk/docs/Cellulitis%20guidelines,%20CREST,%2005.pdf.
11. Liu C, Bayer A, Cosgrove SE, Daum RS, Fridkin SK, Gorwitz RJ, et al. Clinical practice guidelines by the Infectious Diseases Society of America for the treatment of methicillin-resistant Staphylococcus aureus infections in adults and children. *Clin Infect Dis* 2011;52:e18-e55.
12. Ruhe JJ, Menon A. Tetracyclines as an oral treatment option for patients with community onset skin and soft tissue infections caused by methicillin-resistant Staphylococcus aureus. *Antimicrob Agents Chemother* 2007;51:3298-303.
13. UK Dermatology Clinical Trials Network's PATCH Trial Team, Thomas K, Crook A, Foster K, Mason J, Chalmers J, et al. Prophylactic antibiotics for the prevention of cellulitis (erysipelas) of the leg: results of the UK Dermatology Clinical Trials Network's PATCH II trial. *Br J Dermatol* 2012;166:169-78.
14. King MD, Humphrey BJ, Wang YF, Kourbatova EV, Ray SM, Blumberg HM. Emergence of community-acquired methicillin-resistant Staphylococcus aureus USA 300 clone as the predominant cause of skin and soft-tissue infections. *Ann Intern Med* 2006;144:309-17.

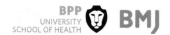

15 Moran GJ, Krishnadasan A, Gorwitz RJ, Fosheim GE, McDougal LK, Carey RB, et al. Methicillin-resistant S aureus infections among patients in the emergency department. *N Engl J Med* 2006;355:666-74.

16 Otter JA, French GL. Molecular epidemiology of community-associated meticillin-resistant Staphylococcus aureus in Europe. *Lancet Infect Dis* 2010;10:227-39.

17 Halpern J, Holder R, Langford NJ. Ethnicity and other risk factors for acute lower limb cellulitis: a UK-based prospective case-control study. *Br J Dermatol* 2008;158:1288-92.

18 Dupuy A, Benchikhi H, Roujeau JC, Bernard P, Vaillant L, Chosidow O, et al. Risk factors for erysipelas of the leg (cellulitis): case-control study. *BMJ* 1999;318:1591-4.

19 Jorup-Rönström C, Britton S. Recurrent erysipelas: predisposing factors and cost of prophylaxis. *Infection* 1987;15:105-6.

20 Keeley VL. Lymphoedema and cellulitis: chicken or egg? *Br J Dermatol* 2008;158:1175-6.

21 Ko DS, Lerner R, Klose G, Cosimi AB. Effective treatment of lymphedema of the extremities. *Arch Surg* 1998;133:452-8.

22 David CV, Chira S, Eells SJ, Ladrigan M, Papier A, Miller LG, et al. Diagnostic accuracy in patients admitted to hospitals with cellulitis. *Dermatol Online J* 2011;17:1.

23 Chan YL, Liao HC, Tsay PK, Chang SS, Chen JC, Liaw SJ. C-reactive protein as an indicator of bacterial infection of adult patients in the emergency department. *Chang Gung Med J* 2002;25:437-45.

24 Perl B, Gottehrer NP, Ravesh D, Schlesinger Y, Rudensky B, Yinnon AM. Cost-effectiveness of blood cultures for adult patients with cellulitis. *Clin Infect Dis* 1999;29:1483-8.

25 Hook EW 3rd, Hooton TM, Horton CA, Coyle MB, Ramsey PG, Turck M. Microbiologic evaluation of cutaneous cellulitis in adults. *Arch Intern Med* 1986;146:295-7.

26 Holzapfel L, Jacquet-Francillon T, Rahmani J, Achard P, Marcellin E, Joffre T, et al. Microbiological evaluation of infected wounds of the extremities in 214 adults. *J Accid Emerg Med* 1999;16:32-4.

27 Rabuka CE, Azoulay LY, Kahn SR. Predictors of a positive duplex scan in patients with a clinical presentation compatible with deep vein thrombosis or cellulitis. *Can J Infect Dis* 2003;14:210-4.

28 Tayal VS, Hasan N, Norton HJ, Tomaszewski CA. The effect of soft-tissue ultrasound on the management of cellulitis in the emergency department. *Acad Emerg Med* 2006;13:384-8.

29 Rahmouni A, Chosidow O, Mathieu D, et al. MR imaging in acute infectious cellulitis. *Radiology* 1994;192:493-6.

30 Kilburn SA, Featherstone P, Higgins B, Brindle R. Interventions for cellulitis and erysipelas. *Cochrane Database Syst Rev* 2010;6:CD004299.

31 Forcade NA, Parchman ML, Jorgensen JH, Du LC, Nyren NR, Treviño LB, et al. Prevalence, severity, and treatment of community-acquired methicillin-resistant Staphylococcus aureus (CA-MRSA) skin and soft tissue infections in 10 medical clinics in Texas: a South Texas Ambulatory Research Network (STARNet) Study. *J Am Board Fam Med* 2011;24:543-50.

32 Stevens DL, Bisno AL, Chambers HF, Everett ED, Dellinger P, Goldstein EJ, et al. Practice guidelines for the diagnosis and management of skin and soft-tissue infections. *Clin Infect Dis* 2005;41:1373-1406.

33 Marwick C, Broomhall J, McCowan C, Phillips G, Gonzalez-McQuire S, Akhras K, et al. Severity assessment of skin and soft tissue infections: cohort study of management and outcomes for hospitalized patients. *J Antimicrob Chemother* 2011;66:387-97.

34 Eron L. J. Infections of skin and soft tissues: outcome of a classification scheme. *Clin Infect Dis* 2000;31:287.

35 Chapman AL, Dixon S, Andrews D, Lillie PJ, Bazaz R, Patchett JD. Clinical efficacy and cost-effectiveness of outpatient parenteral antibiotic therapy (OPAT): a UK perspective. *J Antimicrob Chemother* 2009;64:1316-24.

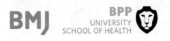

HIV testing and management of newly diagnosed HIV

Michael Rayment, consultant[1], David Asboe, consultant[2], Ann K Sullivan, consultant[2]

[1]Homerton Sexual Health Services, Homerton University Hospital NHS Foundation Trust, London E9 6SR, UK

[2]Directorate of HIV/GU Medicine, Chelsea and Westminster Hospital NHS Foundation Trust, London, UK

Correspondence to: M Rayment michaelrayment@nhs.net

Cite this as: BMJ 2014;349:g4275

DOI: 10.1136/bmj.g4275

http://www.bmj.com/content/349/bmj.g4275

HIV infection in the United Kingdom remains a public health challenge; in 2012 an estimated 98 400 people were living with HIV infection, with 1 in 5 cases undiagnosed. The prognosis for those with a diagnosis of HIV is broadly excellent. Most patients with newly diagnosed HIV infection should prepare for a normal, healthy, and productive lifespan.

UK guidance on HIV testing,[1] published in 2008, encouraged the normalisation and expansion of HIV testing. As a result more testing is now being undertaken in non-specialist settings, with an increase now being seen in the number of cases being diagnosed outside specialist services.

The purpose of this review is to provide an evidence based summary to support primary and secondary care clinicians in delivering HIV testing and to guide them in the initial management of patients with newly diagnosed HIV infection. Although we focus on the situation in the UK, many of the principles apply to populations worldwide. Globally, undiagnosed and late stage diagnosed HIV infection is a feature of many epidemics in the developed world. Some countries face different problems. In the United States, for example, poor linkage to (and retention in) specialist care of patients with known HIV infection is a greater problem than in western Europe. Guidance for a specific country must be responsive to the specifics of the epidemiology of HIV infection and clinical outcomes within the local health system.

What is the current epidemiology of HIV infection in the UK?
The advent of combination antiretroviral therapy has transformed the prognosis of patients with HIV infection. People with a diagnosis of HIV infection before moderate to severe immunosuppression occurs should now anticipate a normal life expectancy.[2]

The prevalence of HIV infection in the UK has risen steadily and, in 2012, stood at an estimated 98 400 people (1.5/1000 population). The epidemic remains concentrated in, but is not restricted to, higher risk groups—men who have sex with men, and heterosexuals from areas of high endemicity, notably sub-Saharan Africa. There is also notable variation in prevalence geographically, with most people living with HIV residing in large urban centres.[3] In 2012, more than 6000 people were newly diagnosed as having HIV infection, an increase on 2011. The highest number of annual diagnoses ever was recorded in men who have sex with men (MSM), at 3250 (51% of total). Heterosexuals comprised 45% of all new diagnoses in 2012.[3] Of these, 52% were believed to have acquired their infection in the UK (including 48% of heterosexuals born abroad)—a figure that has risen from 27% in 2002.[4]

Timely linkage to care and excellent clinical outcomes are consistently shown in the UK, with 95% of people with a diagnosis currently accessing specialist care, of whom 88% are receiving antiretroviral therapy. Eighty six per cent of this group has an undetectable viral load—a surrogate marker of treatment success.[3]

Why diagnose the undiagnosed, and why the hurry?
The epidemiology of HIV in the UK remains marred by a stubborn undiagnosed fraction, and by a high proportion of late diagnoses.

Undiagnosed HIV infection
An estimated 22% of people living with HIV infection do not know their status (ranging from 18% in men who have sex with men to 30% in male heterosexuals).[3] Undiagnosed HIV infection contributes disproportionately to ongoing transmission, with onward infection up to 3.5 times greater in this group based on mathematical modelling and behavioural and surveillance data.[5] Knowledge of status reduces risk behaviours and allows partners to access testing.[6] Importantly, in several observational studies antiretroviral therapy has been shown to reduce transmission[7][8] and in one randomised controlled trial was definitively shown to reduce transmission from index case to partner by up to 96%.[9] Access to antiretroviral therapy is contingent on knowledge of status.

Late diagnosis of HIV infection
European consensus of late HIV diagnosis was arrived at in 2009 and defined as a CD4 count at diagnosis of <350 cells/μL.[10] It is generally agreed across international guidelines that all patients ought to have started antiretroviral therapy before their CD4 count has fallen below this threshold (although some guidelines promote starting substantially earlier). By this definition, 47% of patients in the UK in 2012 had a late diagnosis.[3] This fraction declined from 58% in 2003. Late diagnosis remains more common among older age groups (>50 years), black and minority ethnic groups, and male heterosexuals. CD4 count at diagnosis is a strong predictor of short term and long term mortality, with patients whose CD4 count is <350 cells/μL being 10 times more likely to die in the first year after diagnosis than those with CD4 counts >350 cells/μL (fig 1).[3]

Reducing the number of cases of undiagnosed and late diagnosed HIV is thus likely to yield individual and public health benefits. The main barrier to HIV treatment in the UK, and also therefore prevention, remains timely diagnosis. Broadening access to HIV testing is a key strategy.

SUMMARY POINTS

- HIV testing is the gateway to both HIV treatment and HIV prevention
- Patients with a diagnosis of HIV infection before moderate to severe immunosuppression occurs should plan for a normal life expectancy with effective access to antiretroviral therapy
- The UK HIV epidemic continues to grow and remains marred by a high proportion of cases (50%) diagnosed at a late stage in the clinical course of the infection, and a persistent undiagnosed fraction (22% of patients living with HIV are unaware of their status)
- Every clinician can, and should, offer patients an HIV test in line with national guidelines
- Primary HIV infection should be considered, and an HIV test offered to all patients with a mononucleosis-like illness
- All patients living with HIV infection should be encouraged to disclose their HIV status to other healthcare providers, especially their general practitioner

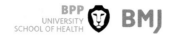

List of HIV indicator conditions

Body system/specialty	AIDS defining conditions	Other conditions where HIV testing should be routinely offered
Respiratory	Tuberculosis, pneumocystis	Bacterial pneumonia, aspergillosis
Neurology	Cerebral toxoplasmosis, primary cerebral lymphoma, cryptococcal meningitis, progressive multifocal leucoencephalopathy	Aseptic meningitis/encephalitis, cerebral abscess, space occupying lesion of unknown cause, Guillain-Barré syndrome, transverse myelitis, peripheral neuropathy, dementia, leucoencephalopathy
Dermatology	Kaposi's sarcoma	Severe or recalcitrant seborrhoeic dermatitis, severe or recalcitrant psoriasis, multidermatomal or recurrent herpes zoster
Gastroenterology	Persistent cryptosporidiosis	Oral candidiasis; oral hairy leukoplakia; chronic diarrhoea of unknown cause; weight loss of unknown cause; salmonella, shigella, or campylobacter enteritis; hepatitis B infection; hepatitis C infection
Oncology	Non-Hodgkin's lymphoma	Anal cancer or anal intraepithelial dysplasia, lung cancer, seminoma, head and neck cancer, Hodgkin's lymphoma, Castleman's disease
Gynaecology	Cervical cancer	Vaginal intraepithelial neoplasia, cervical intraepithelial neoplasia grade II or more
Haematology		Any unexplained blood dyscrasia including: thrombocytopenia, neutropenia, lymphopenia
Ophthalmology	Cytomegalovirus retinitis	Infective retinal diseases including herpesviruses and toxoplasma, any unexplained retinopathy
Ear, nose, and throat		Lymphadenopathy of unknown cause, chronic parotitis, lymphoepithelial parotid cysts
Other		Mononucleosis-like syndrome (primary HIV infection), pyrexia of unknown origin, any lymphadenopathy of unknown cause, any sexually transmitted infection

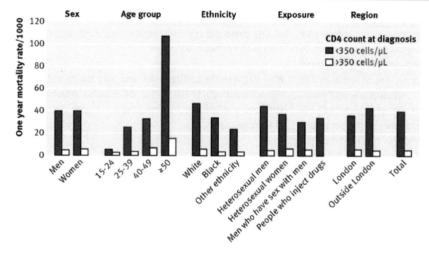

Fig 1 One year mortality (per 1000 population) by CD4 count in people with newly diagnosed HIV, 2010. Adapted from Public Health England. HIV in the United Kingdom, 2013 report[3]

Who should be tested for HIV infection in the UK?

UK national HIV testing guidelines were published in 2008 (box 1).[1] This guidance has since been ratified by the National Institute for Health and Care Excellence and by a parliamentary select committee in 2011.[11 12]

The three strata of the guidelines are designed to normalise, destigmatise, and expand HIV testing. Routine testing is recommended for all patients presenting to any healthcare service if they belong to a higher risk group, have certain medical conditions (known as HIV indicator conditions), or are accessing care in certain clinical and geographical settings (box 1 and fig 2). Routine testing means that the recommendation to test is made to all, as a matter of course.

What conditions should prompt general practitioners to consider testing for HIV?

The UK guidelines are designed to be applicable to primary care, with the recommendation of routine screening for all adults registering for or accessing care in high prevalence areas, plus targeted testing for those in higher risk groups based on demography and risk factors. Regarding diagnostic testing for indicator diseases, relatively few data are currently available on the predictive value of testing in these conditions and identifying HIV infection, but prospective studies are in progress in secondary and primary care settings. A UK retrospective case-control study of 939 cases and 2576 controls accessing primary care did identify that 12 of the 37

BOX 1 SUMMARY OF UK NATIONAL HIV TESTING GUIDELINES, 2008[1]

Who can test?

- It should be within the competence of any doctor, midwife, nurse, or trained healthcare worker to obtain consent for and to conduct an HIV test

Who should be offered a test?

- Universal HIV testing is recommended in all of the following settings:
- Genitourinary medicine or sexual health clinics
- Antenatal services
- Termination of pregnancy services
- Drug dependency programmes
- Healthcare services for those with a diagnosis of tuberculosis, hepatitis B, hepatitis C, and lymphoma
- An HIV test should be considered in the following settings where the prevalence of diagnosed HIV in the local population (primary care trust/local authority) exceeds 2/1000 population (see fig 2)
- All men and women registering in general practice
- All general medical admissions
- HIV testing should be also routinely offered and recommended to all:
- Patients presenting for healthcare where HIV, including primary HIV infection, enters the differential diagnosis (table)
- Patients with a diagnosis of a sexually transmitted infection
- Sexual partners of men and women known to be positive for antibodies to HIV
- Men who have disclosed sexual contact with other men
- Female sexual contacts of men who have sex with men
- Patients reporting a history of injecting drug use
- Men and women known to be from a country of high HIV prevalence (>1%)*
- Men and women who report sexual contact abroad or in the UK with people from countries of high HIV prevalence

*Data available at www.unaids.org

---

non-AIDS indicator conditions were significantly associated with subsequent HIV diagnosis; most strongly were bacterial pneumonia (odds ratio 47.7, 95% confidence interval 5.6 to 404.0), oral candidiasis (29.4, 6.9 to 125.5), and herpes zoster (25.4, 8.4 to 76.1).[13] Signs and symptoms most associated with HIV were weight loss (13.4, 5.0 to 36.0), pyrexia of unknown origin (7.2, 2.8 to 18.7), and diarrhoea (one or two

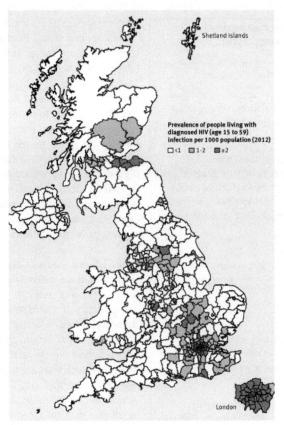

Fig 2 Routine HIV testing in high prevalence areas: prevalence of diagnosed HIV infection by area of residence in population aged 15-59 years, 2012. In areas of high prevalence of diagnosed HIV infection UK national guidelines recommend expanding HIV testing among people admitted to hospital and new registrants to general practice. In 2012, 64 of 326 (20%) local authorities had a diagnosed prevalence above the ≥2/1000 threshold. All but one of the 33 London local authorities had a prevalence above this threshold. Outside London, the five local authorities with the highest prevalence and which were above ≥2/1000 were Brighton and Hove, Salford, Manchester, Blackpool, and Luton. Adapted from Public Health England. HIV in the United Kingdom, 2013 report[3]

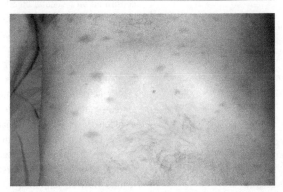

Fig 3 Maculopapular rash of primary HIV infection

consultations). Notably, 74.2% of HIV cases (n=697) presented with none of the HIV indicator conditions before diagnosis. Thus a combined testing approach is likely to be optimal. Until more data from prospective studies are available, we would recommend the routine offer of an HIV test to all such patients independent of risk factors. Knowledge of risk factors, including the taking of a sexual history may inform this process but should not influence the decision not to test. We would also strongly recommend routine HIV testing in primary care (and emergency departments and medical admissions units) in patients presenting with mononucleosis-

like illnesses, given the possibility of primary HIV infection in the differential diagnosis.

Testing in primary HIV infection

Primary HIV infection or seroconversion illness occurs in up to 80% of people with HIV infection, within 2-4 weeks of exposure to the virus. Such individuals frequently present to primary and secondary care settings with a variety of non-specific symptoms (commonly fever, rash, ulceration, myalgia, pharyngitis, and aseptic meningitis; fig 3) that may mimic other acute infections, notably infectious mononucleosis. Relatively few clinical features are specific, but the presence of oral or genital ulceration is suggestive of primary HIV infection.

Diagnosing primary HIV infection presents an important potential opportunity to make an HIV diagnosis early in the clinical course of HIV infection. On a public health level, a major proportion of new HIV infections are probably acquired from patients who are seroconverting, or have recently seroconverted, as a result of behavioural and virological factors that facilitate transmission.[14] Diagnosing primary HIV infection may help reduce onward transmission by alerting patients to their status.[15] There may also be benefit at the individual level from starting antiretroviral therapy in this context in some patients, and antiretroviral therapy may reduce onward transmission.[16]

The most important predictor of primary HIV infection being diagnosed is suspicion by the patient or clinician.[17][18] All clinicians should make a risk assessment by taking a sexual/HIV exposure history in patients presenting with mononucleosis-like syndromes. Men reporting sex with men should be considered at higher risk, in particular. A fourth generation test should be requested, which is likely to be positive for p24 antigen (a virally derived protein of early infection, the presence of which is detected by fourth generation HIV tests, see fig 4) depending on the duration of the illness. If the test result is negative and clinical suspicion is high, then a repeat test should be performed one or two weeks later. Alternatively, the patient could be referred to specialist services where testing for HIV viral load may be considered.

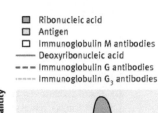

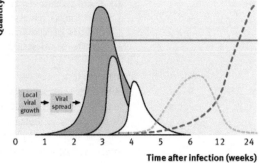

Fig 4 Typical evolution of viral and serological markers after exposure to HIV. Viral markers: RNA=ribonucleic acid; DNA=deoxyribonucleic acid; Ag=antigen. Immunological markers: IgM=immunoglobulin M antibodies; IgG=immunoglobulin G antibodies. Adapted from Murphy and Parry[19]

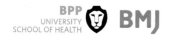

BOX 2 BASELINE INVESTIGATIONS AT FIRST SPECIALIST ASSESSMENT OF A PATIENT WITH NEWLY DIAGNOSED HIV BY CATEGORIES

HIV markers

- CD4 T cell count (absolute and percentage); HIV viral load (repeat to confirm baseline in 1-3 months); HIV genotypic drug resistance test; determination of HIV-1 subtype

Biochemistry

- Renal function (and calculated estimated glomerular filtration rate by modification of diet in renal disease); liver function tests (bilirubin, alanine transaminase, aspartate transaminase, albumin, γ-glutamyl transferase); bone profile (corrected calcium, phosphate, alkaline phosphatase)

Haematology

- Full blood count

Urinalysis

- Dipstick test for blood, protein, glucose; urine protein:creatinine ratio

Metabolic assessment

- Lipid profile and glucose (cholesterol, high density lipoprotein cholesterol:cholesterol ratio, triglycerides; repeat fasted if random measures above reference ranges)

Serology

- Syphilis; hepatitis A (total or IgG); hepatitis B surface antigen, core antibody, surface antibody; hepatitis C antibody (followed by hepatitis C RNA polymerase chain reaction if antibody detected); toxoplasma serology (if CD4 count <200 cells/μL); measles IgG; varicella IgG (unless patient gives reliable history of chickenpox or herpes zoster); rubella IgG in women of childbearing age; schistosoma serology (if >1 month spent in sub-Saharan Africa)

Tuberculosis screening

- Interferon γ releasing assay recommended to screen for latent infection (decision to screen depends on country of origin, CD4 count, and time already spent receiving antiretroviral therapy)

Stool sample

- Ova, cysts, and parasites (if from, or spent >1 month in, tropics)

Imaging

- Chest radiography not recommended routinely unless: signs and symptoms of current or previous chest disease, history of injecting drug use, risk of tuberculosis

Additional

- Sexual health screen, cervical cytology in females, cardiovascular risk assessment (for example, Joint British Societies' guidelines on cardiovascular disease; QRISK), fracture risk assessment in those aged >50

Who can test?

Any doctor, nurse, midwife, or other trained healthcare provider can offer an HIV test. A lengthy pretest discussion is not necessary. Obtaining consent from a patient for an HIV test should follow the same procedure as that for any other medical investigation. Briefly, it is essential that the patient is made aware of the benefits of accepting an HIV test, the meaning of various test results, and how they will obtain their result and from whom.

If patients decline a test, the reasons why they have made that choice should be explored to ensure that these are not due to incorrect beliefs about the virus or the consequences of testing. If concerns about insurance are a disincentive to testing, this should be challenged. The code of practice from the Association of British Insurers has clearly stated since 1994 that questions about whether anyone has ever had an HIV test or a negative test result should not be asked. Applicants should, however, declare any positive test results (as applies to any other condition).

The outcome of the pretest discussion should be recorded in the case notes. Written consent is not required. In the UK, there is no specific guidance from the General Medical Council relating to consent for infectious diseases—this was repealed in 2006. Testing for HIV should fall within generic good medical practice for obtaining consent as outlined in the GMC guidance document "Consent: patients and doctors making decisions together."

Which HIV test should be used?

Two methods are routinely used to test for HIV: a laboratory based screening assay on a blood sample obtained by venepuncture, or a rapid point of care test. The recommended laboratory based screening assay is one that tests for HIV antibody and p24 antigen simultaneously (p24 antigen is a virally derived protein detectable in the early stages of HIV infection). Such tests are termed fourth generation assays. The "window period" (the time after exposure to HIV before which the antigen or antibody can be reliably detected) is shorter than for older antibody only assays, meaning that most patients will test positive within four weeks of exposure. HIV RNA quantitative assays (viral load tests) are not recommended for screening because of the possibility of false positive results. They also offer only a marginal advantage over fourth generation assays for detecting primary infection (fig 4). Samples that are "reactive" on the screening assay will then be confirmed using a total of three independent assays. These assays should be able to distinguish between HIV-1 and HIV-2 and between HIV antibodies and antigen. A test result positive for antibodies to HIV should only be issued once the serological pattern is confirmed on a second blood sample. Indeterminate results do occur, and patients should be referred to specialist services for discussion and further testing.

Point of care tests yield a "near patient" result within 30 seconds to 30 minutes. Biological samples usually comprise capillary blood ("finger prick") or oral fluid (saliva). Most tests only detect anti-HIV antibodies, and the manufacturer stated window period is usually 6-12 weeks. All commercially available tests have reasonable specificities, but this is always lower than with fourth generation assays: screening in lower prevalence settings may reduce the positive predictive value of these tests. All reactive point of care results must be confirmed with standard serological tests.

How should patients obtain their results?

A mechanism needs to be in place for patients to obtain their results in a timely fashion, with explicit guidance for those with non-negative test results. Patients who are HIV negative could obtain their test results in several ways: telephone, email, or short message service.

For specific patient populations it may be preferable to deliver the result directly to the patient: all patients with a non-negative result, inpatients, vulnerable patients or those with mental health problems or anxiety, and patients where English is not their first language.

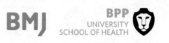

Ensuring safe governance of results

A clear mechanism must be established to ensure that all results—negative and non-negative—are appropriately acted on. This may be facilitated by working collaboratively with pathology or specialist services, but the ultimate responsibility for following up test results rests with the ordering clinician.

Ensuring appropriate transfer to care, and collaborative working with specialist services

Many successful testing ventures involve collaborative working with local specialist services (for example, sexual health/genitourinary medicine, infectious diseases, virology). Specialty services may provide training, facilitate results governance, and develop pathways to specialist care with the test provider. A clear pathway should be developed for the management of patients with reactive or positive results, perhaps involving expedited appointments with specialist physicians, nurses, or sexual health advisers. Patients may also be directed to online information resources and third sector providers.

How often should a patient be offered an HIV test?

How often patients are offered an HIV test will depend on the indication for the test. For opportunistic screening this depends on the patient's level of ongoing risk. Guidance from Public Health England and the British Association for Sexual Health and HIV recommends that men who have sex with men have an HIV test annually, and three monthly if they have sex with new and casual partners; and that black African men and women have an HIV test if they have unprotected sex with new or casual partners.[3] It may be prudent to refer patients at ongoing risk of HIV infection to sexual health services. For indicator disease based testing, a single test should be sufficient to rule out HIV infection, with the exception of testing in patients with suspected primary HIV infection where consideration needs to be given to testing outside of the window period.

Management of patients with newly diagnosed HIV

How do I deal with a "reactive" HIV test result?

The full initial assessment of a patient with newly diagnosed HIV infection is likely to be undertaken in specialist care. However, an increasing number of non-specialist primary and secondary care clinicians will deliver and manage "reactive" HIV test results and deal with the need for immediate patient education and management. It is essential that robust pathways are developed between testing venues and specialist care centres. The clinical context is clearly important, as is the original indication for the HIV test, which will dictate the urgency of referral to specialist care.

The clinician delivering the result should be able to present the following points of information to patients:

The meaning of a reactive screening test and the process of confirming the result—Patients should be advised that a reactive screening test result is a "non-negative" outcome. They should be told that false reactive results do occur and that further tests are needed to verify whether this means that they are positive for antibodies to HIV.

The clinical course of HIV infection: acquisition/ transmission, how HIV causes disease, the clinical trajectory of untreated HIV infection—Consider telling patients that HIV is a virus transmitted from human to human primarily through sexual contact or by sharing injecting equipment. Explain that the virus attacks the immune system over many years, which can leave the body vulnerable to serious infections or cancers.

Modern HIV treatment in general terms: availability of antiretroviral therapy, indications for treatment, excellent prognosis—Explain that you will refer the patient to a specialist clinic. Tell him or her that HIV remains incurable, but that excellent and safe treatments are now available that can keep them fit and well. Mention that people living with HIV today should expect to live a long and healthy life with access to treatment.

An initial assessment ought also to be made about the immediate risk of HIV infection to others:

Is a sexual partner at risk of infection?—If sexual exposure has occurred within the preceding 72 hours, consider urgent evaluation and provision of post-exposure prophylaxis if appropriate. Condom use should be discussed and strongly recommended.

Patients with reactive HIV screening test results: how do I know if this is a true positive result?

An initial non-negative screening test result is defined as a "reactive" result. A positive result can only be issued once a second confirmatory test, undertaken on a separate sample, has been obtained. Patients with a reactive screening test result should be advised of this, taking into account the risk factors and clinical context. A reactive test result in the context of a patient admitted with possible *Pneumocystis jiroveci* pneumonia clearly carries a greater value than, for example, a reactive test result in a low risk patient screened as a new registrant to general practice in a high prevalence area. The second sample will confirm or refute the diagnosis and will differentiate between HIV-1 and HIV-2 infection. Close liaison with the laboratory may be required in the context of indeterminate or non-specific results, and referral to specialist care could also be considered.

What is the best way to deliver a positive test result?

A reactive or confirmed positive test result should ideally be delivered face to face by the team or clinician who tested the patient, in a confidential environment and using clear language (aided by an interpreter if necessary). The result should not be shared with third parties unless explicit consent has been given. Small qualitative studies exploring the psychological impact and engagement in care for those with newly diagnosed HIV infection support this face to face approach.[20][21][22] Timely access to specialist multidisciplinary care (for example, sexual health advisers) is beneficial.

All patients with newly diagnosed HIV infection should be seen by a specialist HIV clinician within two weeks; sooner if they have HIV attributable symptoms or other acute needs.[1]

What happens at a first consultation with an HIV specialist?

The first consultation provides an opportunity to perform a thorough medical, psychological, and social review, to educate the patient about the clinical course and treatment of HIV, and to request the investigations that will form the basis of future monitoring of the disease.

The medical history

A detailed medical, psychological, and social history should be performed at baseline. A thorough systems review may guide the physical examination and further investigations.

Mental health problems are a risk factor for HIV infection, and depression and anxiety are common in patients living with HIV. UK guidelines recommend screening with questions such as "During the last month, have you often been bothered by feeling down, depressed, or hopeless?"[23]

A sexual history and drug use history should be undertaken to identify the risk of HIV acquisition and partners at risk. These discussions inform partner notification processes and provide an opportunity to discuss evidence based interventions to reduce transmission to susceptible partners (such as condom use, post-exposure prophylaxis, and the use of antiretroviral therapy as a prevention tool). A full sexual health screen should be performed, as sexually transmitted infections facilitate HIV transmission (and acquisition),[24] and co-infection is common. Surveillance data show that 19% of all people with newly diagnosed HIV infection in 2012 were co-diagnosed as having an acute sexually transmitted infection (29% in men who have sex with men).[3] Advice on safer sex should be revisited, and all patients must be counselled on the legal aspects of HIV transmission and disclosure, including "reckless transmission."[25]

Women living with HIV should have a gynaecological and obstetric history taken, and future requirements for pregnancy or contraception should be discussed. All women should have annual cytology, as cytological abnormalities and invasive cervical cancer are more prevalent in women living with HIV, although this is related to the degree of immunosuppression, and antiretroviral therapy is likely to reduce this risk.[26] Patients living with HIV infection, especially men who have sex with men, are also at increased risk of anal cancer, despite antiretroviral therapy.[27] Anal cytology is sensitive at detecting anal dysplasia but lacks specificity,[28] and it remains uncertain whether screening with cytology or high resolution anoscopy is cost effective.[29] UK guidelines do not currently recommend routine screening for anal cancer, but this may be revised in the light of new evidence.[23]

Physical examination

A full physical examination should be undertaken, with particular emphasis on the reticuloendothelial system, skin, and mucous membranes. The extent of examination will also be dictated by the degree of immunosuppression. For example, dilated fundoscopy should be performed in all patients with a confirmed CD4 count <50 cells/µL to exclude cytomegalovirus retinitis.

Baseline investigations

Several baseline investigations are performed (box 2).

The absolute CD4 count is the most useful single surrogate marker of HIV stage and progression.[23] In patients with untreated HIV infection, the likelihood of developing an AIDS defining condition increases exponentially as the CD4 count decreases, particularly with a count of <200 cells/µL.[10] In one study, compared with patients starting highly active antiretroviral therapy with a CD4 count of <50 cells/µL, adjusted hazard ratios for progression to AIDS or death over three years in higher CD4 count groups were 0.74 for 50-99 cells/µL, 0.52 for 100-199 cells/µL, 0.24 for 200-349 cells/µL, and 0.18 for ≥350 cells/µL.[30] Primary HIV infection is associated with a high plasma viral load.[31] This declines substantially 3-6 months after infection to a nearly steady level "set point." It is predominately used to monitor response to antiretroviral therapy. Other tests are also carried out to look for evidence of related liver, kidney, and cardiovascular disease.

Interventions in the initial assessment

Beyond a comprehensive clinical assessment and patient education on the clinical course and treatment of HIV infection, including the excellent prognosis, other things to be discussed may include initiation of partner notification; general advice on health—maintaining a healthy lifestyle, support for smoking cessation, exercise, and nutrition; the increased risk of many comorbidities; social and occupational considerations, with referral to occupational health services if indicated; and provision of immunisation.

Partner notification

Partner notification is the process of informing the sexual partners of someone with a diagnosis of a sexually transmitted infection of their risk of exposure, and of facilitating their evaluation and treatment. An individual may wish to defer disclosure to partners, and some delay may be acceptable if there is no ongoing risk. Attempts to encourage and support disclosure and testing of contacts should be revisited regularly. Some patients will already have a partner known to be HIV positive, but in many cases elicited contacts will require testing. Relatively few prospective trials have been undertaken comparing the effectiveness of different methods of partner notification about HIV, but all reported strategies have high rates of case finding.[32] A recent national audit in the UK showed that among contacts who underwent testing, 21% were subsequently diagnosed as having HIV infection[33]—this figure compares to approximately 3% in men who have sex with men attending genitourinary services[3] and strongly supports the value of partner notification in effectively detecting undiagnosed HIV infection.

Immunisation

Influenza vaccination should be provided annually, and vaccination with the 23 valent pneumococcal vaccine is recommended every 5-10 years. Those who are non-immune to hepatitis A, hepatitis B, measles, and varicella should all be vaccinated (plus rubella in women of childbearing potential). Some live vaccines are contraindicated or limited by CD4 count (see the British HIV Association immunisation guidelines[34]).

How can patients be encouraged to disclose their HIV status to other healthcare professionals?

Many patients historically have sought all of their medical care through their HIV centre. However, increasingly general practitioners are responsible for many aspects of the medical care of patients who have HIV. Most patients consent to disclosure of HIV status to their general practitioners. The benefits of increased and enhanced primary care involvement include:

- improved access to and coordination of care
- enhanced management of comorbidities and risk reduction
- experience in managing mental health problems
- experience in managing an aging population
- avoidance of drug-drug interactions
- appropriate management of unrelated medical problems.

It is important that regular, effective, two way communication between the HIV centre and primary care is established. Such communication will help establish a comprehensive list of prescribed drugs, highlight and safely manage important potential drug interactions, and recommend appropriate health screening (for example, cardiovascular disease risk assessment and cervical cytology), which takes account

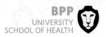
BOX 3 CURRENT INDICATIONS FOR STARTING ANTIRETROVIRAL THERAPY IN THE UK[35]

Chronic HIV infection

- Patients meeting any of the following criteria should start antiretroviral therapy:
- CD4 count <350 cells/μL
- AIDS defining illness, irrespective of CD4 count
- HIV related comorbidity, including HIV associated nephropathy, idiopathic thrombocytopenic purpura, symptomatic HIV associated neurocognitive disorders, irrespective of CD4 count
- Co-infection with hepatitis B or hepatitis C virus if the CD4 count is <500 cells/μL
- Non-AIDS defining malignancies requiring immunosuppressive chemotherapy or radiotherapy

Patients presenting with AIDS or a major bacterial infection

- Patients presenting with an AIDS defining infection or with a serious bacterial infection and CD4 count <200 cells/μL should start antiretroviral therapy within two weeks

Primary HIV infection

- Patients with primary HIV infection meeting any of the following criteria should start antiretroviral therapy
- Neurological involvement
- Any AIDS defining illness
- Confirmed CD4 count <350 cells/μL

Treatment to reduce HIV transmission

- It is recommended that the evidence showing treatment with antiretroviral therapy lowers the risk of transmission if discussed with all patients, and an assessment of the current risk of transmission to others is made at the time of this discussion. If a patient with a CD4 count >350 cells/μL then wishes to start antiretroviral therapy to reduce the risk of transmission to partners, this decision should be respected and antiretroviral therapy started

Adapted from the British HIV Association guidelines for treatment of HIV-1 positive adults with antiretroviral therapy 2012 (updated November 2013)

SOURCES AND SELECTION CRITERIA

We undertook a review of the literature using Medline, Embase, and the Cochrane database of systematic reviews using a variety of search terms relating to HIV testing, HIV epidemiology, and the management of newly diagnosed HIV infection. We also consulted national clinical guidelines from the British HIV Association, the British Association for Sexual Health and HIV, and the National Institute for Health and Care Excellence. We reviewed conference abstracts from national and international conferences in the specialty area from 2006 to the present. Where possible, we cite the highest quality strata of evidence.

QUESTIONS FOR FUTURE RESEARCH

- Can we use routine surveillance data to measure the effectiveness of wider HIV testing?
- How can we assess the effectiveness and the sustainability of routine and diagnostic testing across the breadth of settings proposed in the testing guidelines?
- What about other strategies to diagnose HIV infection, such as home testing?

of differences in protocol resulting from differences in HIV status or antiretroviral therapy.

When will my patient start antiretroviral therapy?

A full review of current indications to start antiretroviral therapy is beyond the scope of this review, but box 3 summarises the current 2012 British HIV Association guidelines.[35] Antiretroviral therapy is recommended before the CD4 count is <350 cells/μL, in all AIDS defining illnesses (irrespective of CD4 count), in the context of HIV related comorbidity (including HIV associated nephropathy, idiopathic thrombocytopenic purpura, symptomatic HIV associated neurocognitive disorders, irrespective of CD4 count) and in co-infection with hepatitis B or C virus if the CD4 count is <500 cells/μL. Antiretroviral therapy should also be recommended for non-AIDS defining malignancies requiring immunosuppressive chemotherapy or radiotherapy. Antiretroviral therapy is also indicated during primary HIV infection in specific circumstances.

Figure 3 was provided courtesy of David Hawkins and Medical Illustrations Department, Chelsea and Westminster Hospital, London, UK.

ADDITIONAL EDUCATIONAL RESOURCES

Resources for healthcare professionals

- British HIV Association HIV testing guidelines (www.bhiva. org/HIVTesting2008.aspx)—freely accessible; national guidance document
- Public Health England HIV/STI surveillance (www.hpa.org. uk/Publications/InfectiousDiseases/HIVAndSTIs/)—freely accessible; national surveillance data on HIV and sexually transmitted infections plus recommendations and policy documents, updated regularly
- National AIDS Trust prevention and testing policy documents (www.nat.org.uk/Information-and-Resources/New%20 publications.aspx#preventionandtesting)—freely accessible; advocacy and policy documents from the National AIDS Trust
- HIV in Europe, HIV indicator conditions: guidance for implementing HIV testing in adults in healthcare settings (www.hiveurope.eu/LinkClick.aspx?fileticket=b8rDoBh 8NjM=&tabid=37)—freely accessible; guidance for the implementation of routine HIV testing in indicator conditions across European healthcare settings

Resources for patients

- National AIDS Trust: information for patients (www.nat. org.uk/HIV-Facts.aspx)—freely accessible; patient centred resources on all aspects of HIV testing, prevention, and specialist care
- Terrence Higgins Trust "My HIV" resource (www.tht.org.uk/ myhiv)—freely accessible; self management and information for patients living with HIV
- Positively UK, resources for patients (http://positivelyuk. org/)—freely accessible; patient focused resources and stories for patients living with HIV, and their partners
- NHS Choices, HIV testing (www.nhs.uk/Conditions/HIV/Pages/ Diagnosispg.aspx)—freely accessible; guidance for patients on how and why to access HIV testing in the National Health Service

Contributors: MR, DA, and AKS conceived the content of the article. MR wrote the first draft of the article, and all authors reviewed it. AKS is the guarantor.

Competing interests: We have read and understood the BMJ Group policy on declaration of interests and declare the following interests: none.

Provenance and peer review: Commissioned; externally peer reviewed.

Patient consent: Obtained.

1 British HIV Association. British Association for Sexual Health and HIV (BASHH), the British HIV Association (BHIVA), and the British Infection Society (BIS) guidelines for HIV testing. 2008. www.bhiva.org/ HIVTesting2008.aspx.
2 May MT, Gompels M, Delpech V, Porter K, Orkin C, Kegg S, et al. Impact on life expectancy of HIV-1 positive individuals of CD4+ cell count and viral load response to antiretroviral therapy: UK cohort study. AIDS 2014; published online 19 Feb.
3 Health Protection Agency. HIV in the United Kingdom: 2013 report. www.hpa.org.uk/Publications/InfectiousDiseases/HIVAndSTIs/1311HIVin theUk2013report/.
4 Rice BD, Elford J, Yin Z, Delpech VC. A new method to assign country of HIV infection among heterosexuals born abroad and diagnosed with HIV. AIDS 2012;26:1961-6.
5 Phillips AN, Cambiano V, Nakagawa F, Brown AE, Lampe F, Rodger A, et al. Increased HIV incidence in men who have sex with men despite high levels of ART-induced viral suppression: analysis of an extensively documented epidemic. PLoS One 2013;8:e55312.
6 Marks G, Crepaz N, Janssen RS. Estimating sexual transmission of HIV from persons aware and unaware that they are infected with the virus in the USA. AIDS 2006;20:1447-50.
7 Reynolds SJ, Makumbi F, Nakigozi G, Kagaayi J, Gray RH, Wawer M, et al. HIV-1 transmission among HIV-1 discordant couples before and after the introduction of antiretroviral therapy. AIDS 2011;25:473-7.
8 Donnell D, Baeten JM, Kiarie J, Thomas KK, Stevens W, Cohen CR, et al. Heterosexual HIV-1 transmission after initiation of antiretroviral therapy: a prospective cohort analysis. Lancet 2010;375:2092-8.
9 Cohen MS, Smith MK, Muessig KE, Hallett TB, Powers KA, Kashuba AD. Antiretroviral treatment of HIV-1 prevents transmission of HIV-1: where do we go from here? Lancet 2013;382:1515-24.

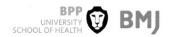

10   Antinori A, Coenen T, Costagiola D, Dedes N, Ellefson M, Gatell J, et al. Late presentation of HIV infection: a consensus definition. *HIV Med* 2011;12:61-4.

11   National Institute for Health and Care Excellence. Increasing the uptake of HIV testing among black Africans in England. (Public Health Guidance PH33.) 2011. www.nice.org.uk/guidaance/PH33.

12   National Institute for Health and Care Excellence. Increasing the uptake of HIV testing among men who have sex with men. (Public Health Guidance PH34.) 2011. http://guidance.nice.org.uk/PH34.

13   Damery S, Nichols L, Holder R, Ryan R, Wilson S, Warmington S, et al. Assessing the predictive value of HIV indicator conditions in general practice: a case-control study using the THIN database. *Br J Gen Pract* 2013;63:e370-7.

14   Pao D, Fisher M, Hué S, Dean G, Murphy G, Cane PA, et al. Transmission of HIV-1 during primary infection: relationship to sexual risk and sexually transmitted infections. *AIDS* 2005;19:85-90.

15   Fox J, White PJ, Macdonald N, Weber J, McClure M, Fidler S, et al. Reductions in HIV transmission risk behaviour following diagnosis of primary HIV infection: a cohort of high-risk men who have sex with men. *HIV Med* 2009;10:432-8.

16   SPARTAC Trial Investigators, Fidler S, Porter K, Ewings F, Frater J, Ramjee G, et al. Short-course antiretroviral therapy in primary HIV infection. *N Engl J Med* 2013;368:207-17.

17   Sudarshi D, Pao D, Murphy G, Parry J, Dean G, Fisher M. Missed opportunities for diagnosing primary HIV infection. *Sex Transm Infect* 2008;84:14-6.

18   Sharrocks K, Jones CB, Naftalin C, Darling D, Fisher M, Fidler S, et al. Missed opportunities for identifying primary HIV within genitourinary medical/HIV services. *Int J STD AIDS* 2012;23:540-3.

19   Murphy G, Parry JV. Assays for the detection of recent infections with human immunodeficiency virus type 1. *Euro Surveill* 2008;13:pii:18966.

20   Hult JR, Maurer SA, Moskowitz JT. "I'm sorry, you're positive": a qualitative study of individual experiences of testing positive for HIV. *AIDS Care* 2009;21:185-8.

21   Myers T, Worthington C, Aguinaldo JP, Haubrich DJ, Ryder K, Rawson B. Impact on HIV test providers of giving a positive test result. *AIDS Care* 2007;19:1013-9.

22   Anderson M, Elam G, Gerver S, Solarin I, Fenton K, Easterbrook P. "It took a piece of me": initial responses to a positive HIV diagnosis by Caribbean people in the UK. *AIDS Care* 2010;22:1493-8.

23   Asboe D, Aitken C, Boffito M, Booth C, Cane P, Fakoya A, et al. British HIV Association guidelines for the routine investigation and monitoring of adult HIV-1-infected individuals 2011. *HIV Med* 2012;13:1-44.

24   Fleming DT, Wasserheit JN. From epidemiological synergy to public health policy and practice: the contribution of other sexually transmitted diseases to sexual transmission of HIV infection. *Sex Transm Infect* 1999;75:3-17.

25   British HIV Association. HIV transmission, the law and the work of the clinical team. January 2013. www.bhiva.org/Reckless-HIV-Transmission-2013.aspx.

26   Moore AL, Sabin CA, Madge S, Mocroft A, Reid W, Johnson MA. Highly active antiretroviral therapy and cervical intraepithelial neoplasia. *AIDS* 2002;16:927-9.

27   Piketty C, Selinger-Leneman H, Grabar S, Duvivier C, Bonmarchand M, Abramowitz L, et al. Marked increase in the incidence of invasive anal cancer among HIV-infected patients despite treatment with combination antiretroviral therapy. *AIDS* 2008;22:1203-11.

28   Berry JM, Palefsky JM, Jay N, Cheng S-C, Darragh TM, Chin-Hong PV. Performance characteristics of anal cytology and human papillomavirus testing in patients with high-resolution anoscopy-guided biopsy of high-grade anal intraepithelial neoplasia. *Dis Colon Rectum* 2009;52:239-47.

29   Czoski-Murray C, Karnon J, Jones R, Smith K. Cost-effectiveness of screening high-risk HIV-positive men who have sex with men (MSM) and HIV-positive women for anal cancer. *Health Tech Assess* 2010;14:iii-iv, ix-x, 1-101.

30   Egger M. Prognostic importance of initial response in HIV-1 infected patients starting potent antiretroviral therapy: analysis of prospective studies. *Lancet* 2003;362:679-86.

31   Sabin CA, Devereux H, Phillips AN, Hill A, Janossy G, Lee CA, et al. Course of viral load throughout HIV-1 infection. *J Acquir Immune Defic Syndr* 2000;23:172-7.

32   Ferreira A, Young T, Mathews C, Zunza M, Low N. Strategies for partner notification for sexually transmitted infections, including HIV. *Cochrane Database Syst Rev* 2013;10:CD002843.

33   British HIV Association, British Association for Sexual Health and HIV. Joint National Audit of the British HIV Association and the British Society for Sexual Health and HIV, 2013. HIV partner notification processes and outcomes. www.bhiva.org/documents/ClinicalAudit/FindingsandReports/PNsummaryResultsWeb.pptx.

34   Geretti AM, BHIVA Immunization Writing Committee, Brook G, Cameron C, Chadwick D, Heyderman RS, et al. British HIV Association guidelines for immunization of HIV-infected adults 2008. *HIV Med* 2008;9.795-848.

35   Williams I, Churchill D, Anderson J, Boffito M, Bower M, Cairns G, et al. British HIV Association guidelines for the treatment of HIV-1-positive adults with antiretroviral therapy 2012. *HIV Med* 2012;13(Suppl 2):1-85.

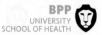

HIV infection, antiretroviral treatment, ageing, and non-AIDS related morbidity

Steven G Deeks, professor of medicine[1], Andrew N Phillips, professor of epidemiology[2]

[1]Positive Health Program, San Francisco General Hospital, University of California, San Francisco, CA 94131, USA

[2]HIV Epidemiology and Biostatistics Group, Department of Primary Care and Population Sciences, and Royal Free Centre for HIV Medicine, Royal Free and University College Medical School, University College London, London NW3 2PF

Correspondence to: S G Deeks, 995 Potero Avenue, San Francisco, CA 94110, USA sdeeks@php.ucsf.edu

Cite this as: BMJ 2009;338:a3172

DOI: 10.1136/bmj.a3172

http://www.bmj.com/content/338/bmj.a3172

More than 25 antiretroviral drugs from six therapeutic classes are now available for the management of HIV infection (box 1). Most patients who take medication achieve durable and perhaps lifelong viral suppression, so the classic AIDS related conditions are becoming less common. However, treated patients do not have completely restored health. Compared with people without HIV infection, patients with the infection who are treated with antiretrovirals have increased risk for several "non-AIDS" complications, many of which are commonly associated with ageing (box 2). This risk is particularly evident in patients whose CD4+ T cell counts are below normal during long term treatment, but it is also seen to some extent in those with higher CD4+ T cell counts. As a consequence of the changing spectrum of HIV associated disease, the medical management of HIV infection is evolving—a lower proportion of time is now spent managing drug resistance and short term toxicities and a higher proportion is spent managing these premature age associated complications. This review discusses the evidence that the major complications of "treated" HIV disease—including cardiovascular disease, malignancy, renal disease, liver disease, bone disease, and perhaps neurological complications, which are phenomena of the normal ageing process—occur at an earlier age in the HIV infected population. The implications for clinical management are also discussed.

Untreated HIV infection increases the risk of non-AIDS related events

Overall mortality in HIV infected people dropped dramatically when combination treatment was introduced. This decline was largely due to the prevention of AIDS related events, but was also due to a decrease in non-AIDS associated events and deaths.[1] [2] In a 5472 patient study of continuous treatment versus intermittent treatment (the SMART study), people who interrupted treatment when CD4+ T cell counts were over 350 cells ×10⁶/l and restarted it when they fell below 250 cells ×10⁶/l had a higher risk of dying than those who were treated continuously. Much of the benefit of antiretroviral therapy resulted from the prevention of events not previously thought to be HIV related, including myocardial infarction, cancer, renal failure, and liver disease.[2] The importance of this study cannot be overstated—it showed that HIV disease is associated with higher risk of several non-AIDS complications (including cardiovascular disease, renal disease, and liver disease) and that antiretroviral therapy reduces the risks of these events.

Can antiretroviral treatment fully restore health in most patients?

Although effective antiretroviral treatment prevents AIDS and non-AIDS related morbidity and mortality, treatment does not fully restore health. In a population based cohort study that included all HIV infected patients in Denmark and a larger number of matched non-HIV infected controls, overall life expectancy for those with HIV increased dramatically after the introduction of combination antiretroviral treatment but was lower than that in the uninfected population.[3] Similar findings were reported in a more recent study of 14 distinct cohorts.[4] In the French population, mortality in HIV infected patients approached that in uninfected patients only if treatment could durably increase peripheral CD4+ T cell counts into the normal range.[5] All these studies had limitations (limited follow-up, inability to control for all confounding variables), but the consistency of the findings are hard to ignore.

Low CD4+ T cell counts during treatment predict non-AIDS events

Further evidence that treatment often fails to restore health completely comes from studies showing that the peripheral CD4+ T cell count during long term antiretroviral treatment is a consistent predictor of non-AIDS related events. For example, among long term treated patients followed in the FIRST study, a lower CD4+ T cell count on treatment was associated with a higher immediate risk of cardiovascular disease, renal disease, liver disease, and cancer.[6] Non-AIDS events were more common than AIDS events in treated patients whose CD4+ T cell count was greater than 200 cells ×10⁶/l. The implications of this study and others are clear—even patients treated successfully are at risk for significant morbidity and mortality if their peripheral blood CD4+ T cell count is below normal.

How effective is antiretroviral therapy in restoring normal CD4+ T cell counts?

Once effective therapy is started, the peripheral CD4+ T cell count increases by about 50 cells ×10⁶/l over the first three months of treatment and then by 50-100 cells ×10⁶/l year until the cell count is normal (most studies define this as 500 cells ×10⁶/l, even though the average count in HIV uninfected people is often higher). Most effectively treated patients will eventually achieve a normal CD4+ T cell count, although it can take several years to achieve this outcome in those who delay treatment until their CD4+ T cell count is very low. One recent multicentre study found that about a third of patients who started treatment with a CD4+ cell

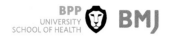

BOX 1 ANTIRETROVIRAL DRUGS CURRENTLY AVAILABLE

Nucleoside and nucleotide analogues

- Abacavir
- Didanosine
- Emtricitabine
- Lamivudine
- Stavudine
- Tenofovir
- Zidovudine

Non-nucleoside reverse transcriptase inhibitors

- Delavirdine
- Efavirenz
- Etravirine
- Nevirapine

Protease inhibitors

- Atazanavir
- Darunavir
- Fosamprenavir
- Indinavir
- Lopinavir
- Nelfinavir
- Ritonavir
- Saquinavir
- Tipranavir

CCR5 antagonists

- Maraviroc

Integrase inhibitors

- Raltegravir

BOX 2 NON-AIDS RELATED COMPLICATIONS THAT MAY BE MORE COMMON PATIENTS WITH HIV

- Hypertension
- Diabetes mellitus and insulin resistance
- Cardiovascular disease
- Pulmonary hypertension
- Cancer
- Osteopenia and osteoporosis
- Liver failure
- Kidney failure
- Peripheral neuropathy
- Frailty
- Cognitive decline and dementia

count below 200 cells ×10⁶/l failed to achieve a normal count after up to 10 years of otherwise effective treatment.[7]

Which non-AIDS related diseases are affected?

Cardiovascular disease

Much attention is turning to cardiovascular diseases because patients treated with antiretroviral drugs now live longer and have to deal with the complications of ageing. Also, HIV infected adults generally have higher rates of certain cardiovascular risk factors (such as smoking) and other comorbid conditions than non-infected people. Nevertheless, HIV disease and antiretroviral treatment seem to be causally associated with early heart disease, even after controlling for age and traditional cardiovascular risk factors.

Although the epidemiology and pathogenesis of HIV associated cardiovascular disease are complex and controversial, two consistent trends have emerged. Firstly, the risk of cardiovascular events is higher in untreated than treated HIV infection, probably because inflammation is increased in untreated infection.[8] Secondly, some antiretroviral drugs have direct effects on cardiovascular disease. For example, prolonged exposure to protease inhibitors is associated with hyperlipidaemia, insulin resistance, and a higher rate of cardiovascular disease events.[9] Abacavir—a commonly used nucleoside analogue—seems to increase the risk of heart disease,[10] perhaps because of its proinflammatory effect. The beneficial effects of treatment overwhelm its potential negative effects, however.

An important question remains—does the negative effect of HIV disease on the cardiovascular system persist during effective treatment, even if drugs that have no known cardiovascular toxicity are used? Several cohort studies have suggested that this is the case, but they could not fully account for drug toxicity or for the presence of traditional risk factors (particularly smoking). Perhaps the strongest evidence for a persistent effect of HIV disease is the consistent link between a lower CD4+ T cell count (on treatment) and a higher risk of cardiovascular disease. Given the strong and consistent association between inflammation and suboptimal CD4+ T cell gains,[11] persistent proatherogenic inflammation during treatment may be the main cause of suboptimal CD4+ T cell gains and early heart disease.

Cancer

The advanced immunodeficiency associated with untreated HIV infection greatly increases the risk of Kaposi's sarcoma and non-Hodgkin's lymphoma. HIV infected patients also have an increased risk of other cancers—including lung cancer, skin cancer, colorectal cancer, prostate cancer, and anal cancer—which is unlikely to be entirely the result of a higher prevalence of smoking and other confounding factors.[12]

The higher rate of cancer in patients with treated HIV infection is probably partly caused by persistent immunodeficiency. In a large cohort of treated patients, a low CD4+ T cell count was strongly associated with a higher risk of developing a non-AIDS associated cancer.[13] Transplant patients have comparable risks to those with HIV, which supports the idea that long term immunosuppression is causally associated with cancer in HIV infected patients.

Liver and renal disease

Liver disease is common in HIV infected adults, partly because of high rates of chronic viral hepatitis and alcohol misuse, as well as long term exposure to potentially hepatoxic antiretroviral drugs. HIV infection is also probably harmful. In the SMART study, people who interrupted (or delayed) treatment were more likely to develop liver failure than those who did not.[2] Although antiretroviral therapy is probably protective in HIV disease, it does not seem completely to reverse any persistent harm. In one cohort, treated patients with a low CD4+T cell count had a much higher risk of dying from liver disease.[14]

The link between HIV disease, antiretroviral treatment, and renal disease is complex. Compared with a matched population of HIV uninfected US veterans, infected people are more likely to develop chronic kidney failure. This difference was seen in black but not white people and persisted after controlling for traditional risk factors.[15] Similarly, HIV infected people have higher levels of cystatin C (a measure of glomerular filtration rates) and mircoalbuminuria than well matched HIV uninfected adults.[16] The SMART study

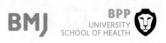

found that patients on intermittent treatment had a non-significantly higher risk of kidney failure than those on continuous treatment.[2] Thus, untreated HIV infection seems to cause kidney dysfunction through an unknown mechanism, in addition to directly causing nephropathy. It is still unclear whether renal function continues to deteriorate once a patient is on effective treatment.

Other diseases

Most research has focused on non-AIDS events that are easy to observe and adjudicate in observational settings (such as myocardial infarction, cancer, kidney failure, and liver failure). Emerging data suggest that other diseases, including pulmonary artery hypertension[17] and bone disease,[18] are more common in HIV infected patients than in age matched uninfected people. There is also a concern that HIV associated neurological disease persists or even progresses during otherwise effective long term combination treatment.[19] It has also been suggested that "frailty" is higher in HIV infected people than in uninfected ones.[20]

The effect of untreated and treated HIV infection on gastrointestinal function is the focus of intense investigation. Acute HIV infection has a dramatic effect on the mucosal lining of the gastrointestinal tract—CD4+ T cells are rapidly and possibly irreversibly lost. The loss of mucosal integrity results in chronic translocation of microbial products into the systemic circulation; this may contribute to the persistent inflammation and non-AIDS related morbidity that occurs in untreated, and to a lesser extent, treated HIV infection.[21] Whether these changes to the gastrointestinal mucosa contribute to gastrointestinal disease is unclear.

Immunological ageing

The immune system has persistent defects even after years of treatment mediated viral suppression. Many are similar to those seen in normal ageing, but they occur at an earlier age than normal.[22] Persistent abnormalities include low CD4:CD8 ratio, low naive:memory cell ratio, expansion of CD28− effector T cells, reduced T cell repertoire, and reduced responsiveness to vaccines. Most of these abnormalities are seen only in patients who start treatment in late stage disease (CD4 nadir <200 cells ×10⁶/l). The link between accelerated immunological ageing and age associated complications is not known.

Why are treated patients still at risk for premature morbidity and mortality?

The data tell a consistent story—antiretroviral treated patients remain at risk for premature morbidity and mortality compared with HIV uninfected patients. The mechanism for this risk is almost certainly multifactorial. For example, HIV infected patients often have several other chronic comorbid conditions that may contribute to the increased risk of severe non-AIDS morbidity. In a large study comparing HIV infected veterans with sex and age matched uninfected veterans, those with HIV disease were more likely to have comorbid conditions such as liver disease, kidney disease, substance misuse, and multimorbidity.[23] Hypertension, diabetes, and dyslipidaemia are also more common in HIV infected people.[24] The heightened risk for age associated diseases is also the result of residual immunodeficiency and inflammation, as shown by the prognostic value of the CD4+ T cell count and

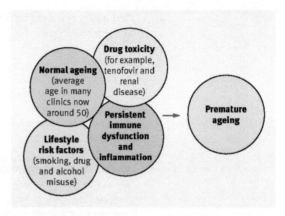

In treated patients who achieve durable suppression of the HIV virus, natural ageing, drug specific toxicity, lifestyle factors, persistent inflammation, and perhaps residual immunodeficiency are causally associated with premature development of many complications normally associated with ageing, including cardiovascular disease, cancer, and osteoporosis or osteopenia

other immunological markers in treated patients (figure).[8] Finally, antiretroviral drug toxicity also contributes to this risk.

What are the clinical implications?

The success of antiretroviral treatment means that HIV infected people live longer and must deal with a series of age related diseases. It may be unrealistic to expect treated patients to achieve a normal lifespan free of any premature disease, and further management considerations are important.

Firstly, high CD4+ T cell counts consistently reduce the risk of non-AIDS associated morbidity and mortality, so most guidelines now recommend treatment before CD4+ T cell counts fall below 350 cells ×10⁶/l. A trial of the risks and benefits of starting treatment in people with a CD4+ T cell count above 500 ×10⁶/l, rather than deferring until the count is 350 cells ×10⁶/l, is ongoing.

Secondly, HIV infected people may be disproportionately affected by the complications of ageing, so look for these diseases in patients presenting with symptoms of cardiovascular disease, cerebral vascular events, and cancer.

Thirdly, HIV is an independent risk factor for cardiovascular disease, so aggressive preventive care should be considered in all infected patients. Given the complex nature of HIV and cardiovascular disease, several focused guidelines have been published.[25]

Fourthly, because of the increased risk of cancer, aggressive screening should be considered. One expert panel recommends aggressive screening for anal and cervical cancer, while others argue for earlier implementation of screening colonoscopy.

Fifthly, many antiretroviral drugs have complex pharmacological interactions. Because polypharmacy is common in HIV infected patients (and will become more so as patients age), they need access to a clinical pharmacologist with expertise in the management of HIV. Interactive web based resources are available for clinicians (additional educational resources box).

Finally, some of the more difficult to diagnose complications of ageing—including osteopenia, frailty, and declining mental acuity—may be more prevalent in HIV infected patients than in uninfected people. This might

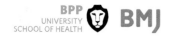

affect quality of life and the ability to work, even if obvious disease is not present.

Conclusion

The care of patients with HIV will probably become more complex as patients grow older and confront unique challenges. Cardiologists, oncologists, gastroenterologists, endocrinologists, geriatricians, and other specialists will be increasingly called on to help manage this complex disease.

SOURCES AND SELECTION CRITERIA

We searched Medline for terms related to HIV and age associated conditions, including "ag(e)ing", "cancer", "cardiovascular disease", "frailty", and "guidelines". We also considered presentations made at international conferences in 2007 and 2008. Given the nature of the questions at hand, we relied primarily on observational data generated from established ongoing cohort studies. One large randomised clinical trial (SMART) was highly informative, however, and was the basis for much of the discussion.

ADDITIONAL EDUCATIONAL RESOURCES

Resources for healthcare professionals

- US Department of Health and Human Services (http://aidsinfo.nih.gov/contentfiles/AdultandAdolescentGL.pdf)—Guideline on the use of antiretroviral drugs in HIV-1 infected adults and adolescents

- US Department of Health and Human Services (www.aidsinfo.nih.gov/contentfiles/Adult_OI.pdf)—Guidelines on the prevention and treatment of opportunistic infections

- World Health Organization (www.who.int/hiv/pub/guidelines/adult/en/index.html)—Antiretroviral therapy for HIV infection in adults and adolescents

- British HIV Association (www.bhiva.org/cms1191541.aspx)—Treatment of HIV-1 infection with antiretroviral drugs

- British HIV Association (www.bhiva.org/cms1221367.asp)—HIV associated malignancies

- Drug-drug interactions (www.hivinsite.org/InSite?page=ar-00-02; www.drug-interactions.com)—Databases outlining multiple possible drug interactions with HIV associated drugs

Resources for patients

- The Body (www.thebody.com)—Comprehensive website that covers emerging concerns for patients living with HIV

- Project Inform (www.projectinform.org)—Comprehensive website aimed at patient education and patient advocacy

- HIV Insite (www.hivinsite.org)—Extensive information on HIV and AIDS treatment, prevention, and policy from the University of California San Francisco

---

Contributors: SGD did the review, drafted the manuscript, and finalised the manuscript. ANP contributed to intellectual content, worked on revising the content, and approved the final version.

Competing interests: None declared.

Provenance and peer review: Commissioned; externally peer reviewed.

1 Mocroft A, Brettle R, Kirk O, Blaxhult A, Parkin JM, Antunes F, et al. Changes in the cause of death among HIV positive subjects across Europe: results from the EuroSIDA study. *AIDS* 2002;16:1663-71.

2 El-Sadr WM, Lundgren JD, Neaton JD, Gordin F, Abrams D, Arduino RC, et al. CD4+ count-guided interruption of antiretroviral treatment. *N Engl J Med* 2006;355:2283-96.

3 Lohse N, Hansen AB, Pedersen G, Kronborg G, Gerstoft J, Sorensen HT, et al. Survival of persons with and without HIV infection in Denmark, 1995-2005. *Ann Intern Med* 2007;146:87-95.

4 The Antiretroviral Therapy Cohort Collaboration. Life expectancy of individuals on combination antiretroviral therapy in high-income countries: a collaborative analysis of 14 cohort studies. *Lancet* 2008;372:293-9.

5 Lewden C, Chene G, Morlat P, Raf Filig F, Dupon M, Dellamonica P, et al. HIV-infected adults with a CD4 cell count greater than 500 cells/mm³on long-term combination antiretroviral therapy reach same mortality rates as the general population. *J Acquir Immune Defic Syndr* 2007;46:72-7.

6 Baker JV, Peng G, Rapkin J, Abrams DI, Silverberg MJ, MacArthur RD, et al. CD4+ count and risk of non-AIDS diseases following initial treatment for HIV infection. *AIDS* 2008;22:841-8.

7 Kelly CF, Kitchen CM, Hunt PW, Rodriguez B, Hecht FM, Kitahata M, et al. Incomplete peripheral CD4+ cell count restoration among long-term antiretroviral treated HIV infected patients. *Clin Infect Dis* (in press).

8 Kuller LH, Tracy R, Belloso W, De Wit S, Drummond F, Lane HC, et al. Inflammatory and coagulation biomarkers and mortality in patients with HIV infection. *PLoS Med* 2008;5:e203.

9 Friis-Moller N, Reiss P, Sabin CA, Weber R, Monforte A, El-Sadr W, et al. Class of antiretroviral drugs and the risk of myocardial infarction. *N Engl J Med* 2007;356:1723-35.

10 Sabin CA, Worm SW, Weber R, Reiss P, El-Sadr W, Dabis F, et al. Use of nucleoside reverse transcriptase inhibitors and risk of myocardial infarction in HIV-infected patients enrolled in the D:A:D study: a multi-cohort collaboration. *Lancet* 2008;371:1417-26.

11 Hunt PW, Martin JN, Sinclair E, Bredt B, Hagos E, Lampiris H, et al. T cell activation is associated with lower CD4+ T cell gains in human immunodeficiency virus-infected patients with sustained viral suppression during antiretroviral therapy. *J Infect Dis* 2003;187:1534-43.

12 Kirk GD, Merlo C, O'Driscoll P, Mehta SH, Galai N, Vlahov D, et al. HIV infection is associated with an increased risk for lung cancer, independent of smoking. *Clin Infect Dis* 2007;45:103-10.

13 Monforte A, Abrams D, Pradier C, Weber R, Reiss P, Bonnet F, et al. HIV-induced immunodeficiency and mortality from AIDS-defining and non-AIDS-defining malignancies. *AIDS* 2008;22:2143-53.

14 Weber R, Sabin CA, Friis-Moller N, Reiss P, El-Sadr WM, Kirk O, et al. Liver-related deaths in persons infected with the human immunodeficiency virus: the D:A:D study. *Arch Intern Med* 2006;166:1632-41.

15 Choi AI, Rodriguez RA, Bacchetti P, Bertenthal D, Volberding PA, O'Hare AM. Racial differences in end-stage renal disease rates in HIV infection versus diabetes. *J Am Soc Nephrol* 2007;18:2968-74.

16 Odden MC, Scherzer R, Bacchetti P, Szczech LA, Sidney S, Grunfeld C, et al. Cystatin C level as a marker of kidney function in human immunodeficiency virus infection: the FRAM study. *Arch Intern Med* 2007;167:2213-9.

17 Hsue PY, Deeks SG, Farah HH, Palav S, Ahmed SY, Schnell A, et al. Role of HIV and human herpesvirus-8 infection in pulmonary arterial hypertension. *AIDS* 2008;22:825-33.

18 Arnsten JH, Freeman R, Howard AA, Floris-Moore M, Lo Y, Klein RS. Decreased bone mineral density and increased fracture risk in aging men with or at risk for HIV infection. *AIDS* 2007;21:617-23.

19 McCutchan JA, Wu JW, Robertson K, Koletar SL, Ellis RJ, Cohn S, et al. HIV suppression by HAART preserves cognitive function in advanced, immune-reconstituted AIDS patients. *AIDS* 2007;21:1109-17.

20 Desquilbet L, Jacobson LP, Fried LP, Phair JP, Jamieson BD, Holloway M, et al. HIV-1 infection is associated with an earlier occurrence of a phenotype related to frailty. *J Gerontol A Biol Sci Med Sci* 2007;62:1279-86.

21 Brenchley JM, Price DA, Schacker TW, Asher TE, Silvestri G, Rao S, et al. Microbial translocation is a cause of systemic immune activation in chronic HIV infection. *Nat Med* 2006;12:1365-71.

22 Appay V, Rowland-Jones SL. Premature ageing of the immune system: the cause of AIDS? *Trends Immunol* 2002;23:580-5.

23 Goulet JL, Fultz SL, Rimland D, Butt A, Gibert C, Rodriguez-Barradas M, et al. Aging and infectious diseases: do patterns of comorbidity vary by HIV status, age, and HIV severity? *Clin Infect Dis* 2007;45:1593-601.

24 Triant VA, Lee H, Hadigan C, Grinspoon SK. Increased acute myocardial infarction rates and cardiovascular risk factors among patients with HIV disease. *J Clin Endocrinol Metab* 2007;92:2506-12.

25 Hsue PY, Squires K, Bolger AF, Capili B, Mensah GA, Temesgen Z, et al. Screening and assessment of coronary heart disease in HIV-infected patients. *Circulation* 2008;118:e41-7.

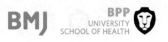

Ebola virus disease

Nicholas J Beeching, senior lecturer (honorary consultant)[1][2], Manuel Fenech, specialist trainee in infectious diseases[2], Catherine F Houlihan, clinical research fellow[3]

[1]Liverpool School of Tropical Medicine, Royal Liverpool University Hospital, Liverpool, UK

[2]Royal Liverpool University Hospital, Liverpool, UK

[3]London School of Hygiene and Tropical Medicine, London, UK

Correspondence to: N J Beeching
nicholas.beeching@rlbuht.nhs.uk

Cite this as: BMJ 2014;349:g7348

DOI: 10.1136/bmj.g7348

http://www.bmj.com/content/349/bmj.g7348

This clinical review has been developed for *The BMJ* in collaboration with BMJ Best Practice, based on a regularly updated web/mobile topic that supports evidence-based decision making at the point of care. To view the complete and current version, please refer to the Ebola virus infection topic on the BMJ Best Practice website.

Ebola virus disease is a severe, often fatal, zoonotic filovirus infection (fig 1). There are five species: *Zaire ebolavirus*, *Sudan ebolavirus*, *Taï Forest ebolavirus*, *Bundibugyo ebolavirus*, and *Reston ebolavirus*.[1]

Zaire ebolavirus is responsible for the current outbreak in west Africa, the largest outbreak since the virus was discovered in 1976 (fig 2).

Transmission occurs by close contact with body fluids of infected patients. The incubation period after infection is usually 5-9 days, with a range of 1-21 days in 95% or more of patients,[2][3] and patients are not considered infectious until they develop symptoms. The initial presentation is non-specific, which makes early clinical diagnosis difficult. Human infection carries a high case fatality rate depending on the species of Ebola virus and quality of supportive care available.[4][5]

Ebola virus infection (formerly Ebola haemorrhagic fever) is part of a group of diseases known as viral haemorrhagic fevers.[6]

What causes it?

The virus is thought to be initially acquired by exposure to body fluids or tissue from infected animals, such as bats and non-human primates; however, the natural reservoir and mode of transmission to humans has not been confirmed.[7][8] Laboratory testing of reservoir competence shows that successful infection is possible in bats and rodents, but not in plants or arthropods.[9][10][11][12] Animal to human transmission may occur during hunting and consumption of the reservoir species or infected non-human primates. The practice of butchering or eating bush meat or food contaminated with bat faeces (three species of tree roosting bats have been implicated as a reservoir) is also thought to contribute.

Human to human transmission occurs through contact with body fluids from infected patients.[13] In early epidemics, the re-use of non-sterile injections was responsible for many healthcare associated transmissions.[14] However, although this remains a risk, most cases result from close physical contact or contact with body fluids (such as sweat, blood, faeces, vomit, saliva, genital secretions, urine, and breast milk) of infected patients. In a study of viral shedding in various body fluids, Ebola virus was isolated from saliva, breast milk, stool, tears, and semen up to 40 days after the onset of illness,[15][16][17] confirming the possibility of delayed sexual transmission. Virus may be found in urine during recovery, and the duration of this phenomenon needs further study.[18]

Infection through inhalation is possible in non-human primates, but there is no evidence for airborne transmission in humans.[19]

Outside endemic areas, Ebola virus infection is rare and is usually imported.[20] Travellers from affected areas, and laboratory scientists and others working with potentially infected materials and animals, are at high risk.

What is the pathophysiology of this infection

Although there have been major advances in elucidating the pathogenesis of Ebola virus infection, most of the studies were performed in non-human primate and rodent models.[8] This is because of the difficulties in conducting human studies in poorly resourced settings where these infections naturally occur.

The virus genome consists of a single 19 kb strand of negative sense RNA with seven viral genes that are transcribed by the viral RNA dependent RNA polymerase present in the virion. The single strand of RNA is covered by helically arranged viral nucleoproteins NP and VP30, which are linked by matrix proteins VP24 and VP4 to the lipid bilayer that coats the virion.[21]

Tissue invasion occurs through infected fluid coming into contact with breaks in the mucosa or skin. This can occur with animal to human or human to human transmission. Monocytes, macrophages, and dendritic cells are the preferred replication sites for filoviruses on initial infection. Infected cells migrate to the regional lymph nodes, liver, and spleen, thereby disseminating the infection. Ebola virus has a wide cell tropism and can infect a variety of cell types.[8][21] It also has the remarkable ability to modulate the expression of genes involved in the host immune response, causing lymphocyte apoptosis and attenuation of the protective effects of interferon.[22][23]

The host immune response is crucial and dictates the outcome of infection. Progression to severe disease occurs when the virus triggers expression of a host of pro-inflammatory cytokines, including interferons; interleukins (ILs) such as IL-2, IL-6, IL-8, and IL-10; interferon inducible protein; and tumour necrosis factor α (TNF-α).[8][21][24] This causes endothelial activation and reduced vascular integrity, release of tissue factor (with associated onset of coagulopathy), and increased nitric oxide levels (with associated hypotension).[25] Thrombocytopenia is most commonly caused by loss of platelets from damaged tissue or more generalised virus induced disseminated intravascular coagulation, where

THE BOTTOM LINE

- Ebola virus disease is a severe, often fatal, zoonotic infection caused by a virus of the Filoviridae family (genus *Ebolavirus*)
- Human to human transmission occurs through contact with body fluids from infected patients. The incubation period after infection is 1-21 days and patients are not considered infectious until they develop symptoms
- Initial stages of infection are non-specific, which makes the differential diagnosis broad. A history of exposure and clinical suspicion of infection should prompt isolation
- Management is currently focused on supportive care and infection control. Healthcare workers should familiarise themselves with local guidance
- Case fatality rates range from 30% to 90%
- Because of the high likelihood of infected people travelling, all countries should have tested and practised protocols ready for screening and managing patients

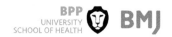
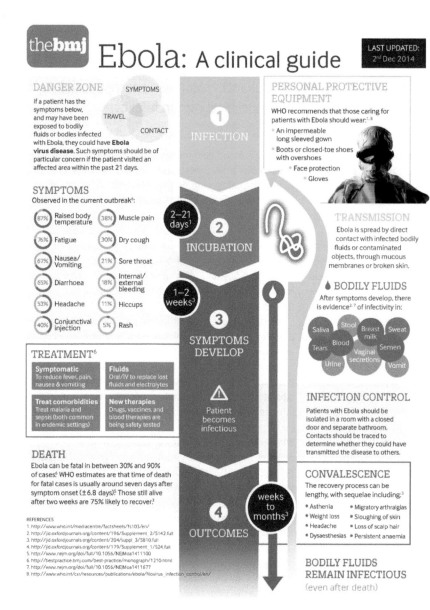

Fig 1 Infographic on Ebola virus disease

Fig 2 Map of Ebola virus outbreaks 1976-2014 (Centers for Disease Control and Prevention)

Early diagnosis hinges on identifying patients who are at risk. Case definitions developed by WHO and the US Centers for Disease Control and Prevention (CDC) are based on a history of exposure and clinical evidence of illness (for example, fever, headache, and myalgia). In the current epidemic areas, history of exposure is now less useful.

Screening ensures the quick identification of potential cases that need immediate isolation and investigation. People who are asymptomatic and have epidemiological risk factors may need to be monitored (for example, twice daily temperature readings) for the duration of the incubation period, depending on their risk of exposure. This ensures rapid recognition of symptoms and immediate isolation.

Contacts

Contacts of infected patients (including healthcare workers and household contacts) are at risk of infection if they were exposed to the patient's body fluids without protective equipment within the past 21 days.[2] [3] Brief interactions, such as walking past a person or moving through a hospital, do not constitute close contact.

Epidemiological risk factors are divided into high risk, some risk, low (but not zero) risk, and no identifiable risk categories.

A contact is defined by WHO as someone who has slept in the same household as a patient; had direct physical contact with the patient during the illness or at the funeral; touched the patient's body fluids, clothes, or bed linens during the illness; or been breast fed by the patient (babies).[27]

What infection prevention and control measures are used?
Boxes 1 and 2 list infection prevention and control measures for healthcare workers and people living in affected areas. If infection is suspected on the basis of initial screening, immediate isolation is warranted before any further investigations. This is crucial to reduce contact with other patients and healthcare workers while the patient is being investigated. Isolation measures should be continued until the patient has tested negative.[28]

coagulation factors are depleted.[26] Disseminated intravascular coagulation, along with acute hepatic impairment, predisposes the patient to bleeding complications. Other complications of severe disease include acute kidney injury, hepatitis, and pancreatitis.[21] An early antibody response, along with reduced lymphocyte depletion, is associated with effective viral clearance and survival.[16]

The development of shock is still not well understood. Many factors may contribute, including bacterial sepsis, possibly through gut translocation of bacteria; a direct effect of the virus; disseminated intravascular coagulation; and haemorrhage.[23]

How are people at risk identified?
Ebola virus infection is transmitted mainly through close physical contact with infected patients. There is no evidence of a risk of infection before symptoms develop, but late diagnosis delays effective patient isolation, allowing for potential transmission of the infection among contacts. Screening and active case finding are therefore essential to avoid or stop an epidemic.

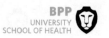

 BMJ

BOX 1 INFECTION CONTROL MEASURES FOR HEALTHCARE WORKERS

- Wear protective clothing
- Practise proper infection control and sterilisation measures
- Isolate suspected patients from each other (if possible), and patients with confirmed disease from those with suspected disease
- Avoid direct contact with bodies of people who have died from Ebola, or suspected Ebola. During epidemics, avoid direct contact with any dead body
- Notify health officials if you have direct contact with the body fluids of an infected patient

BOX 2 INFECTION CONTROL MEASURES FOR PEOPLE IN AFFECTED AREAS

- Practise careful hygiene (for example, wash hands with soap and water, alcohol based hand sanitiser, or diluted chlorine)
- Avoid contact with body fluids
- Do not handle items that have come into contact with an infected person's body fluids (such as clothes, medical equipment, and needles)
- Avoid funeral or burial rituals that require handling of the body of someone who has died from proven or suspected Ebola
- Avoid contact with non-human primates and bats, including body fluids or raw meat prepared from these animals
- Avoid hospitals in west Africa in which infected patients are being treated
- Returning travellers, including healthcare workers, should follow national policy for surveillance and should monitor their health for 21 days and seek medical attention if symptoms develop, especially fever

Personal protective equipment

The highest risk facing healthcare workers when looking after infected patients is inadvertently touching their own faces or neck under the face shield during patient care, and removing (doffing) personal protective equipment (PPE; shown in fig 3).

Healthcare workers should understand the following basic principles of using PPE:

Donning—PPE must be donned correctly in the proper order before entering the patient care area. Because PPE cannot be adjusted while in the patient care area, care should be taken to ensure it is as comfortable as possible before entering and that no skin is exposed. Donning activities must be directly observed by a trained observer and a final check performed before entering the patient care area

During patient care—PPE must remain in place and be worn correctly for the duration of exposure to potentially contaminated areas. PPE should not be adjusted during patient care. Healthcare workers should regularly disinfect gloved hands using an alcohol based hand rub or chlorinated water, particularly after handling body fluids. If there is a partial or total breach in PPE (such as gloves separating from sleeves to leave exposed skin, a tear in an outer glove, or a needlestick) during patient care, the healthcare worker must move immediately to the doffing area to assess the exposure and implement the facility exposure plan, if indicated

Doffing—Removal of used PPE is a high risk process that requires a structured procedure, a trained observer, and a designated area for removal to ensure protection. PPE must be removed slowly and deliberately in the correct

sequence to reduce the possibility of self contamination or other exposure. A stepwise process should be developed and used during training and daily practice.[29]

The importance of a "buddy" when inside the patient care area, and during donning and doffing, to ensure safe practice cannot be overstated, together with guidance from independent monitors if available.

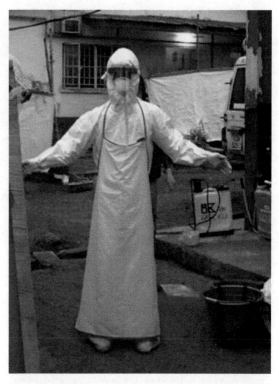

Fig 3 Healthcare worker in personal protective equipment at an Ebola treatment centre in Sierra Leone, 2014 (with permission from Chris Lane, Public Health England/WHO)

What other measures are needed if Ebola virus disease is suspected?

If infection is suspected, the patient should be isolated and all healthcare workers in contact with the patient should wear personal protective equipment.

Contact tracing (family, friends, and work colleagues) is essential. People who have been exposed to Ebola virus within the past 21 days and who are asymptomatic need to be monitored for the duration of the incubation period with twice daily temperature readings to ensure rapid recognition of symptoms. If symptoms are detected immediate isolation is essential.[30]

Healthcare workers suspected of being infected should be isolated and treated in the same way as any other patient until a negative diagnosis is confirmed.[31] If exposure to body fluids from a patient with suspected infection has occurred, the person should immediately wash affected skin surfaces with soap and water and irrigate mucous membranes with copious amounts of water.

The patient's home and any personal belongings that might have been contaminated (such as clothes, linens, eating utensils, and medical material) should be disinfected or disposed of (usually by incineration). In epidemic areas, the patient's home is sprayed with 0.5% chorine solution.

What are the clinical features?

The case definition for Ebola virus infection is very broad and includes a long list of possible differential diagnoses (fig 4).

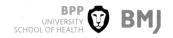

Condition	Differentiating signs/symptoms	Differentiating tests
Malaria infection	Most common cause of non-specific febrile illness in returning travellers Inadequate or no malaria chemoprophylaxis There are no differentiating signs and symptoms Malaria infection and Ebola virus infection may co-exist	Giemsa stained thick and thin blood smears: positive for *Plasmodium* species Rapid diagnostic tests: positive for *Plasmodium* species. *Plasmodium ovale* not always detected by some rapid diagnostic tests
Other viral haemorrhagic fevers	There are no differentiating signs and symptoms Epidemiological features can help differentiate between the viral haemorrhagic fevers Marburg virus: exposure to bats, caves, or mining[32] Crimean Congo haemorrhagic fever (CCHF): animal butchering, tick bite, or exposure to animals[33] Lassa fever: exposure to rats in endemic areas[34]	Reverse transcriptase-polymerase chain reaction (RT-PCR): positive for infective virus
Typhoid infection	There are no differentiating signs and symptoms	Blood or stool culture: positive for *Salmonella enterica*
Rickettsial infections	Includes murine typhus, African tick bite fever, and epidemic typhus[6] Eschar is typical Variable lymphadenopathy or discrete rash (or both)	Serology: positive for *Rickettsia* species Eschar PCR: positive for *Rickettsia* species
Dengue fever	There are no differentiating signs and symptoms	Serology: positive IgM or IgG Non-structural protein (NS1) detection: positive RT-PCR: positive
Measles	Unvaccinated There are no differentiating signs and symptoms in prodromal phase Koplik's spots (red spots with bluish-white central dot) on buccal mucosa Rash typically starts on face and spreads craniocaudally	Serology: positive for measles virus
Leptospirosis	There are no differentiating signs and symptoms; however, a history of exposure may be helpful Exposure to contaminated water or soil contaminated by infected rodents[35] More common in tropical climates	PCR: positive Serology: positive
Seasonal influenza infection	Respiratory signs and symptoms (for example, cough, nasal congestion) are more common	Viral culture or PCR: detection of seasonal influenza virus or viral RNA Full blood count: normal
Gastroenteritis	In the correct epidemiological context, this can present in a similar way to Ebola virus infection. However, features such as rash, conjunctival injection, and prostration are very rare in gastroenteritis	Stool culture, PCR, or rapid antigen testing: positive
Sepsis	Bacterial sepsis with an unclear origin is a common presentation in developing countries. Often turns out to be deep abdominal infection, upper urinary tract infection, endocarditis, or discitis Diarrhoea is often absent	Blood cultures: positive

Fig 4 Differential diagnosis. Confirmatory tests should be performed before, or in tandem with, differentiating tests if Ebola virus infection is suspected

History

The initial assessment of a patient with suspected Ebola hinges on two main factors: epidemiological risk (for example, living or working in, or arrival from, an endemic area such as west Africa in the past 21 days) and presence or history of a fever in the past 24 hours. Apart from healthcare workers, people who work with primates or bats from endemic areas or with high risk clinical samples are also at high risk.

A detailed history helps to clarify the level of risk for infection and to assess the possibility of other causes of an acute febrile syndrome (fig 5). Because malaria is still the most common cause of febrile illness in returning travellers,

the presence of risk factors for acquiring malaria should be assessed (for example, living or working in, or arriving from, an endemic area; inadequate or absent chemoprophylaxis; not using insecticides or bed nets).[36] Infection control risk should be assessed. Having determined that a patient may be infected, the doctor needs to determine how infectious the patient currently is. For example, the absence of vomiting or diarrhoea reduces the risk of transmission, whereas uncontrolled diarrhoea greatly increases the risk.

Precautionary isolation procedures and use of PPE are mandated in symptomatic patients who may be at risk of infection until the infection is confirmed or excluded. It is extremely important to minimise the risk of transmission while investigating patients (see later).[28 37]

Symptoms

There are typically three phases of illness, starting with a few days of non-specific fever, headache, and myalgia, followed by a gastrointestinal phase in which diarrhoea and vomiting, abdominal symptoms, and dehydration are prominent. In the second week, the patient may recover or deteriorate, with a third phase of illness including collapse, neurological manifestations, and bleeding, which is often fatal.[38]

The most common symptoms reported between symptom onset and case detection in the 2014 outbreak were fever (87.1%), fatigue (76.4%), loss of appetite (64.5%), vomiting (67.6%), diarrhoea (65.6%), headache (53.4%), abdominal pain (44.3%), and unexplained bleeding (18%) (box 3).[3] The high frequency of vomiting and diarrhoea means that patients are often dehydrated and hypovolaemic, particularly if they present late.

BOX 3 TYPICAL SYMPTOMS OF EBOLA VIRUS DISEASE[4]

- Fever ≥37.5°C*
- Fatigue
- Nausea or vomiting
- Diarrhoea
- Headache
- Abdominal pain
- Myalgia
- Prostration
- Sore throat
- Unexplained bleeding or bruising
- Spontaneous abortion or miscarriage
- Hiccups
- Rash

*The temperature threshold for "fever" level varies between different guidelines.[39]

Children present with similar symptoms to adults; however, younger children are reported to have more respiratory (such as cough and dyspnoea) and gastrointestinal symptoms, but less bleeding and neurological signs, than adults.[40 41] Anecdotally, children under 4 years present initially with more subtle symptoms before developing a fever and are often diagnosed late.

Physical examination

A full physical examination should be undertaken with precautionary isolation procedures and use of PPE. The aim of examination is to exclude a focus for sepsis while looking for signs of viral haemorrhagic fever (such as conjunctival injection, purpuric rash, or other signs of bleeding).

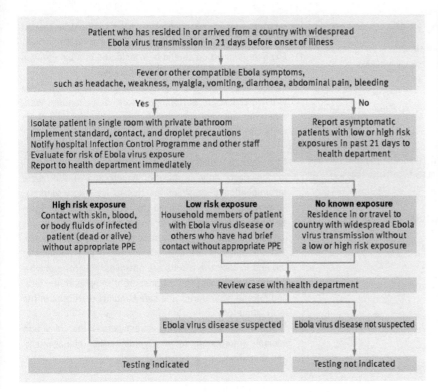

Fig 5 Diagnostic pathway for the investigation of suspected Ebola virus infection (produced by the BMJ Evidence Centre)

Vital signs should be taken:

Fever ($\geq$37.5°C)—Fever is the presenting symptom in about 90% of patients,[3 39 42] and its presence is enough to raise concern in the appropriate epidemiological context. Wide variations in body temperature are seen during the course of illness, with normothermia or hypothermia occurring in the later stages of fatal infection.[40 43 44] Some patients initially have a low grade fever with no other symptoms

Blood pressure—Hypotension is a feature of preterminal disease and shock. It is underdocumented in field studies, owing to a lack of measuring equipment in endemic areas[43]

Pulse rate—Bradycardia may be present in the initial stages of illness, whereas tachycardia may be seen in the later stages of fatal infections[43]

Respiratory rate—Tachypnoea, along with tachycardia, correlates with a more severe or advanced infection. It is more likely to be caused by respiratory compensation of a metabolic acidosis than respiratory involvement.[43]

Other possible findings include a maculopapular rash, bleeding, hiccups, hepatomegaly, lymphadenopathy, and neurological signs (box 4).[43]

Multi-organ dysfunction is common in advanced infection and includes acute kidney injury, pancreatitis, adrenal failure, and liver damage. Hepatitis is common, with aspartate aminotransferase (AST) higher than alanine aminotransferase (ALT), although jaundice is rare.[23] Renal dysfunction is common in advanced disease but can be reversed with adequate fluid resuscitation in the initial stages.[23] In early disease it may be caused by dehydration, but in later stages it may be a consequence of disseminated intravascular coagulation or direct damage to the kidneys by the Ebola virus.[23 43] Massive bleeding, typically in the gastrointestinal tract (for example, bloody diarrhoea or melaena), is usually seen only in fatal cases.[43] Internal bleeding may be missed if there are no external signs.

Signs that indicate severe or advanced infection include hiccups, hypotension, tachycardia, hepatomegaly, splenomegaly, confusion, and seizures.

How is it investigated?

All specimens should be collected according to strict protocols.

Initial investigations

The main confirmatory test for Ebola virus infection is a positive Ebola RT-PCR.[48] This test should be ordered in all patients with suspected Ebola infection while the patient is isolated. The results of RT-PCR are available 24-48 hours before those of enzyme linked immunosorbent assay (ELISA) testing. In Western settings, Ebola RT-PCR may be available only in regional or national reference laboratories that have a high level of biosafety precautions (category 4 facilities).[8] In epidemic settings and some European countries, category 4 laboratories are set up locally, and RT-PCR is available four hours after the sample has arrived. Viral RNA can be detected in the patient's blood by RT-PCR from day 3 to days 6-17 of symptoms. A positive result implies that the patient is potentially infectious, particularly if there is active diarrhoea, vomiting, or bleeding. If negative, the test should be repeated within 48 hours because viral load can be low and undetectable early in the illness. Negative tests should also be repeated to rule out the diagnosis (or confirm resolution of infection) if there is a strong suspicion of Ebola.[31] Higher viral load correlates with adverse outcome.[5 24 38 47 49]

The choice of whether to test for Ebola depends on the patient's history and the risk of infection (fig 5).

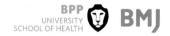

BOX 5 OTHER USEFUL INVESTIGATIONS WHEN DIAGNOSING EBOLA VIRUS DISEASE

Antigen capture enzyme linked immunosorbent assay (ELISA) testing

- A useful diagnostic test with high specificity, although it is not universally available
- Most likely to give a positive result on days 3-6 of symptoms and can give widely variable results from days 7-16[17]
- Can be used to confirm the diagnosis along with a positive reverse transcriptase-polymerase chain reaction result

Full blood count

- Decreasing platelet count with marked lymphopenia can be seen in the initial stages of infection but is not diagnostic. This is often followed by neutrophil leucocytosis in the later stages in patients who eventually recover, along with normalisation of thrombocytopenia. Leucocytosis may persist and show immature forms
- Patients with severe disease may show a progressive decline in platelet count as a manifestation of disseminated intravascular coagulation (DIC)
- Haemoglobin may be low in patients with bleeding manifestations[43]

Coagulation studies

- Prolonged prothrombin time or activated partial thromboplastin time is associated with more severe infection and bleeding manifestations such as DIC
- D-dimer values are four times higher on days 6-8 of infection in patients who die than in those who survive[50]

Renal function and serum electrolytes

- Raised serum creatinine or urea and abnormal electrolytes may indicate acute kidney injury; this may be seen at the end of the first week of infection[51]
- Some studies found hypokalaemia (associated with vomiting and diarrhoea) in about half of cases
- Hypocalcaemia has been associated with fatal infection
- Haematuria and proteinuria may also be seen in severe disease
- Oliguria that does not respond to fluid resuscitation is a poor prognostic sign[43]

Arterial blood gases

- Arterial or venous blood lactate, pH, and bicarbonate can help identify the degree of systemic hypoperfusion and guide fluid resuscitation in acutely ill patients with signs of sepsis[52]
- Raised lactate is a marker of tissue hypoperfusion and is an indicator of shock.

Liver function tests

- Both ALT and AST are usually raised; most studies show that AST rises more than ALT—this is more suggestive of systemic tissue damage rather than hepatocellular injury
- The AST:ALT ratio peaked at 15:1 on days 6-8 of infection in fatal cases compared with days 5:1 in non-fatal cases[43 45 50]
- Bilirubin, γ-glutamyl transferase, and alkaline phosphatase are often slightly raised. Greatly raised ALT and severe jaundice suggests an alternative diagnosis (such as viral hepatitis)

Serum amylase

- High concentrations have been reported in several studies and indicate the presence of pancreatitis, an indicator of severe infection[43]

Blood cultures

- Negative blood cultures are helpful because they rule out other non-viral infectious causes (such as sepsis or enteric fever)

Ebola specific IgM and IgG antibodies

- Useful in later stages of infection
- IgM antibodies can appear in serum as early as day 2 after infection but results are variable up to day 9. They become negative between 30 and 168 days after symptom onset
- An IgG response develops between days 6 and 18 and can persist for several years
- A positive IgM or a rising IgG titre is strong evidence of recent Ebola virus infection[17]

Chest radiography

- Useful in patients with respiratory symptoms
- Pulmonary infiltrates are not typical of infection and suggest an alternative (or comorbid) diagnosis
- May be difficult to arrange in an isolation unit and should be ordered judiciously to avoid contamination[53]

Malaria is still the most common cause of fever in people who live or work in, or travellers who have returned from, an endemic area and should be ruled out.[36] If a malaria rapid diagnostic test is positive, malaria should be treated while keeping in mind the possibility of a dual infection. Ebola virus infection should be considered in a patient who does not respond to antimalarial therapy.

It is recommended that confirmatory tests for Ebola virus infection are performed before, or in tandem with, differentiating tests for other suspected conditions if Ebola virus infection is suspected.

Other investigations

In the past, only a malaria screen and RT-PCR were recommended because of the risk to laboratory workers. However, it is now recognised that other investigations can be done safely according to recommended guidelines, as long as the laboratory is informed of the sample in advance, and the samples are correctly packaged and retained at the end in case the results are positive.[28 42] Local protocols should be clear about safe transport of samples to the local and referral laboratories and safe handling on receipt in the local laboratory.

Box 5 outlines additional investigations that may add valuable information to help guide further management, and that should be ordered if possible.

How is it managed?

The mainstay of treatment is early recognition of infection, coupled with effective isolation and best available supportive care in a hospital setting.

High case fatality rates may be related to the supportive care available in resource poor rural settings where outbreaks have occurred They reflect the difficulties that patients in these settings have in accessing basic medical care in a healthcare structure that is overwhelmed.[3 5]

During the 2014 outbreak, comprehensive supportive care—including organ support in intensive care units—was available to cases imported to developed countries such as Spain, Italy, Switzerland, Germany, France, Norway, the UK, and the US.[18 54 55] Despite this, deaths still occurred because of the lack of specific effective treatments.

There is active debate about the suitability of moving patients with advanced disease and a poor prognosis to intensive care, where the risk for nosocomial infection may be high.[52 56 57] However, failure to provide full supportive care to those with suspected (not confirmed) infection may result in substandard care for these patients, who may later be shown to have a treatable disease such as malaria. Local hospital protocols should consider how this situation should be handled for patients with suspected infection before possible transfer to the intensive care unit, and for those who have already been transferred there.[52 56 57]

Isolation and infection control

Patients identified as being at risk of infection should immediately be isolated in a room with private bathroom facilities.

All attending healthcare personnel must wear PPE that conforms with published protocols (fig 3).[29 58] All contaminated materials (such as clothes and bed linens) should be treated as potentially infectious.

Specimens for laboratory investigations (such as Ebola RT-PCR, full blood count, serum creatinine and urea, liver function tests, arterial blood gases, coagulation studies, blood cultures, and investigations for other conditions such as malaria) should be collected and sent off according to local and national protocols. Judicious selection of

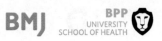

investigations is needed to reduce the risk of transmission to laboratory workers and other healthcare personnel. Early placement of a central line (if possible) allows blood to be taken and fluids to be given while minimising the risk of needlestick injuries.

Fluid and electrolyte replacement

Vomiting and diarrhoea are common, so patients are often dehydrated and hypovolaemic, particularly if they present late. This is probably the cause of the high case fatality rates because essential clinical monitoring (temperature, respiratory rate, pulse rate, blood pressure, and fluid input and output) is often difficult in resource poor settings.

Oral rehydration solutions can be used for patients who can tolerate oral administration and who are not severely dehydrated.

The volume of intravenous fluids needed should be assessed on the basis of the clinical examination (level of dehydration, signs of shock) and fluid losses (volume of diarrhoea or vomitus, or both). Large volumes of fluid replacement (>10 L/day) may be needed in febrile patients with diarrhoea.[18]

Access to point of care tests in the isolation facility means that the patient's biochemical status can be monitored more efficiently and reduces the risks associated with specimen transport.[5] [52] Electrolyte monitoring should be performed daily. More frequent monitoring can be considered if large volumes of intravenous fluids are being given or if severe biochemical abnormalities are present. High blood lactate values are a reliable measure of hypoperfusion and can help guide fluid resuscitation.[52] In patients with anuria who do not respond to fluid resuscitation, renal replacement therapy has been used,[18] [55] [59] although there are no trial data to support its effectiveness.

Major bleeding is uncommon, but is seen in advanced infection that is usually fatal. When available, platelet and plasma transfusions should be given according to local protocols.[60]

Symptomatic management

The following management strategies are recommended:

Fever and pain—Fever and pain should be treated with paracetamol first. Opioid analgesics (such as morphine) are preferable for more severe pain. Non-steroidal anti-inflammatory drugs (including aspirin) should be avoided because of the associated increased risk of bleeding and potential for nephrotoxicity[31]

Nausea and vomiting—Oral or intravenous antiemetics (such as ondansetron and metoclopramide) are recommended[31]

Heartburn, dysphagia, and upper abdominal pain—An antacid or proton pump inhibitor (such as omeprazole) may be beneficial[31]

Seizures—Although uncommon, seizures can be seen in advanced disease and pose a risk to healthcare workers because they increase the risk of contact with the patient's body fluids. Contributing factors (such as high temperature, hypoperfusion, and electrolyte disturbances) must be recognised and corrected. A benzodiazepine can be used to abort the seizure and can be given intramuscularly or rectally if intravenous access is unavailable. An anticonvulsant (such as phenobarbital) can be given for repeated seizures[31]

Agitation—Although uncommon, agitation can occur in advanced disease. It may be associated with encephalopathy or may be a direct effect of the virus on the brain. Judicious use of a sedative (such as haloperidol or a benzodiazepine) will help to keep the patient calm and prevent needlestick injuries in healthcare workers[31]

Sepsis and septic shock—Management follows the same principles as for bacterial sepsis.[61] It should include broad spectrum antibiotics (such as ceftriaxone, piperacillin-tazobactam, or meropenem) in the first hour after sending blood cultures, rapid intravenous fluid resuscitation with assessment of response, appropriate airway management and oxygen administration, and monitoring of urine output preferably by urethral catheterisation. Broad spectrum antibiotics in these patients are used to target the presumed translocation of gut organisms. This is not backed by any evidence. Blood cultures are difficult to perform safely in infected patients.

In the absence of a response to initial management, inotropic support should be considered, preferably through a central venous catheter in an intensive care unit where invasive monitoring enables more aggressive correction of fluids, electrolytes, and acid-base balance.[52] [54]

Malaria should be tested for and treated with appropriate antimalarial therapy. In endemic settings all patients in Ebola treatment centres are treated for malaria routinely.[5] [38] [47]

Are there any emerging treatments?

Although experimental treatments for Ebola virus infection are under development, they have not yet been fully tested for safety or effectiveness.[62] [63]

Convalescent whole blood or plasma

There is limited evidence from past outbreaks that transfusion of blood from convalescent patients might be beneficial in the acute phase of infection and may reduce mortality.[46] [63] Trials are planned.[62] [64]

ZMapp

The best known emerging treatment so far, ZMapp, is a combination of three humanised monoclonal antibodies targeted at three Ebola virus glycoprotein epitopes and is engineered for expression in tobacco plants.[62] [63] [65] [66] Before the current 2014 outbreak, ZMapp had proved protective when given to non-human primates 24-48 hours after infection. Another study showed that the drug could rescue non-human primates when treatment was started up to five days after infection.[67] It has not yet been tested in humans for safety or efficacy; however, very limited stock (seven doses) was made available to infected patients during the current outbreak, and only one patient died. Despite its potential, numbers are too small to make any conclusions about the drug's safety and efficacy. More doses are not currently available to conduct larger trials, but development is being accelerated with support from the US government.[68]

TKM-Ebola

TKM-Ebola consists of a combination of small interfering RNAs that target Ebola virus RNA polymerase L, formulated with lipid nanoparticle technology. It has been shown to be protective in non-human primates and is effective against Marburg virus in guinea pigs and monkeys.[62] [63] [66] [69] [70] [71] The US Food and Drug Administration has granted expanded

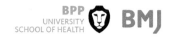

access to this drug under an Investigational New Drug application. Under emergency protocols, it has been given to a small number of patients.

Brincidofovir
Formerly known as CMX-001, brincidofovir is currently undergoing phase III trials for the treatment of cytomegalovirus and adenovirus. It also shows activity against Ebola virus in vitro. The drug has been used in patients with Ebola virus infection in the US under Emergency Investigational New Drug applications approved by the FDA. Trials are planned in the near future in west Africa.[62 63 64]

Favipiravir
Formerly known as T-705, favipiravir selectively inhibits viral RNA dependent RNA polymerase. It is active against influenza viruses, West Nile virus, yellow fever virus, foot and mouth disease virus, as well as other flaviviruses, arenaviruses, bunyaviruses, and alphaviruses. The drug is approved in Japan for influenza pandemics and is effective against Ebola virus in mouse models.[62 63 72] Human trials are due to start in west Africa.[64]

BCX-4430
BCX-4430 is an adenosine analogue that is active against Ebola virus in rodents. It is thought to act through the inhibition of viral RNA dependent RNA polymerase. It is active against flaviviruses, bunyaviruses, arenaviruses, and paramyxoviruses. The drug has been shown to be protective in non-human primates and rodents, even when given 48 hours after infection with filoviruses[63 73]; however, no human studies have been performed.

AVI-7537
AVI-7537 consists of antisense phosphorodiamidate morpholino oligomers (PMOs) that target the Ebola virus VP24 gene. It confers a survival benefit to Ebola virus infected non-human primates.[63 74] AVI-6002 consists of two PMOs (AV-7537 and AV-7539, which targets the VP35 gene). AV-6002 has undergone phase I clinical studies.

Other agents
Interferons have been used in the past, with uncertain benefit.[16 63] Therapeutic agents used for other diseases, such as amiodarone, clomiphene, and chloroquine, inhibit Ebola virus interactions with human cells in models, and amiodarone will shortly be trialled in west Africa.[62 75]

Vaccines
Two experimental vaccines are currently undergoing trials.[62 63] cAd3-ZEBOV is a chimpanzee derived adenovirus vector with an Ebola virus gene inserted.[76] Trials are under way in the United Kingdom, United States, Switzerland, and some African countries. rVSV-ZEBOV is an attenuated vesicular stomatitis virus with one of its genes replaced by an Ebola virus gene. Human trials have started in the US.

What is the prognosis?
The natural clinical course of Ebola virus infection varies markedly between the different viral species and according to the level of supportive medical care available. The most lethal species is *Zaire ebolavirus*, which has a reported case fatality rate of up to 90%. The rate in the current 2014 outbreak is less than this and is estimated at 60-70%, although accurate data are biased by poor record keeping and registration.[3] Most epidemics have occurred in resource poor settings with little supportive care, and the case fatality rate in high income settings could be less than 40%.[52] Mortality is higher in younger children (<5 years) and adults over 40 years than in adolescents and young adults.[3 5 38 40 41 47 51] An observational study during an outbreak in 1995 showed a marked decrease in the case fatality rate from 93% to 69% between the initial and final phases of the outbreak.[77] This suggests that later cases were recognised earlier and possibly received higher quality care. Pregnant women have a high incidence of miscarriage and the infection is almost always fatal in these women.[38 78 79 80]

Infection course
Patients who die tend to develop clinical signs early on in the infection, with death, usually attributed to shock and multi-organ failure, typically occurring between days 6 and 16 (median 9 days) from symptom onset.[19 81 82] Patients who eventually recover exhibit isolated fever for several days with improvement typically around days 6-11. A high viral load at presentation is correlated with mortality.[5 24 38 47 49] Biomarkers as prognostic indicators require further study.[51 81]

Recovery and convalescence
Patients who live through the second week of infection have more than a 75% chance of surviving.[43] Patients are usually discharged from the isolation facility when they are ambulant, able to self care, have no serious symptoms (such as diarrhoea, vomiting, or bleeding), and have two negative Ebola RT-PCR results taken 48 hours apart.[47]

Patients who survive usually have a protracted recovery characterised by asthenia, weight loss, and migratory arthralgia. Skin desquamation and transient hair loss are also common. Late manifestations during convalescence are uncommon but include uveitis, orchitis, myelitis, parotitis, pancreatitis, hepatitis, psychosis, hearing loss and tinnitus.[44] The cause of these manifestations is unclear but they might be related to immune complex phenomena.

Survivors of infection probably have lifetime immunity to the same strain of Ebola virus. Such patients have therefore been invaluable in caring for those with active infections.

What advice should patients be given during recovery?
Patients should be educated about the likely course of convalescence and the possibility of long term complications. There are no specific requirements for monitoring after discharge; however, eligible patients may be asked to donate blood from 28 days after discharge to be used in the treatment of patients with active infection.

Male patients should be reminded about the importance of using condoms to prevent sexual transmission in the three months after resolution of infection.[15 16 17] Women should be advised not to breast feed during infection.[15]

Survivors and orphans of those who died from the disease face stigma and ostracism in many communities. This—along with substantial associated psychological disturbance—was reported after previous outbreaks,[83 84] and it is an increasing problem in the 2014 outbreak.

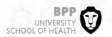

The authors thank Adam Mitchell, clinical editor and drug editor, BMJ Best Practice, for his extensive editorial support on this topic.

Competing interests: NJB is an author of several references cited in this monograph. NJB is partially supported by a National Institute of Health Research grant to the Health Protection Unit in Emerging Infections and Zoonoses, a partnership between the University of Liverpool, the Liverpool School of Tropical Medicine, and Public Health England.

Provenance and peer review: Not commissioned; externally peer reviewed.

This clinical review series has been developed for The BMJ in collaboration with BMJ Best Practice (http://bestpractice.bmj.com), an independent product produced by BMJ Publishing Group Limited. BMJ Best Practice comprises web/mobile topics that support evidence-based decision making at the point of care. Peer review of the content in this clinical review was carried out exclusively according to BMJ Best Practice's own, independent process (http://bestpractice.bmj.com/best-practice/marketing/how-is-best-practice-produced.html). This adaptation of a BMJ Best Practice topic for a clinical review in The BMJ uses only a portion of content from the latest available web version of BMJ Best Practice. BMJ Best Practice is updated on an ongoing basis, and the content of any BMJ Best Practice topic is expected to change periodically including subsequent to its publication as a clinical review in The BMJ. To view the complete and current versions of all BMJ Best Practice topics, please refer to the BMJ Best Practice website (http://bestpractice.bmj.com).

Content from BMJ Best Practice is intended to support, aid and supplement the expertise, discretion and judgment of licensed medical health professionals who remain solely responsible for decisions regarding diagnosis and treatment of their patients. Content from BMJ Best Practice is not intended to function as a substitute for a licensed medical health professional's judgment. BMJ Best Practice reflects evidence available to its authors and licensors prior to publication. The BMJ relies on its authors to confirm the accuracy of the information presented to reflect generally accepted practices. While The BMJ seeks to ensure BMJ Best Practice is up to date and accurate, it does not warrant that is the case. Content from BMJ Best Practice is supplied on an "as is" basis and any statements made to the contrary are void. BMJ Best Practice does not endorse drugs, diagnose patients, or recommend therapy. The full disclaimer applicable to BMJ Best Practice can be found at http://bestpractice.bmj.com/best-practice/marketing/disclaimer.html.

1 Centers for Disease Control and Prevention. About Ebola virus disease. 2014. www.cdc.gov/.
2 WHO. Are the Ebola outbreaks in Nigeria and Senegal over? 2014. www.who.int/.
3 WHO Ebola Response Team. Ebola virus disease in West Africa: the first 9 months of the epidemic and forward projections. N Engl J Med 2014;371:1481-95.
4 Centers for Disease Control and Prevention. Ebola fact sheet. 2014. www.cdc.gov/.
5 Bah EI, Lamah MC, Fletcher T, Jacob ST, Brett-Major DM, Sall AA, et al. Clinical presentation of patients with Ebola virus disease in Conakry, Guinea. N Engl J Med 2014; published online 5 Nov. doi:10.1056/NEJMoa1411249.
6 Hensley LE, Wahl-Jensen V, McCormick JB, Rubins KH. Viral hemorrhagic fevers. In: Cohen J, Powderly W, Opal S, eds. Infectious diseases. 3rd ed. Mosby; 2010:1231-7.
7 Peters CJ, LeDuc JW. An introduction to Ebola: the virus and the disease. J Infect Dis 1999;179(suppl 1):9-16.
8 Feldmann H, Geisbert TW. Ebola haemorrhagic fever. Lancet 2011;377:849-62.
9 Swanepoel R, Smit SB, Rollin PE, Formenty P, Leman PA, Kemp A, et al. Studies of reservoir hosts for Marburg virus. Emerg Infect Dis 2007;13:1847-51.
10 Peterson AT, Bauer JT, Mills JN. Ecologic and geographic distribution of filovirus disease. Emerg Infect Dis 2004;10:40-7.
11 Swanepoel R, Leman PA, Burt FJ, Zachariades NA, Braack LE, Ksiazek TG, et al. Experimental inoculation of plants and animals with Ebola virus. Emerg Infect Dis 1996;2:321-5.
12 Reiter P, Turell M, Coleman R, Miller B, Maupin G, Liz J, et al. Field investigations of an outbreak of Ebola hemorrhagic fever, Kikwit, Democratic Republic of the Congo, 1995: arthropod studies. J Infect Dis 1999;179(suppl 1):S148-54.
13 Dowell SF, Mukunu R, Ksiazek TG, Khan AS, Rollin PE, Peters CJ. Transmission of Ebola hemorrhagic fever: a study of risk factors in family members, Kikwit, Democratic Republic of the Congo, 1995. Commission de Lutte contre les Epidémies à Kikwit. J Infect Dis 1999;179(suppl 1):S87-91.
14 Report of an International Commission. Ebola haemorrhagic fever in Zaire, 1976. Bull World Health Organ 1978;56:271-93.
15 Bausch DG, Towner JS, Dowell SF, Kaducu F, Lukwiya M, Sanchez A, et al. Assessment of the risk of Ebola virus transmission from bodily fluids and fomites. J Infect Dis 2007;196(suppl 2):S142-7.
16 Emond RT, Evans B, Bowen ET, Lloyd G. A case of Ebola virus infection. BMJ 1977;2:541-4.
17 Rowe AK, Bertolli J, Khan AS, Mukunu R, Muyembe-Tamfum JJ, Bressler D, et al. Clinical, virologic, and immunologic follow-up of convalescent Ebola hemorrhagic fever patients and their household contacts, Kikwit, Democratic Republic of the Congo. Commission de Lutte contre les Epidémies à Kikwit. J Infect Dis 1999;179(suppl 1):S28-35.
18 Kreuels B, Wichmann D, Emmerich P, Schmidt-Chanasit J, de Heer G, Kluge S, et al. A case of severe Ebola virus infection complicated by gram-negative septicemia. N Engl J Med 2014; published online 22 Oct.
19 Mahanty S, Bray M. Pathogenesis of filoviral haemorrhagic fevers. Lancet Infect Dis 2004;4:487-98.
20 Beeching NJ, Fletcher TE, Hill DR, Thomson GL. Travellers and viral haemorrhagic fevers: what are the risks? Int J Antimicrob Agents 2010;36(suppl 1):S26-35.
21 Ramanan P, Shabman RS, Brown CS, Amarasinghe GK, Basler CF, Leung DW. Filoviral immune evasion mechanisms. Viruses 2011;3:1634-49.
22 Ramanan P, Edwards MR, Shabman RS, Leung DW, Endlich-Frazier AC, Borek DM, et al. Structural basis for Marburg virus VP35-mediated immune evasion mechanisms. Proc Natl Acad Sci U S A 2012;109:20661-6.
23 Fletcher T, Fowler RA, Beeching NJ. Understanding organ dysfunction in Ebola virus disease. Intensive Care Med 2014;40:1936-9.
24 Sanchez A, Lukwiya M, Bausch D, Mahanty S, Sanchez AJ, Wagoner KD, et al. Analysis of human peripheral blood samples from fatal and nonfatal cases of Ebola (Sudan) hemorrhagic fever: cellular responses, virus load, and nitric oxide levels. J Virol 2004;78:10370-7.
25 Zapata JC, Cox D, Salvato MS. The role of platelets in the pathogenesis of viral hemorrhagic fevers. PLoS Negl Trop Dis 2014;8:e2858.
26 Leroy EM, Baize S, Volchkov VE, Fisher-Hoch SP, Georges-Courbot MC, Lansoud-Soukate J, et al. Human asymptomatic Ebola infection and strong inflammatory response. Lancet 2000;355:2210-5.
27 WHO. Case definition for Ebola or Marburg virus disease. 2014. www.who.int/.
28 Fletcher TE, Brooks TJ, Beeching NJ. Ebola and other viral haemorrhagic fevers. BMJ 2014;349:g5079.
29 Centers for Disease Control and Prevention. Guidance on personal protective equipment to be used by healthcare workers during management of patients with Ebola virus disease in U.S. hospitals,

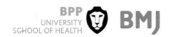

including procedures for putting on (donning) and removing (doffing). 2014. www.cdc.gov/.

30 Centers for Disease Control and Prevention. Interim guidance for monitoring and movement of persons with Ebola virus disease exposure. 2014. www.cdc.gov/.

31 WHO. Clinical management of patients with viral haemorrhagic fever: a pocket guide for the front-line health worker. 2014. http://apps.who.int/.

32 Public Health England. Marburg virus disease: origins, reservoirs, transmission and guidelines. 2014. www.gov.uk.

33 Public Health England. Crimean-Congo haemorrhagic fever: origins, reservoirs, transmission and guidelines. 2014. www.gov.uk.

34 Public Health England. Lassa fever: origins, reservoirs, transmission and guidelines. 2014. www.gov.uk.

35 Hartskeerl RA, Collares-Pereira M, Ellis WA. Emergence, control and re-emerging leptospirosis: dynamics of infection in the changing world. Clin Microbiol Infect 2011;17:494-501.

36 Mendelson M, Han PV, Vincent P, von Sonnenburg F, Cramer JP, Loutan L, et al. Regional variation in travel-related illness acquired in Africa, March 1997-May 2011. Emerg Infect Dis 2014;20:532-41.

37 Centers for Disease Control and Prevention. Case definition for Ebola virus disease (EVD). 2014. www.cdc.gov/.

38 Chertow DS, Kleine C, Edwards JK, Scaini R, Giuliani R, Sprecher A. Ebola virus disease in West Africa—clinical manifestations and management. N Engl J Med 2014;371:2054-7.

39 Dananché C, BénetT, Vanhems P. Ebola: fever definitions might delay detection in non-epidemic areas. Lancet 2014;384:1743.

40 Mupere E, Kaducu OF, Yoti Z. Ebola haemorrhagic fever among hospitalised children and adolescents in northern Uganda: epidemiologic and clinical observations. Afr Health Sci 2001;1:60-5.

41 Peacock G, Uyeki TM, Rasmussen SA. Ebola virus disease and children: what pediatric health care professionals need to know. JAMA Pediatr 2014; published online 17 Oct.

42 Public Health England. Ebola virus disease: clinical management and guidance. 2014. www.gov.uk/government/collections/ebola-virus-disease-clinical-management-and-guidance

43 Kortepeter MG, Bausch DG, Bray M. Basic clinical and laboratory features of filoviral hemorrhagic fever. J Infect Dis 2011;204(suppl 3):S810-6.

44 Bwaka MA, Bonnet MJ, Calain P, Colebunders R, De Roo A, Guimard Y, et al. Ebola hemorrhagic fever in Kikwit, Democratic Republic of the Congo: clinical observations in 103 patients. J Infect Dis 1999;179(suppl 1):S1-7.

45 Formenty P, Hatz C, Le Guenno B, Stoll A, Rogenmoser P, Widmer A. Human infection due to Ebola virus, subtype Côte d'Ivoire: clinical and biologic presentation. J Infect Dis 1999;179(suppl 1):S48-53.

46 Roddy P, Howard N, Van Kerkhove MD, Lutwama J, Wamala J, Yoti Z, et al. Clinical manifestations and case management of Ebola haemorrhagic fever caused by a newly identified virus strain, Bundibugyo, Uganda, 2007-2008. PLoS One 2012;7:e52986.

47 Schieffelin JS, Shaffer JG, Goba A, Gbakie M, Gire SK, Colubri A, et al; KGH Lassa Fever Program; Viral Hemorrhagic Fever Consortium; WHO Clinical Response Team. Clinical illness and outcomes in patients with Ebola in Sierra Leone. N Engl J Med 2014;371:2092-100.

48 WHO. Laboratory guidance for the diagnosis of Ebola virus disease: interim recommendations. 2014. www.who.int/.

49 Towner JS, Rollin PE, Bausch DG, Sanchez A, Crary SM, Vincent M, et al. Rapid diagnosis of Ebola hemorrhagic fever by reverse transcription-PCR in an outbreak setting and assessment of patient viral load as a predictor of outcome. J Virol 2004;78:4330-41.

50 Rollin PE, Bausch DG, Sanchez A. Blood chemistry measurements and D-Dimer levels associated with fatal and nonfatal outcomes in humans infected with Sudan Ebola virus. J Infect Dis 2007;196(suppl 2):S364-71.

51 McElroy AK, Erickson BR, Flietstra TD, Rollin PE, Nichol ST, Towner JS, et al. Biomarker correlates of survival in pediatric patients with ebola virus disease. Emerg Infect Dis 2014;20:1683-90.

52 Fowler RA, Fletcher T, Fischer WA 2nd, Lamontagne F, Jacob S, Brett-Major D, et al. Caring for critically ill patients with Ebola virus disease. Perspectives from West Africa. Am J Respir Crit Care Med 2014;190:733-7.

53 Auffermann WF, Kraft CS, Vanairsdale S, Lyon GM 3rd, Tridandapani S. Radiographic imaging for patients with contagious infectious diseases: how to acquire chest radiographs of patients infected with the Ebola virus. AJR Am J Roentgenol 2014; published online 17 Nov.

54 Parra JM, Salmerón OJ, Velasco M. The first case of Ebola virus disease acquired outside Africa. N Engl J Med 2014; published online 19 Nov.

55 Lyon GM, Mehta AK, Varkey JB, Brantly K, Plyler L, McElroy AK, et al; the Emory Serious Communicable Diseases Unit. Clinical care of two patients with Ebola virus disease in the United States. N Engl J Med 2014 published online 12 Nov. doi:10.1056/NEJMoa1409838.

56 Decker BK, Sevransky JE, Barrett K, Davey RT, Chertow DS. Preparing for critical care services to patients with Ebola. Ann Intern Med 2014; published online 23 Sep.

57 Canadian Critical Care Society, Canadian Association of Emergency Physicians, Association of Medical Microbiology and Infectious Diseases of Canada. Ebola clinical care guidelines: guide for clinicians in Canada. 2014. http://cccsnew.businesscatalyst.com/.

58 European Centre for Disease Prevention and Control. Epidemiological update: outbreak of Ebola virus disease in West Africa. 2014. www.ecdc.europa.eu.

59 Connor MJ Jr, Kraft C, Mehta AK, Varkey JB, Lyon GM, Crozier I, et al. Successful delivery of RRT in Ebola virus disease. J Am Soc Nephrol 2014; published online 14 Nov.

60 Wada H, Thachil J, Di Nisio M, Mathew P, Kurosawa S, Gando S, et al. Guidance for diagnosis and treatment of DIC from harmonization of the recommendations from three guidelines. J Thromb Haemost 2013; published online 4 Feb.

61 Dellinger RP, Levy MM, Rhodes A, Annane D, Gerlach H, Opal SM, et al. Surviving sepsis campaign: international guidelines for management of severe sepsis and septic shock: 2012. Crit Care Med 2013;41:580-637.

62 Bishop BM. Potential and emerging treatment options for Ebola virus disease. Ann Pharmacother 2014; published online 20 Nov.

63 WHO. Potential Ebola therapies and vaccines. 2014. http://www.who.int/csr/resources/publications/ebola/potential-therapies-vaccines/en/.

64 Gulland A. Clinical trials of Ebola therapies to begin in December. BMJ 2014;349:g6827.

65 Zhang Y, Li D, Jin X, Huang Z. Fighting Ebola with ZMapp: spotlight on plant-made antibody. Sci China Life Sci 2014;57:987-8.

66 Goodman JL. Studying "secret serums": toward safe, effective Ebola treatments. N Engl J Med 2014;371:1086-9.

67 Qiu X, Wong G, Audet J, Bello A, Fernando L, Alimonti JB, et al. Reversion of advanced Ebola virus disease in nonhuman primates with ZMapp. Nature 2014;514:47-53.

68 McCarthy M. US signs contract with ZMapp maker to accelerate development of the Ebola drug. BMJ 2014;349:g5488.

69 Thi EP, Mire CE, Ursic-Bedoya R, Geisbert JB, Lee AC, Agans KN, et al. Marburg virus infection in nonhuman primates: therapeutic treatment by lipid-encapsulated siRNA. Sci Transl Med 2014;6:250ra116.

70 Geisbert TW, Lee AC, Robbins M, Geisbert JB, Honko AN, Sood V, et al. Postexposure protection of non-human primates against a lethal Ebola virus challenge with RNA interference: a proof-of-concept study. Lancet 2010;375:1896-905.

71 Choi JH, Croyle MA. Emerging targets and novel approaches to Ebola virus prophylaxis and treatment. BioDrugs 2013;27:565-83.

72 Furuta Y, Takahashi K, Shiraki K, Sakamoto K, Smee DF, Barnard DL, et al. T-705 (favipiravir) and related compounds: novel broad-spectrum inhibitors of RNA viral infections. Antiviral Res 2009;82:95-102.

73 Warren TK, Wells J, Panchal RG, Stuthman KS, Garza NL, Van Tongeren SA, et al. Protection against filovirus diseases by a novel broad-spectrum nucleoside analogue BCX4430. Nature 2014;508:402-5.

74 Iversen PL, Warren TK, Wells JB, Garza NL, Mourich DV, Welch LS, et al. Discovery and early development of AVI-7537 and AVI-7288 for the treatment of Ebola virus and Marburg virus infections. Viruses 2012;4:2806-30.

75 Turone F. Doctors trial amiodarone for Ebola in Sierra Leone. BMJ 2014;349:g7198.

76 Ledgerwood JE, DeZure AD, Stanley DA, Novik L, Enama ME, Berkowitz NM, et al; the VRC 207 Study Team. Chimpanzee adenovirus vector Ebola vaccine - preliminary report. N Engl J Med 2014; published online 26 Nov. doi:10.1056/NEJMoa1410863.

77 Sadek RF, Khan AS, Stevens G, Peters CJ, Ksiazek TG. Ebola hemorrhagic fever, Democratic Republic of the Congo, 1995: determinants of survival. J Infect Dis 1999;179(suppl 1):S24-7.

78 Mupapa K, Mukundu W, Bwaka MA, Kipasa M, De Roo A, Kuvula K, et al. Ebola hemorrhagic fever and pregnancy. J Infect Dis 1999;179(suppl 1):S11-2.

79 Jamieson DJ, Uyeki TM, Callaghan WM, Meaney-Delman D, Rasmussen SA. What obstetrician-gynecologists should know about Ebola: a perspective from the Centers for Disease Control and Prevention. Obstet Gynecol 2014; published online 8 Sep.

80 Association of Women's Health, Obstetric and Neonatal Nurses. Ebola: caring for pregnant and postpartum women and newborns in the United States: AWHONN practice brief number 3. J Obstet Gynecol Neonat Nurs 2014; published online 24 Nov. doi:10.1111/1552-6909.12518.

81 Leroy EM, Gonzalez JP, Baize S. Ebola and Marburg haemorrhagic fever viruses: major scientific advances, and a relatively minor public health threat for Africa. Clin Microbiol Infect 2011;17:964-76.

82 McElroy AK, Erickson BR, Flietstra TD, Rollin PE, Nichol ST, Towner JS, et al. Ebola hemorrhagic fever: novel biomarker correlates of clinical outcome. J Infect Dis 2014;210:558-66.

83 De Roo A, Ado B, Rose B, Guimard Y, Fonck K, Colebunders R. Survey among survivors of the 1995 Ebola epidemic in Kikwit, Democratic Republic of Congo: their feelings and experiences. Trop Med Int Health 1998;3:883-5.

84 Locsin RC, Barnard A, Matua AG, Bongomin B. Surviving Ebola: understanding experience through artistic expression. Int Nurs Rev 2003;50:156-66.

Related links

thebmj.com
• Get CME/CPD credits for this article

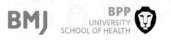

Infectious mononucleosis

Paul Lennon, specialist registrar[1], Michael Crotty, general practitioner[2],
John E Fenton, professor[1]

[1]Department of Otolaryngology, Head and Neck Surgery, University Hospital Limerick, Dooradoyle, Limerick, Ireland, and Graduate Entry Medical School, University of Limerick, Ireland

[2]General Practice, Synergy Medical Clinic, Sherwood Park, Edmonton, Alberta, Canada

Correspondence to: P Lennon paullennon81@gmail.com

Cite this as: BMJ 2015;350:h1825

DOI: 10.1136/bmj.h1825

http://www.bmj.com/content/350/bmj.h1825

Infectious mononucleosis is commonly seen in both the community and the hospital setting. Patients usually present with a sore throat and often presume that an antibiotic is required. It is therefore important to dispel the many myths relating to the condition with appropriate patient education. Knowledge of the clinical course of the disease, as well as potential complications, is paramount. In an information age, difficult questions may arise for a general practitioner, emergency doctor, or trainee in ear, nose, and throat medicine. The aim of this review is to assist those who encounter infectious mononucleosis in the adolescent and adult population.

What is infectious mononucleosis and what causes it?

It would be most accurate to consider infectious mononucleosis as a non-genetic syndrome, defined by the classic triad of fever, pharyngitis, and cervical lymphadenopathy, where lymphocytosis is also present. For many doctors the terms Epstein-Barr virus and infectious mononucleosis are synonymous. Epstein-Barr virus causes approximately 90% of the cases of infectious mononucleosis, with the remainder due largely to cytomegalovirus, human herpesvirus 6, toxoplasmosis, HIV, and adenovirus.[1] [W4] The World Health Organization's ICD-10 (international classification of diseases, 10th revision) has four subheadings for infectious mononucleosis (or B27 in the manual[W5]): infectious mononucleosis associated with Epstein-Barr virus (B27.0), cytomegalovirus infectious mononucleosis (B27.1), other infectious mononucleosis (B27.8), and infectious mononucleosis unspecified (27.9). To confuse things further the multiple synonyms for infectious mononucleosis (glandular fever, monocytic angina, Pfeiffer's disease, Filatov's disease, Drusenfieber, and even the kissing disease) are still included in ICD-9, which will be in use in the United States until 1 October 2015.[W6]

The Epstein-Barr virus is a ubiquitous herpesvirus, with more than 90% of the world's population infected by adulthood.[W7] The virus is one of our most effective parasites[W8] and remains as a lifelong, latent infection, by integrating itself into the life cycle of healthy B lymphocytes.[2] [W9] There is persistent low grade replication and the virus is shed intermittently into pharyngeal secretions, particularly saliva, through which it is transmitted.[W10] [W11] These low titres of infectious virus account for the low to moderate contagiousness of the disease and the apparent requirement of intimate contact for disease transmission.[W12] During an active infection the viral load may be increased, and therefore some precautions about contact should be mentioned (cough etiquette, hand hygiene, kissing, sharing food or utensils); however, as most of the population is positive for Epstein-Barr virus, special precautions against transmission are not necessary in most cases.[W13] Childhood infection, which is usually subclinical, is associated with poor hygiene and over-crowding. In lower socioeconomic groups most of the population will have acquired immunity by adolescence.[3] After an incubation period of four to seven weeks,[W14] Epstein-Barr virus infection of adolescents or adults results in infectious mononucleosis in up to 70% of cases.[4] Most symptoms tend to resolve in two to four weeks, although approximately 20% of patients continue to mention a sore throat at one month.[W15] In one study, patients with severe infectious mononucleosis who were admitted to hospital for intravenous hydration required a significantly longer stay than those admitted with bacterial tonsillitis. Reactivation of Epstein-Barr virus may occur in immunocompromised patients[W17] and, rarely, in immunocompetent patients, which may lead to Epstein-Barr virus associated lymphoproliferative conditions. These are a heterogeneous group of diseases that often need to be treated with chemotherapy.[W18] Diagnoses depend on the specific disease but are often associated with an increased viral load.[W19] Chronic active Epstein-Barr virus infection is a rare condition that is typified by severe, chronic, or recurrent infectious mononucleosis-like symptoms after a well documented primary infection with Epstein-Barr virus in a previously healthy person.[5] Chronic active Epstein-Barr virus infection is occasionally associated with the development of lymphoma.[W20]

How is it diagnosed?

Infectious mononucleosis may account for as little as 1% of patients who present with a sore throat to their doctor.[W21] Non-specific prodromal symptoms of fever, chills, and malaise may be seen in infectious mononucleosis. These symptoms may also be present in cases of viral pharyngitis, commonly caused by rhinovirus, adenovirus, and coronavirus. Whereas these viruses generally give rise to symptoms of a common cold,[W21] clinically infectious mononucleosis should be suspected in anyone who presents with fever, pharyngitis, and cervical lymphadenopathy (the classic triad).[W22] Lymphadenopathy may be prominent in both the anterior and the posterior triangles of the neck, which distinguishes infectious mononucleosis from bacterial tonsillitis (where the lymphadenopathy is usually limited to the upper anterior cervical chain). These signs were found in 98% of patients with a diagnosis of infectious mononucleosis.[6] Other common physical signs include palatal petechiae (25-50%), splenomegaly (8%),[W15] hepatomegaly (7%), and jaundice (6-8%),[W23] with a transitory derangement of liver function tests (in particular increased aspartate aminotransferase and alanine aminotransferase levels, returning to normal after 20 days) seen in 80-90% of patients.[7] Anecdotally,

---

THE BOTTOM LINE

- Infectious mononucleosis is a clinical diagnosis, caused by Epstein-Barr virus in 90% of cases, although in some patients (pregnancy, high risk HIV population) further investigations are warranted

- Treatment should be supportive, with steroids given only in cases of airway compromise

- Treatment with antiviral agents has yet to be shown to be of benefit

- Patients wanting to return to contact sports before one month should undergo abdominal ultrasonography to rule out splenomegaly

- Splenic rupture should be considered with any abdominal pain in infectious mononucleosis

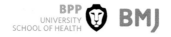

Table 1 Diagnostic tests for infectious mononucleosis

Tests	Sensitivity (%)	Specificity (%)	Comment
Infectious mononucleosis			
Full blood count:			
L/WCC >50%+10% atypical lymphocytes[w75]	61	95	An increase in lymphocyte count tends to lead to a greater specificity but poorer sensitivity[8]
L/WCC >35%	84	72	
Monospot	71-98	91-99	Results vary between different available commercial kits[w76]
Antibody to VCA or EBNA	97	94	May have replaced monospot as standard investigation in some countries
Bacterial tonsillitis			
Antistreptolysin O titre			Peak value 3-6 weeks after infection, and thus not of value in acute setting
Throat swab	78	99	Delay of 2-3 days for result[w77]
Rapid streptococcal[w78] antigen test	84	94	Increased cost

L/WCC=lymphocyte to white cell count ratio; VCA=antiviral capsid antigen; EBNA=Epstein-Barr virus nuclear antigen.

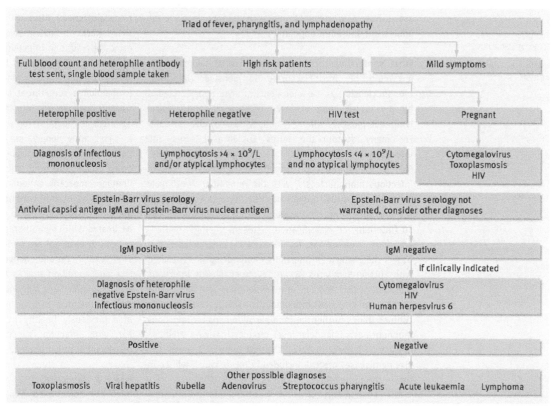

Fig 1 Algorithm for diagnosing infectious mononucleosis

a "whitewash"' exudate on the tonsils may also help to distinguish infectious mononucleosis from the more speckled exudate of bacterial tonsillitis and the erythema of a viral pharyngitis that is void of exudate. In the primary care setting a clinical diagnosis alone may be sufficient to allow adequate management of a patient. However, should a definitive diagnosis be sought, the Hoagland criteria state that in patients presenting with clinically suspected infectious mononucleosis and at least a 50% lymphocytosis (10% atypical), the diagnosis should be confirmed by the heterophile antibody (monospot) test.[6] Using a lower rate of lymphocytosis[w24 w25] has been shown to give a greater rate of false negative results (table 1).[8 w26 w27] The heterophile test may also be falsely negative in up to 25% of adults in the first week of symptoms.[1 6] It is not always necessary to definitively diagnose a cause for infectious mononucleosis, but specific antibody tests are available. Patients are considered to have a primary Epstein-Barr virus infection if they are positive for antiviral capsid antigen IgM but do not have antibodies to Epstein-Barr virus nuclear antigen, which would suggest past infection. Levels of antiviral capsid antigen IgG will also increase in the acute phase and persist for the rest of the patient's life, whereas the antiviral capsid antigen IgM will disappear after 4-6 weeks. The presence of antiviral capsid antigen IgG and Epstein-Barr virus nuclear antigen suggest past infection.[9] A recent review found that real time polymerase chain reaction and measurement of Epstein-Barr virus viral load provide useful tools for the early diagnosis of infectious mononucleosis in cases with inconclusive serological results.[10] In a small number of cases, where the patient is either pregnant or in a high risk group for HIV infection (injecting drug user or men who have sex with men), further testing for cytomegalovirus, HIV, and other possible causes for infectious mononucleosis should be undertaken.[w28 w29] Figure 1 presents an algorithm for diagnosing infectious mononucleosis.[w30]

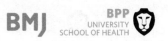

Table 2 Infectious mononucleosis and chronic fatigue syndrome (CFS)

Study	No of participants	Age of cohort (years)	% of patients with a diagnosis of CFS
White 1998[w49]	104	>16	9
Buchwald 2000[w79]	150	>16	12
Candy 2003[w46]	62	>16	11
Petrersen 2005[15]	1318	>16	0
Hickie 2006[w80]	68	>16	7.3
Moss-Morris 2011[w50]	246	>16	7.8
Katz 2009[w81]	301	12-18	13

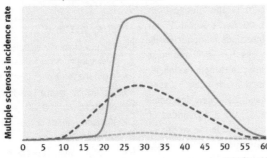

—— Late Epstein-Barr virus infection with infectious mononucleosis

- - - Early Epstein-Barr virus infection without infectious mononucleosis

······ No Epstein-Barr virus infection

Fig 2 Incidence of multiple sclerosis by Epstein-Barr virus infection. Adapted from Thacker et al 2006[19]

How is it treated?

Infectious mononucleosis is a viral illness in most cases, and as such it can be treated with rest, hydration, analgesia, and antipyretics. Inadvertent treatment with ampicillin results in a fine macular rash in 90% of patients.[w8] This should be distinguished from an urticarial rash seen in an allergic reaction. Studies have shown that symptoms experienced by patients are more severe for infectious mononucleosis than for bacterial tonsillitis.[w16] Antiviral treatment with aciclovir has been shown to significantly decrease the rate of oropharyngeal Epstein-Barr virus shedding.[w31] Some early trials found a significant positive overall effect in cases of infectious mononucleosis treated with aciclovir[w32] and that it was useful in severe cases, with airway compromise. However, a meta-analysis of five studies found no evidence to support its use in the acute setting: an improvement in oropharyngeal symptoms was observed in 25 out of 59 (42.4%) patients treated with aciclovir and in 18 out of 57 (31.6%) control patients (odd ratio 1.6, 95% confidence interval 0.7 to 3.6; P=0.23).[11] Other antiviral treatments such as valaciclovir and ganciclovir[w33] have shown some promise in the treatment of severe infectious mononucleosis and its complications and immunocompromised people. Two trials are in progress,[w2] but at present the routine use of both drugs is not advocated.[w34] Anaerobic antibacterial agents such as metronidazole have been suggested to hasten recovery in infectious mononucleosis by suppression of the oral anaerobic flora that contribute to the inflammatory process.[w35] This finding was borne out in some clinical studies,[w36-w41] with a recent randomised controlled trial showing the beneficial effects of metronidazole in severe infectious mononucleosis by shortening hospital stays.[12] Larger trials may be required before the use of metronidazole is routinely recommended.

Are steroids of use in the treatment of infectious mononucleosis?

Several early reports supported the use of corticosteroids in the treatment of infectious mononucleosis.[w42] Further trials showed these effects to be short lived, with no significant difference between the control and intervention arm.[w43] A Cochrane review was therefore undertaken, which concluded that there was insufficient evidence and the trials were too few, heterogeneous, and of poor quality to recommend steroid treatment for symptom control in glandular fever.[13] Another more recent Cochrane review concluded that corticosteroids increased the likelihood of both resolution and improvement of pain in participants with sore throat[14]; however, this review excluded publications on patients with a diagnosis of infectious mononucleosis. Steroid treatment should be considered in cases of airway emergency, in an attempt to temporise or preclude the need for intubation or tracheotomy.[w44] Despite these guidelines, the use of corticosteroids remains widespread on a day to day basis.[w45] Several reports have mentioned the adverse effects of corticosteroid use in infectious mononucleosis, including cases of peritonsillar cellulitis, acute onset diabetes mellitus, and neurological sequelae.[w46]

Does infectious mononucleosis lead to chronic fatigue syndrome?

Chronic fatigue syndrome is defined as severe fatigue and disabling musculoskeletal and cognitive symptoms without another explanation that lasts for at least six months and results in severe impairment in daily functioning.[w47] There has been much debate about the cause of this disorder. Some authors suggest that it is precipitated by an acute infection, such as infectious mononucleosis, as many patients relate the onset of their illness to an initial infection from which they never recovered.[w48] Prospective studies have reported an incidence of chronic fatigue syndrome of 7.3-12% in adults six months after infectious mononucleosis.[w49 w50] However, the relation between chronic fatigue syndrome and infectious mononucleosis is still questionable. A study of over 1300 patients diagnosed as having infectious mononucleosis by serology, found that although 10% of patients reported fatigue none fulfilled the criteria for chronic fatigue syndrome (table 2).[15] The cause of chronic fatigue syndrome is likely to be multifactorial. A trial that compared activity with imposed bed rest in the management of infectious mononucleosis found that those patients who were allowed out of bed as soon as they felt able reported a quicker recovery.[w52] A brief intervention at the time of diagnosis of infectious mononucleosis to allay fears of a prolonged disease may help to prevent the development of chronic fatigue syndrome.[w53] A recent editorial commented that chronic fatigue syndrome is unlikely to be a consequence of Epstein-Barr virus

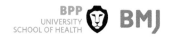

but a heterogeneous family of disorders arising from a constellation of pathophysiological causes.[16]

When is it safe to return to sports?

Splenomegaly, evident on ultrasonography if not on palpation, occurs in almost all cases of infectious mononucleosis, and the risk of splenic rupture has been well established.[w54] A considerable number of 15-21 year olds will have infectious mononucleosis every year,[w16] and many of this population will be involved in contact sports.[w55] Strenuous or contact sports (for example, football, gymnastics, rugby, hockey, lacrosse, wrestling, diving, and basketball) or activities associated with increased intra-abdominal pressure, such as weightlifting, may put athletes at most risk.[w56] Although recommendations of when to return to sport range from three,[w57] four,[w58] eight, and even up to 24 weeks,[w59] no clinical guidelines are specific to infectious mononucleosis. The incidence of splenic rupture is less than 1%[w15] and most occur in the initial three weeks of infectious mononucleosis, although cases have been described much later.[w60] Cases of spontaneous splenic rupture have also been described in the literature and doctors should have a high index of suspicion when abdominal pain is reported in the setting of infectious mononucleosis.[w61] A recent study involved weekly ultrasound examinations until resolution of splenomegaly. A mean increase in splenic length of 33.6% was observed, with a peak in enlargement on average 12.3 days from the onset of clinical symptoms. Most cases of splenomegaly had resolved by 4-6 weeks and there was a predictable rate of splenic regression of approximately 1% each day after reaching peak enlargement.[17] Similar results were reported in another paper, with normalisation of spleens at one month in 84% of participants.[w62] One study recommended that athletes wanting to return to contact sport at 3-4 weeks should have an ultrasound examination to ensure that the spleen had returned to normal size.[w62] A systematic review published in 2014 advocated individualised recommendations for athletes,[18] and future work in this area may concentrate on splenic volume to allow a more accurate assessment of splenomegaly and risk.

Is multiple sclerosis caused by infectious mononucleosis?

There is evidence that a history of infectious mononucleosis significantly increases the risk of multiple sclerosis[19] and that this association is far stronger than with other common childhood infections or afflictions.[w63] A meta-analysis concluded that the risk of multiple sclerosis seems to be greatest in those who were infected with Epstein-Barr virus at a later age (incidence begins to increase in adolescence, peaks around age 25 to 30 years, and declines to nearly zero by age 60) (thus developing infectious mononucleosis), with moderate risk for those infected with Epstein-Barr virus in early childhood, and close to zero risk in those not infected (fig 2).[19] A more recent meta-analysis showed that Epstein-Barr virus is present in 100% of cases of multiple sclerosis and therefore it has been suggested that the virus is not only a risk factor but also a prerequisite of multiple sclerosis.[w64] Whether the association between multiple sclerosis and Epstein-Barr virus demonstrates a causal relation is, however, strongly debated.[w64]

Although controversial, if proponents of the infectious mononucleosis-multiple sclerosis theory are correct, a vaccine against Epstein-Barr virus in theory could eradicate multiple sclerosis. In the only phase II trial of an Epstein-Barr virus vaccine in humans, rates of infectious mononucleosis

SOURCES AND SELECTION CRITERIA

We performed an electronic search through Medline, Scopus, Google Scholar, the Cochrane Database of Systematic Reviews, and the Cochrane central register of controlled trials using the search terms "infectious mononucleosis", "glandular fever", "Epstein-Barr virus", "corticosteroids", and "aciclovir". The search was limited to articles in English. We excluded studies carried out primarily on children. Priority was given to data from meta-analyses, reviews, and randomised controlled trials. Research on infectious mononucleosis was also given priority over articles exclusively relating to Epstein-Barr virus. We also examined guidelines produced by the US Center for Disease Control and Prevention and the UK National Institute for Health and Care Excellence, as well as clinical trials registries of the United States, United Kingdom, and European Union.[w1-w3]

ONGOING RESEARCH

- The use of splenic volume to assess splenomegaly in infectious mononucleosis (proposed)
- Anaerobic antibiotics in infectious mononucleosis (proposed)
- Vaccination against Epstein-Barr virus (proposed—unaware of any active research)
- The pathogenesis of multiple sclerosis (several studies listed on ClinicalTrials.gov)
- Molecular analysis of Epstein-Barr virus related tumours and the role of the virus in ontogenesis (multiple studies listed on ClinicalTrials.gov)

ADDITIONAL EDUCATIONAL RESOURCES

Resources for healthcare professionals

- Candy B, Hotopf M. Steroids for symptom control in infectious mononucleosis. *Cochrane Database Syst Rev* 2006;3:CD004402—a systematic review on the use of steroids in infectious mononucleosis
- Centre of Disease Control and Prevention. Guidelines on laboratory testing for Epstein-Barr virus and infectious mononucleosis (www.cdc.gov/epstein-barr/laboratory-testing.html)—the CDC's guidelines on diagnosing infectious mononucleosis. A thorough list of complications can be found at www.cdc.gov/epstein-barr/hcp.html
- NHS Clinical Knowledge Summaries on glandular fever (http://cks.nice.org.uk/glandular-fever)—a National Health Service resource on infectious mononucleosis
- BMJ best practice guidelines (http://bestpractice.bmj.com/best-practice/monograph/123.html—a helpful online resource from the *BMJ*

Resources for patients

- Medline plus. Infectious mononucleosis (www.nlm.nih.gov/medlineplus/infectiousmononucleosis.html#cat27)
- NHS Choices. Glandular fever (www.nhs.uk/conditions/Glandular-fever/Pages/Introduction.aspx)

TIPS FOR GENERAL PRACTITIONERS

General practitioners may see as many as 10 new cases of infectious mononucleosis a year.[w52] Although most patients will have mild symptoms, referral should be made to a secondary or tertiary centre in the following instances:

- Airway compromise
- Suspected splenic rupture
- Failure of supportive treatments (which may be indicated by the inability to swallow fluids or even saliva, and may occur in approximately 10% of patients)[w23]
- Immunosuppressed or post-transplant patients
- Patients with infectious mononucleosis but negative for Epstein-Barr virus antibodies

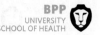

were reduced in adults who were seronegative for Epstein-Barr virus, but the vaccine did not affect the rate of Epstein-Barr virus infection.[w65] The development of a vaccine is challenging for several reasons, not least the long period between primary infection with Epstein-Barr virus and the development of many Epstein-Barr virus related tumours or multiple sclerosis.[20] To add further to the controversy it has been suggested that in lieu of a vaccine, a smaller, but still substantial, number of cases of multiple sclerosis could be prevented by exposing children to Epstein-Barr virus infection before adolescence.[19]

Is there an increased risk of lymphoma or other cancers after infectious mononucleosis?

The association of Epstein-Barr virus with malignancies such as Burkitt's lymphoma[w66] in children and nasopharyngeal carcinoma[w67] are well established. This review, however, focuses on patients presenting with infectious mononucleosis and it can be difficult to differentiate studies on Epstein-Barr virus and infectious mononucleosis about the risk of future malignancies. Two large Scandinavian cohort studies found a 2.55 to 2.83 times increased risk of Hodgkin's lymphoma in patients with a diagnosis of infectious mononucleosis by heterophile antibody tests.[21] [w68] The results were similar in a recent British record linkage paper, which found a 3.44 risk ratio of Hodgkin's lymphoma in the infectious mononucleosis cohort.[22] A review on Epstein-Barr virus related malignancies from 2014 commented that Hodgkin's lymphoma is the only Epstein-Barr virus related malignancy, other than nasopharyngeal carcinoma, for which there is a body of evidence accumulated over time that establishes a strong association.[w69] For other malignancies, a large prospective study found no clear association between a history of clinical infectious mononucleosis and risk of invasive breast cancer,[w70] and one of the cohort studies found that lung cancer was significantly less likely in the cohort with infectious mononucleosis.[w71]

Can infectious mononucleosis cause any complications?

Infectious mononucleosis in most cases resolves over a period of weeks, but may occasionally be exacerbated by a wide variety of complications. Neurological disorders may occur in 1-5% of patients.[w72] Theses include encephalitis, meningoencephalitis, seizures, optic neuritis, sudden sensorineural hearing loss, idiopathic facial palsy, and Guillain-Barré syndrome among others.[w73] Haematological complications are more common, in particular haemolytic anaemia (3%) and thrombocytopenia (25-50%),[w72] but also, rarely, aplastic anaemia, pancytopenia, and agranulocytosis. Other rare acute complications include myocarditis, pericarditits,[w74] pancreatitis, interstitial pneumonia, rhabdomyolysis, and psychological complications ("Alice in Wonderland" syndrome). The strength of association of infectious mononucleosis with many of these complications is based on scattered case reports, and the evidence of causation in many instances is unconvincing.[w72]

Contributors: PL carried out the literature review and was the main writer of the article. He is the lead author and will act as guarantor. MC suggested many of the topics, guided the writing of the review, and helped edit the manuscript. JEF conceived the review, was responsible for a large part of the design of the review, and helped edit the manuscript.

Competing interests: We have read and understood the BMJ policy on declaration of interests and declare the following: none.

Provenance and peer review: Commissioned; externally peer reviewed.

1 Hurt C, Tammaro D. Diagnostic evaluation of mononucleosis-like illnesses. Am J Med2007;120:911 e1-8.
2 Thorley-Lawson DA, Miyashita EM, Khan G. Epstein-Barr virus and the B cell: that's all it takes. Trends Microbiol1996;4:204-8.
3 Schuster V, Kreth HW. Epstein-Barr virus infection and associated diseases in children. I. Pathogenesis, epidemiology and clinical aspects. Eur J Pediatr1992;151:718-25.
4 Tattevin P, Le Tulzo Y, Minjolle S, et al. Increasing incidence of severe Epstein-Barr virus-related infectious mononucleosis: surveillance study. J Clin Microbiol2006;44:1873-4.
5 Macsween KF, Crawford DH. Epstein-Barr virus-recent advances. Lancet Infect Dis2003;3:131-40.
6 Hoagland RJ. Infectious mononucleosis. Prim Care1975;2:295-307.
7 Kofteridis DP, Koulentaki M, Valachis A, et al. Epstein Barr virus hepatitis. Eur J Intern Med2011;22:73-6.
8 Lennon P, O'Neill JP, Fenton JE, et al. Challenging the use of the lymphocyte to white cell count ratio in the diagnosis of infectious mononucleosis by analysis of a large cohort of Monospot test results. Clin Otolaryngol2010;35:397-401.
9 Centers for Disease Control and Prevention. Epstein-Barr virus and infectious mononucleosis, laboratory testing. 2014. www.cdc.gov/epstein-barr/laboratory-testing.html.
10 Vouloumanou EK, Rafailidis PI, Falagas ME. Current diagnosis and management of infectious mononucleosis. Curr Opin Haematol2012;19:14-20.
11 Torre D, Tambini R. Acyclovir for treatment of infectious mononucleosis: a meta-analysis. Scand J Infect Dis1999;31:543-7.
12 Lennon P, O'Neill JP, Fenton JE. Effect of metronidazole versus standard care on length of stay of patients admitted with severe infectious mononucleosis: a randomized controlled trial. Clin Microbiol Infect2014;20:O450-2.
13 Candy B, Hotopf M. Steroids for symptom control in infectious mononucleosis. Cochrane Database Syst Rev 2006;3:CD004402.
14 Hayward G, Thompson MJ, Perera R, et al. Corticosteroids as standalone or add-on treatment for sore throat. Cochrane Database Syst Rev2012;10:CD008268.
15 Petersen I, Thomas JM, Hamilton WT, et al. Risk and predictors of fatigue after infectious mononucleosis in a large primary-care cohort. Q J Med2006;99:49-55.
16 Chronic fatigue syndrome: going viral? Lancet2010;376:930.
17 Hosey RG, Kriss V, Uhl TL, et al. Ultrasonographic evaluation of splenic enlargement in athletes with acute infectious mononucleosis. Br J Sports Med2008;42:974-7.
18 Becker JA, Smith JA. Return to play after infectious mononucleosis. Sports Health2014;6:232-8.
19 Thacker EL, Mirzaei F, Ascherio A. Infectious mononucleosis and risk for multiple sclerosis: a meta-analysis. Ann Neurol2006;59:499-503.
20 Cohen JI, Fauci AS, Varmus H, et al. Epstein-Barr virus: an important vaccine target for cancer prevention. Sci Transl Med2011;3:107fs7.
21 Hjalgrim H, Smedby KE, Rostgaard K, et al. Infectious mononucleosis, childhood social environment, and risk of Hodgkin lymphoma. Cancer Res2007;67:2382-8.
22 Goldacre MJ, Wotton CJ, Yeates DG. Associations between infectious mononucleosis and cancer: record-linkage studies. Epidemiol Infect2009;137:672-80.

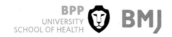

Multidrug resistant tuberculosis

James Millard, clinical lecturer in global health[1], Cesar Ugarte-Gil, epidemiologist[2],
David A J Moore, professor of infectious diseases & tropical medicine[3]

[1]Brighton and Sussex Medical
School, Brighton, UK

[2]Instituto de Medicina Tropical
Alexander von Humboldt,
Universidad Peruana Cayetano
Heredia, Lima, Peru; Department of
International Health, Johns Hopkins
Bloomberg School of Public Health,
Baltimore, USA

[3]TB Centre, London School of
Hygiene and Tropical Medicine,
London WC1E 7HT, UK

Correspondence to: D A J Moore
David.moore@lshtm.ac.uk

Cite this as: BMJ 2015;350:h882

DOI: 10.1136/bmj.h882

http://www.bmj.com/content/350/
bmj.h882

Tuberculosis remains a major cause of morbidity and mortality globally, with an estimated nine million people developing the disease and 1.5 million deaths in 2013; equating to 4100 deaths a day.[1] Nevertheless, considerable gains have been made in international tuberculosis control; incidence rates are decreasing (albeit slowly) and mortality has been reduced by 45% worldwide. The advent of multidrug resistant tuberculosis threatens this progress. In this review we detail the challenges faced globally in the diagnosis, treatment, and control of multidrug resistant tuberculosis and why this matters to high and low burden multidrug resistant tuberculosis settings alike.

What is multidrug resistant tuberculosis?

Rifampicin and isoniazid form the backbone of conventional first line treatment for tuberculosis. Multidrug resistant tuberculosis refers to tuberculosis that is resistant to both rifampicin and isoniazid. This classification is important because treatment outcomes for this group of patients are far worse than for patients with fully drug susceptible or lesser forms of drug resistant tuberculosis.[1][2] Multidrug resistant tuberculosis with additional resistance to any fluoroquinolone (such as ofloxacin or moxifloxacin) and also any one of the three second line injectable agents (amikacin, capreomycin, kanamycin) is designated as extensively drug resistant tuberculosis.

How common is it?

"Missing" patients are a major problem in assessing the burden of tuberculosis globally.[1] Without access to universal drug susceptibility testing, national tuberculosis programmes have to estimate burden by extrapolation from periodic national or subnational surveys. This generates the global estimate of 480 000 cases of multidrug resistant tuberculosis in 2013 (range 350 000-610 000), of which 9% have extensively drug resistant tuberculosis. Out of the estimated 480 000 cases of multidrug resistant tuberculosis in 2013, only 136 000 were reported to the World Health Organization.[1] Globally, the main barrier to diagnosis is the lack of access to drug susceptibility testing in quality assured laboratories. Even among bacteriologically confirmed cases of tuberculosis, few were tested for multidrug resistant tuberculosis, with particularly low levels in the African and South East Asia regions.[1] In the United Kingdom, where all patients with tuberculosis undergo drug susceptibility testing and ascertainment is therefore believed to be almost complete, the reported number of cases remains small but increased from 28 to 81 per year from 2000 to 2012.[3]

What is the prognosis?

An estimated 210 000 deaths (range 130 000-290 000) occur from multidrug resistant tuberculosis worldwide each year, as a consequence of never being diagnosed, the gap between diagnosis and treatment, and poor treatment outcomes. Worldwide, fewer than half of cases achieve treatment success.[1] In the United Kingdom more than 70% of patients with multidrug resistant tuberculosis achieve treatment success, but it has been shown that it is possible to achieve comparable (or even better) outcomes, even in low income settings.[4]

Who is at risk of multidrug resistant tuberculosis?

All patients with tuberculosis should undergo drug susceptibility testing because only testing those perceived to be at risk will miss up to half of multidrug resistant cases.[1] Nevertheless, it is clear that multidrug resistant tuberculosis is more common in some groups, such as the former prison inmate in the example (box 1). In all settings patients who have previously been treated for tuberculosis are at higher risk for multidrug resistant tuberculosis, with recent estimates suggesting that 3.5% of new cases and 20.5% of previously treated cases have multidrug resistant tuberculosis.[1] However, rates of multidrug resistant tuberculosis vary considerably between countries and regions (table) with 27 high burden countries accounting for more than 85% of cases. Worldwide, China, India, and the Russian Federation contribute the largest total number of cases. However, the highest proportions are found in eastern Europe and Central Asia, with around 20% of new cases and 50% of previously treated cases having multidrug resistant tuberculosis. In countries with a high burden of tuberculosis such as South Africa, even a relatively low percentage of multidrug resistant tuberculosis among the large number of cases translates into a high incidence rate when expressed as cases of multidrug resistant tuberculosis per 100 000 population per year.

In the United Kingdom 1.4% of new and 5.7% of previously treated patients have multidrug resistant tuberculosis, with 89% of these patients being born outside the United Kingdom (45% from South Asia, 19% from eastern Europe and 19% from Sub-Saharan Africa).[5] The proportion of multidrug resistant tuberculosis in UK cases of tuberculosis in 2013 did not exceed 6% in most groups. Strikingly, however, for people born in eastern Europe it was over 24%.[4]

Once drug resistance develops the possibility of transmission to other people emerges, with up to half of multidrug resistant tuberculosis cases arising in this way.[1][3]

THE BOTTOM LINE

- Multidrug resistant tuberculosis refers to tuberculosis with resistance to at least rifampicin and isoniazid
- Multidrug resistant tuberculosis is increasingly common; however, there is a large shortfall between the estimated total number of cases and the numbers diagnosed and treated
- Diagnosis is hampered by lack of access to quality assured diagnostics, although newer, rapid molecular and phenotypic methods may go some way to improving this situation
- Compared with drug susceptible tuberculosis, treatment for multidrug resistant tuberculosis requires the use of drug regimens that are prolonged (18-24 months), less efficacious, and noticeably more toxic; new drugs and regimens are becoming available for the first time in decades and ongoing trials should define how best they should be used
- Worldwide, treatment success is only around 50%; however, several settings, including some low income countries, have proved that higher success rates are achievable

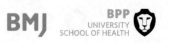

Incidence of tuberculosis and multidrug resistant tuberculosis in selected countries in 2013

Selected countries	No of new cases		% (95% CI) of cases with multidrug resistant tuberculosis	
	Tuberculosis	Multidrug resistant tuberculosis	Newly diagnosed	Retreatment
High burden,* high resistance:†				
Russian Federation	130 000	41 000	19 (14 to 25)	49 (40 to 59)
China	980 000	54 2000	5.7 (4.5 to 7)	26 (22 to 30)
India	2 100 000	61 000	2.2 (1.9 to 2.6)	15 (11 to 19)
South Africa	450 000	6800	1.8 (1.4 to 2.3)	6.7 (5.4 to 8.2)
Non-high burden, high resistance:†				
Belarus	65 000	1790	35 (33 to 37)	55 (52 to 57)
Ukraine	44 000	9400	14 (14 to 15)	32 (31 to 33)
Non-high burden, non-high resistance:				
Peru	38 000	2050	3.9 (3.6 to 4.2)	35 (33 to 37)
United Kingdom	8300	69	1.4 (1 to 1.7)	5.7 (3.2 to 9.4)
United States	11 000	108	1.2 (0.98 to 1.6)	3.9 (1.9 to 7.1)

*22 Countries with highest number of cases of tuberculosis.

†27 Countries with highest number of cases of multidrug resistant tuberculosis.

BOX 1 AN EXAMPLE OF HOW MULTIDRUG RESISTANT TUBERCULOSIS MIGHT PRESENT

A 40 year old man, originally from the Russian Federation and now resident in London, presented to the emergency department of his local hospital with a history of dry cough, fever, and night sweats for several months. His medical history was unremarkable and he had never previously received treatment for tuberculosis. He had spent two years in a Russian prison three years previously. His chest radiograph revealed patchy shadowing in the right upper lobe with several cavities. Sputum was positive for acid fast bacilli and he was prescribed standard first line quadruple tuberculosis treatment as an outpatient, with a combination of rifampicin and isoniazid, pyrazinamide, and ethambutol. Despite this, his symptoms remained and five weeks later the results of a sputum culture confirmed *Mycobacterium tuberculosis* with resistance to rifampicin and isoniazid.

[6][7] In addition, in high incidence settings where reinfection is common, an unknown fraction of previously treated people with tuberculosis will have been infected by multidrug resistant tuberculosis unrelated to their previous infection and thus transmission rates are likely to be systematically underestimated. Other risk factors for multidrug resistant tuberculosis may include being a household contact of a known infected person, younger age, and (putatively) the strain type of tuberculosis.[8][9]

How is it diagnosed?

The diagnosis of multidrug resistant tuberculosis is based on the detection of resistance to rifampicin and isoniazid in the causative organism in a clinical sample, usually sputum. The quality and quantity of the sputum sample can affect test performance.[10] An increasing array of new tools for the diagnosis of multidrug resistance has become available in recent years, for the detection of either phenotypic (growth based) or genotypic (molecular markers) resistance. The use of specific tests in different regions is heterogeneous and most regions will use several different tests in combination.

Phenotypic indirect drug susceptibility testing

Conventional phenotypic tests use methods of indirect drug susceptibility testing. This requires an isolate to be cultured first and then inoculated into solid or liquid media. This leads to a considerable delay until results are available, often several months, therefore results are often not available in a clinically useful timeframe. Automated systems such as the Mycobacteria Growth Indicator Tube 960 (MGIT 960, Becton Dickinson Microbiology Systems, Sparks, MD) speed up culture times through the use of liquid media and automated sensing of culture positivity, but still require subsequent indirect sensitivity testing. High throughput is a major advantage although tempered by relatively high cost and contamination rates.

Phenotypic direct drug susceptibility testing

Phenotypic direct drug susceptibility testing delivers a result direct from inoculation of the sputum sample thus does not need to be subcultured. Samples are inoculated into media containing drugs at specific critical concentrations such that the presence of growth (whether detected by a colour change or visual identification of microscopic growth) is indicative of phenotypic resistance.[11][12] These methods are rapid, non-commercial, and low cost making them well suited to resource constrained settings with a high burden of tuberculosis.[13] Tests endorsed by WHO include microscopic observation drug susceptibility (MODS) and the nitrate reductase assay.

Genotypic drug susceptibility testing

Genotypic methods test for the presence of known resistance mutations associated with multidrug resistant tuberculosis. Two types of geneotypic assay have been endorsed by WHO: molecular beacon assays and line probe hybridisation assays.

WHO has endorsed the use of the molecular beacon assay Xpert MTB/RIF (Cepheid, Sunnyvale, CA) as an initial diagnostic test where multidrug resistant tuberculosis is common.[14] This test is a real time polymerase chain reaction that detects *Mycobacterium tuberculosis* and rifampicin resistance (by identification of mutations in the mycobacterial *rpoB* gene). It is performed directly on sputum, with a turnaround time of two hours, which is a key advantage. Identification of resistance to rifampicin still necessitates subsequent and more extensive drug susceptibility testing of other first line and second line agents, usually by phenotypic (culture based) methods. There are concerns about false negative and false positives test results for rifampicin resistance[15] and the increased frequency of mixed infections in high prevalence settings,[16] so local evaluation of multidrug resistant tuberculosis epidemiology before rollout may be prudent. The higher cost of the test compared with phenotypic testing is also a constraint, particularly since isoniazid susceptibility testing is not assessed. Costs range from $10 (£6; €9) (for low income countries) for each test, to more than $70.[17] [18]

An alternative molecular test platform endorsed by WHO is the line probe assay.[19] This assay exists in two main commercial forms—the INNO-LipA Rif.TB (Fujirebio Europe, Ghent, Belgium), which detects rifampicin resistance, and Genotype MTBDRplus (Hain Lifescience, Nehren, Germany), which identifies rifampicin (through detection of mutations in the rpoB gene) and isoniazid resistance (mutations in the katG and inhA genes).[20] It is performed on cultured isolates or on smear positive sputum samples,[21] and a version is now available (genotype MTBDRsl), although not yet endorsed by WHO, for fluoroquinolone, aminoglycoside, and ethambutol drug susceptibility testing.[22]

As whole genome sequencing becomes increasingly affordable and accessible, the horizon holds potential promise of a single technology that could be utilised simultaneously to detect genotypic resistance to rifampicin and isoniazid and key second line drugs—although some work is needed to characterise a full library of resistance conferring mutations. A useful byproduct of sequencing in this way would be the molecular epidemiological insights yielded into the contribution of transmission (as opposed to reactivation of latent multidrug resistant tuberculosis infection) in different settings.[23]

How is it treated?

Of the 136 000 patients with multidrug resistant tuberculosis reported in 2013, just over 71% (97 000) began treatment.[1] This treatment gap is heterogeneous between countries, with fewer than half of eligible patients enrolled in treatment in the African region. However, these numbers seem to represent progress, particularly in India, Russia, and South Africa, with a more than 150% increase in enrolment to treatment since 2009.[1] Achieving the goal of universal access to the diagnosis and treatment of multidrug resistant tuberculosis requires the strengthening of health services in general. Simply improving rates of treatment initiation in a poor programme is likely to be ineffective and may increase rates of drug resistance and promote transmission.[24]

Recommended drug regimens

Currently recommended treatment for multidrug resistant tuberculosis requires 18-24 months of at least five drugs, none of which are as potent as rifampicin or isoniazid and all of which are more toxic and less well tolerated. Countries with access to quality assured drug susceptibility testing for second line drugs are likely to offer an "individualised" regimen tailored to a patient's resistance pattern. Countries without this facility are likely to offer a "standardised" regimen, which is broadly similar for all patients and based on historical resistance patterns and which drugs have been used in that region. Even in the context of individualised regimens, initial treatment is often empirical (and based on similar principles to standardised treatment), pending second line drug susceptibility testing.[25]

Multidrug resistant tuberculosis should be treated with an injectable agent such as amikacin, kanamycin, or capreomycin (streptomycin is usually not used because of high rates of resistance), a fluoroquinolone (levofloxacin, moxifloxacin, or gatifloxacin are recommended), and at least three other agents with probable activity (ethionamide

or prothionamide, cycloserine, para-aminosalicylic acid). First line agents (that is, pyrazindamide and ethambutol) with retained activity can also be used.

Ideally the injectable agent is administered daily for the first 6-8 months, forming an "intensive phase" of treatment, with the other drugs then continued, forming a "continuation phase."[25] In practice, adverse effects often supervene (see example in box 2) and require stopping the injectable agent, managing side effects or swapping drugs for remaining alternatives.

BOX 2 EXAMPLE OF HOW DRUG SIDE EFFECTS CAN AFFECT TREATMENT

After the symptoms of a 26 year old Swazi woman failed to respond to two months of first line tuberculosis treatment (isoniazid, rifampicin, ethambutol, pyrazinamide) she underwent drug susceptibility testing and was found to have multidrug resistant tuberculosis. Treatment was started with moxifloxacin, kanamycin, ethionamide, and cycloserine, and she continued with pyrazinamide. Early substitution of cycloserine, to which her unbearable initial low mood and irritability was attributed, with para-aminosalicylate sodium replaced neuropsychiatric side effects with profuse diarrhoea. The onset of aminoglycoside induced hearing loss and the prospect of going deaf led to the patient discontinuing treatment after completing only four of 18 months of the regimen.

Challenges to management

Managing the side effects of treatment forms an important part of management and a failure to do so can affect adherence and drive the development of further resistance. Particularly common side effects include local injection site complications, ototoxicity, and nephrotoxicity from the injectable agents; neuropsychiatric symptoms and seizures with cycloserine; and diarrhoea with para-aminosalicylate sodium. Hypothyroidism can occur with ethionamide or prothionamide or para-aminosalicylic acid. Drug induced hepatitis is not uncommon, particularly in association with pyrazinamide. Delivery and monitoring of the drug regimens is complex, and drug stockouts are common and undermine efforts. All regimens are based on cohort data and expert opinion, with a conspicuous absence of randomised controlled trial evidence to inform treatment. However, the available evidence does suggest better outcomes for patients treated with a later generation quinolone, ethionamide or prothionamide, four or more effective drugs in the intensive phase, and three or more effective drugs in the continuation phase.[26] Extensively drug resistant tuberculosis treatment is even more challenging and often relies on drugs with only in vitro or animal data to support their use.

Emerging treatments

For the first time in over 40 years new antituberculosis drugs are becoming available; notably delamanid and bedaquiline, both of which already have a compassionate use role in difficult to treat multidrug resistant tuberculosis and extensively drug resistant tuberculosis. Furthermore there is renewed interest in the efficacy of clofazamine and linezolid. However, an urgent need remains for better regimens rather than new single drugs, and for this reason a handful of phase III trials are in progress. Promising results have been reported with the use of a nine month regimen in Bangladesh and several West African countries, which is now being formally tested in a randomised controlled trial.[27] One view is that some regimens under investigation

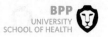

may ultimately be effective for all strains of tuberculosis whether or not susceptible to rifampicin or isoniazid, which would considerably attenuate the importance of the notion of multidrug resistant tuberculosis in global tuberculosis.

What is the role of palliative care?

Some patients with multidrug resistant tuberculosis will, despite apparently adequate treatment, fail to respond and require palliative care. This is particularly a problem for patients with extensively drug resistant tuberculosis. Moreover, there are increasing reports of patients with no treatment options. Only 11 countries with a high burden of multidrug resistant tuberculosis (South Africa the only one outside Europe) reported palliative care facilities as part of their national tuberculosis plan.[1] In high burden countries such as South Africa, where resources for home based palliative care are limited, it has even been suggested that modern day sanatoriums may provide access to palliative care on a large scale, while potentially reducing onward transmission.[28] However this approach has drawn criticism in equal measure, in part because the impact of reducing onward transmission by that stage is likely to be small, and because of potential risks from worsening stigma.[29]

What are the public health implications?

In addition to the complexities of individual case management, there are major public health implications to multidrug resistant tuberculosis. Most transmission is likely to occur before treatment and hence earlier diagnosis is a key determinant in the control of multidrug resistant tuberculosis. There is unlikely to be sufficient bed capacity for full scale-up of hospital based treatment for multidrug resistant tuberculosis and there is increasing evidence for ambulatory, community based treatment that may also reduce the risk of transmission within healthcare settings. Where inpatient admission is required, triage systems, strict infection control practices, building design for improved ventilation (including natural ventilation), and upper room (away from patients and staff) germicidal ultraviolet light all have an important role in reducing transmission. Moreover, in other key transmission hotspots (for example, prisons) there is a need for active intervention to identify cases and reduce transmission.[7]

What are the future directions?

Until relatively recently few national, international, or non-governmental organisations had prioritised multidrug resistant tuberculosis, with a focus instead on drug susceptible tuberculosis.[6] Now multidrug resistant tuberculosis forms a key part in the STOP TB Global Plan to Stop TB 2011-15[30] and has garnered attention at the highest international levels with a World Health Assembly resolution (WHA 62.15) calling on WHO members to provide universal access to multidrug resistant tuberculosis treatment. The STOP TB target is for all patients with newly diagnosed tuberculosis at high risk for multidrug resistance and all previously treated patients to undergo drug susceptibility testing.[30] Achieving global control of multidrug resistant tuberculosis requires timely identification of cases, enrolment into quality assured treatment with relatively short, inexpensive, non-toxic treatment, minimisation of transmission, and accurate epidemiological surveillance. Unfortunately, there are major challenges to achieving each of these steps.

SOURCES AND SELECTION CRITERIA

We searched Medline, Embase, and Scielo with the terms "MDR TB", "Tuberculosis, Multidrug-Resistant". We also reviewed the World Health Organization Global Tuberculosis Report 2014 and other national tuberculosis programme reports. We included data from systematic reviews/meta-analyses, randomised controlled trials, and good quality observational studies focused on multidrug resistant tuberculosis.

ADDITIONAL EDUCATIONAL RESOURCES

Resources for healthcare professionals

- World Health Organization. Multidrug resistant tuberculosis website (www.who.int/tb/challenges/mdr/en/)—Contains several resources, including clinical and programmatic guidelines
- *Lancet Infectious Diseases* March-June 2013—Series of papers covering key areas in tuberculosis, with particular relevance for multidrug resistant tuberculosis

Resources for patients

- Centres for Disease Control. Tuberculosis fact sheet (www.cdc.gov/tb/publications/factsheets/drtb/mdrtb.htm)—Provides information on multidrug resistant tuberculosis

Contributors: All authors contributed equally to the writing and reviewing of all versions of this manuscript. DAJM is the guarantor.

Competing interests: We have read and understood the BMJ policy on declaration of interests and declare the following interests: none.

Provenance and peer review: Commissioned; externally peer reviewed.

1 World Health Organization. Global tuberculosis report 2014. WHO, 2014.
2 Sullivan T, Ben Amor Y. What's in a name? The future of drug-resistant tuberculosis classification. *Lancet Infect Dis* 2013;13:373-6.
3 Anderson LF, Tamne S, Brown T, Watson J, Mullarkey C, Zenner D, et al. Transmission of multidrug-resistant tuberculosis in the UK: a cross-sectional molecular and epidemiological study of clustering and contact tracing. *Lancet Infect Dis* 2014;14:406-15.
4 Furin J, Bayona J, Becerra M, Farmer P, Golubkov A, Hurtado R, et al. Programmatic management of multidrug-resistant tuberculosis: models from three countries. *Int J Tuberc Lung Dis* 2011;15:1294-300.
5 Health Protection Agency. Tuberculosis in the UK 2013 report. HPA, 2013.
6 Keshavjee S, Farmer PE. Tuberculosis, drug resistance, and the history of modern medicine. *N Engl J Med* 2012;367:931-6.
7 Nardell E, Dharmadhikari A. Turning off the spigot: reducing drug-resistant tuberculosis transmission in resource-limited settings. *Int J Tuberc Lung Dis* 2010;14:1233-43.
8 Caminero JA. Multidrug-resistant tuberculosis: epidemiology, risk factors and case finding. *Int J Tuberc Lung Dis* 2010;14:382-90.
9 Faustini A, Hall AJ, Perucci CA. Risk factors for multidrug resistant tuberculosis in Europe: a systematic review. *Thorax* 2006;61:158-63.
10 Peter JG, Theron G, Pooran A, Thomas J, Pascoe M, Dheda K. Comparison of two methods for acquisition of sputum samples for diagnosis of suspected tuberculosis in smear-negative or sputum-scarce people: a randomised controlled trial. *Lancet Resp Med* 2013;1:471-8.
11 Martin A, Panaiotov S, Portaels F, Hoffner S, Palomino JC, Angeby K. The nitrate reductase assay for the rapid detection of isoniazid and rifampicin resistance in *Mycobacterium tuberculosis* : a systematic review and meta-analysis. *J Antimicrob Chemother* 2008;62:56-64.
12 Moore DA, Evans CA, Gilman RH, Caviedes L, Coronel J, Vivar A. Microscopic-observation drug-susceptibility assay for the diagnosis of TB. *N Engl J Med* 2006;355:1539-50.
13 World Health Organization. Noncommercial culture and drug-susceptibility testing methods for screening patients at risk for multidrug-resistant tuberculosis: policy statement. WHO, 2011.
14 World Health Organization. Automated real-time nucleic acid amplification technology for rapid and simultaneous detection of tuberculosis and rifampicin resistance: Xpert MTB/RIF assay for the diagnosis of pulmonary and extrapulmonary TB in adults and children. Policy update. WHO, 2013.
15 Somoskovi A, Deggim V, Ciardo D, Bloemberg GV. Diagnostic implications of inconsistent results obtained with the Xpert MTB/Rif assay in detection of *Mycobacterium tuberculosis* isolates with an rpoB mutation associated with low-level rifampin resistance. *J Clin Microbiol* 2013;51:3127-9.
16 Zetola NM, Shin SS, Tumedi KA, Moeti K, Ncube R, Nicol M, et al. Mixed *Mycobacterium tuberculosis* complex infections and false-negative results for rifampin resistance by GeneXpert MTB/RIF are associated with poor clinical outcomes. *J Clin Microbiol* 2014;52:2422-9.

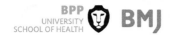

17 Choi HW, Miele K, Dowdy D, Shah M. Cost-effectiveness of Xpert(R) MTB/RIF for diagnosing pulmonary tuberculosis in the United States. *Int J Tuberc Lung Dis* 2013;17(10):1328-35.

18 FIND. Price for Xpert® MTB/RIF and FIND country list. Secondary price for Xpert® MTB/RIF and FIND country list 2013. www.finddiagnostics. org/about/what_we_do/successes/find-negotiated-prices/xpert_mtb_rif.html.

19 World Health Organization. Tuberculosis diagnostics fact sheet. Secondary tuberculosis diagnostics fact sheet. www.who.int/tb/publications/tbDiagnostics_factsheet.pdf?ua=1.

20 Hillemann D, Rusch-Gerdes S, Richter E. Evaluation of the GenoType MTBDRplus assay for rifampin and isoniazid susceptibility testing of *Mycobacterium tuberculosis* strains and clinical specimens. *J Clin Microbiol* 2007;45:2635-40.

21 Raizada N, Sachdeva KS, Chauhan DS, Malhotra B, Reddy K, Dave PV, et al. A multi-site validation in India of the line probe assay for the rapid diagnosis of multi-drug resistant tuberculosis directly from sputum specimens. *PLoS One* 2014;9:e88626.

22 Barnard M, Gey van Pittius NC, van Helden PD, Bosman M, Coetzee G, Warren RM. The diagnostic performance of the GenoType MTBDRplus version 2 line probe assay is equivalent to that of the Xpert MTB/RIF assay. *J Clin Microbiol* 2012;50:3712-6.

23 Koser CU, Bryant JM, Becq J, Török ME, Ellington MJ, Marti-Renom MA, et al. Whole-genome sequencing for rapid susceptibility testing of *M. tuberculosis*. *N Engl J Med* 2013;369:290-2.

24 Chiang CY, Van Deun A, Enarson DA. A poor drug-resistant tuberculosis programme is worse than no programme: time for a change. *Int J Tuberc Lung Dis* 2013;17:714-8.

25 World Health Organization. Guidelines for the programmatic management of drug-resistant tuberculosis 2011. http://whqlibdoc. who.int/publications/2011/9789241501583_eng.pdf.

26 Ahuja SD, Ashkin D, Avendano M, Banerjee R, Bauer M, Bayona JN, et al. Multidrug resistant pulmonary tuberculosis treatment regimens and patient outcomes: an individual patient data meta-analysis of 9,153 patients. *PLoS Med* 2012;9:e1001300.

27 Van Deun A, Maug AK, Salim MA, Das PK, Sarker MR, Daru P, et al. Short, highly effective, and inexpensive standardized treatment of multidrug-resistant tuberculosis. *Am J Resp Crit Care Med* 2010;182:684-92.

28 Dheda K, Migliori GB. The global rise of extensively drug-resistant tuberculosis: is the time to bring back sanatoria now overdue? *Lancet* 2012;379:773-5.

29 Hughes J, Cox H, Ford N. Sanatoria for drug-resistant tuberculosis: an outdated response. *Lancet* 2012;379:2148.

30 Stop TB Partnership. The global plan to stop TB 2011-2015: transforming the fight towards elimination of tuberculosis. WHO, 2010.

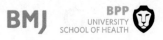

Actinomycosis

V K Wong, specialist registrar in microbiology[1], T D Turmezei, specialist registrar in radiology[2], V C Weston, consultant in microbiology[1]

[1]Queen's Medical Centre, Nottingham NG7 2UH, UK

[2]Addenbrooke's Hospital, Cambridge, UK

Correspondence to: V K Wong
vanessawong@doctors.org.uk

Cite this as: BMJ 2011;343:d6099

DOI: 10.1136/bmj.d6099

http://www.bmj.com/content/343/bmj.d6099

Actinomycosis is a rare, chronic, and slowly progressive granulomatous disease caused by filamentous Gram positive anaerobic bacteria from the Actinomycetaceae family (genus *Actinomyces*).[1] It is often misdiagnosed because it can mimic other conditions such as malignancy and tuberculosis,[2] and a high level of clinical suspicion is needed for an early diagnosis. However, it is readily treatable and curable if the patient is appropriately managed. We review the clinical presentations of actinomycosis, its diagnosis, and approaches to treatment. Our review is based on the findings of randomised controlled trials, prospective analytical and retrospective studies, review articles, and case reports.

How is actinomycosis acquired?

Actinomyces are commensals of the human oropharynx, gastrointestinal tract, and urogenital tract. When tissue integrity is breached through a mucosal lesion they can invade local structures and organs and become pathogenic. Actinomycosis is therefore mainly an endogenous infection.[3] Actinomyces are often isolated with other normal commensals, such as *Aggregatibacter actinomycetemcomitans* (previously *Actinobacillus actinomycetemcomitans*), *Eikenella corrodens*, fusobacteria, bacteroides, capnocytophaga, staphylococci (including *S aureus*), streptococci (including β haemolytic streptococci and *S pneumoniae*), or Enterobacteriaceae, but the precise pattern of organisms depends on the site of infection.[4] Animal studies have suggested that these species help actinomyces establish an infection by inhibiting host defences, although their exact roles are not clear.[W1 W2]

How common is it and who gets it?

Anyone can be infected with actinomyces, but the disease is essentially rare—because of a lack of data, particularly in developing countries, estimates of its incidence are not recent. In the 1970s the incidence in Cleveland, USA, was reported to be one per 300 000, compared with Germany and the Netherlands in the 1960s where it was estimated to be one per million.[1] The Department of Health in the United Kingdom reported that 0.0006% of hospital consultations (71 in total) were for actinomycosis in England between 2002 and 2003.[W3] The incidence of all forms of actinomycosis is thought to have declined in recent years, especially in developed countries as a result of better oral hygiene and susceptibility to a broad range of antibiotics.[1]

A large case series from 1975 found that men were three times more likely to be infected than women,[5] although pelvic actinomycosis mainly affects women who have intrauterine contraceptive devices (IUDs).[6] The authors of another case series suggested that the higher prevalence in men might be explained by poorer oral hygiene and higher rates of oral trauma in men from fistfights, although this has not been substantiated.[7] A 2005 review noted that although actinomycosis affects immunocompromised people, most reported cases have been in immunocompetent people.[8] The components of the immune response that are crucial in the control of actinomycosis and the specific effects (if any) of immunocompromise on the incidence of infection are unclear.[1] Box 1 summarises the risk factors associated with actinomycosis.

How does it present?

Actinomycosis is classified into distinct clinical forms according to the anatomical site infected: orocervicofacial, thoracic, abdominopelvic, central nervous system, musculoskeletal, and disseminated. Of the more than 30 species, *A israelii* is the most common human pathogen and is found in most clinical presentations, but certain species have been linked to particular clinical syndromes. For example, in one study of 1997 cases, *A israelii* and *A gerencseriae* comprised almost 70% of orocervicofacial infections.[11] Less common species include *A naeslundii*, *A odontolyticus*, *A viscosus*, *A meyeri*, *A turicensis*, and *A radingae*.[3 4]

Orocervicofacial actinomycosis is the most common form of the disease and comprises about 50% of all reported cases.[5] It usually follows dental manipulation or trauma to the mouth, although it can arise spontaneously in patients with poor dental hygiene.[W4] Common presenting features include fever and chronic painless or painful soft tissue swelling of the perimandibular region, from which sinus tracts can develop over time.[12] Lesions may develop a firm woody consistency that often leads to a misdiagnosis of malignancy. Regional lymphadenopathy is typically absent until later stages.[8] Infection may also extend into local structures such as bone and muscle. In a retrospective study of 317 patients with cervicofacial actinomycosis, bone infection (periostitis and osteomyelitis) developed in 11.7% of cases.[12] One case study reported involvement of the muscles of mastication, which led to chewing difficulties and trismus.[W5]

Thoracic actinomycosis accounts for 15-20% of cases.[5 13] Infection normally results from aspiration of oropharyngeal secretions, but it can also occur after oesophageal perforation, local spread from cervicofacial or abdominal infection, or from haematogenous spread.[3] A higher incidence has been reported in patients with underlying

---

SUMMARY POINTS

- Although rare, a high level of clinical suspicion is needed to diagnose and cure actinomycosis in patients with indolent, unresolving, or relapsing chronic inflammatory disease
- Actinomyces are commensals that become pathogenic when the mucosa is breached, and co-infection with other organisms is common
- Disease is defined by anatomical location; orocervicofacial disease is the most common, followed by thoracic and abdominopelvic disease
- A mass characteristically enlarges across tissue planes and local tissue invasion may lead to the formation of sinus tracts that can spontaneously heal and recur
- Actinomycosis often mimics other infections and malignancy—clinically and radiologically
- It is generally treated with long term antibiotics, usually penicillin, but surgery may be needed

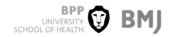

BOX 1 RISK FACTORS ASSOCIATED WITH THE ACQUISITION OF ACTINOMYCES

- Age 20-60 years[9]
- Male sex (except for pelvic actinomycosis, which mainly affects women)[5 6]
- Diabetes[w43 w44]

Immunosuppression

- Steroids[w45]
- Bisphosphonates[w46]
- Leukaemia with chemotherapy[w47 w48]
- HIV[w49]
- Lung and renal transplant receipt[w50 w51]
- Alcoholism[w13 w52]
- Local tissue damage caused by trauma, recent surgery, irradiation[10]

lung disorders, such as emphysema, chronic bronchitis, and bronchiectasis, but the reported series are small.[10 13] Actinomyces are thought to colonise devitalised tissues, which are common in these conditions,[13] although another study reported that actinomycosis did not seem to be caused by the underlying lung disease.[w6] Diagnosis and treatment can be even more challenging if there is coexistent lung disease such as tuberculosis or malignancy.[w7 w8] Initially the clinical picture may be that of pneumonia with a low grade fever, cough, shortness of breath, and chest pain. However, there is usually a longer history of illness and associated weight loss and haemoptysis.[14]

Complications such as empyema necessitans (a rare complication of empyema in which the pleural infection spreads to affect the soft tissues of the chest wall),[w9] pleural effusion,[w10] mediastinal invasion,[w11] and rib destruction[w12] have been reported. Mediastinal disease can progress into the heart, with the most common presentation here being pericarditis.[w13 w14] Myocarditis and endocarditis occur less often, either via extension from the pericardium or by haematogenous spread.[w15 w16]

Abdominopelvic actinomycosis makes up about 20% of cases.[5] Patients who have had acute appendicitis, particularly with perforation, account for most (65%) cases and can present with a right iliac fossa mass.[w17 w18] Other predisposing factors include gastrointestinal perforation, previous surgery, neoplasia, and foreign bodies in the gastrointestinal tract or genitourinary tract, with or without erosion through the mucosal barrier.[15] These infections can be difficult to diagnose because patients may present with non-specific symptoms such as fever, weight loss, and abdominal pain. There may not always be a palpable mass,[16 w19] and fewer than 10% of cases are diagnosed preoperatively.[w20] Infection can spread directly into neighbouring tissues, and sinus tracts may form into the abdominal wall or the perianal region.[1]

Although abdominal disease can spread directly into the pelvis, pelvic actinomycosis is predominantly associated with intrauterine contraceptive devices.[6 16] Patients usually present with a history of prolonged use (>2 years) and symptoms of fever, vaginal discharge, pelvic or abdominal pain, and weight loss.[6 17 18] Although the use of such devices is strongly correlated with intra-abdominal actinomycosis, the duration of use needed to increase the risk of developing infection is not known.[16]

Rare sites of actinomycosis include the central nervous system, bones, muscle tissue, and prosthetic joints. Central nervous system infection usually arises from haematogenous

spread or direct extension of orocervicofacial infection. In one study, the distribution of presentations of 70 cases of central nervous system disease was: brain abscess (67%), meningitis or meningoencephalitis (13%), actinomycoma (7%), subdural empyema (6%), and epidural abscess (6%).[19] For non-meningitic infection, the clinical picture was usually that of a space occupying lesion with symptoms of headache and focal neurological signs related to the anatomical site of disease.

Musculoskeletal infections are usually caused by spread from adjacent soft tissue (75% of cases), but can also be from local trauma (19%) or haematogenous spread (3%).[20] The facial bones, especially the mandible, are the most common sites of bone disease.[12] Actinomycotic infections of hip and knee prostheses have been described, with early presentation suggesting introduction of the organism perioperatively, and late presentation usually indicating haematogenous spread from an extra-articular site.[w21 w22]

Although all species of actinomyces are capable of haematogenous spread, disseminated actinomycosis is exceedingly rare since the development of antibiotics. *A meyeri*, *A israeli*, and *A odontolyticus* are most commonly associated with this clinical syndrome.[21]

How is actinomycosis diagnosed?

Box 2 lists the clinical "warning signs" for actinomycosis; the table outlines important differential diagnoses to consider in each of the clinical syndromes. Making the diagnosis is difficult—a definitive diagnosis depends on isolating the organism from a clinical specimen.

BOX 2 CLINICAL "WARNING SIGNS" OF ACTINOMYCOSIS[1]

- Indolent course
- Chronicity
- Mass-like features
- Development of sinus tracts (which can heal and re-form)
- Progression through tissue planes
- Refractory or relapsing infection after short course of antibiotics

Blood tests

Findings are non-specific. There may be evidence of anaemia, mild leucocytosis, raised erythrocyte sedimentation rate, and raised C reactive protein values.[2 6 13] Alkaline phosphatase concentration may be raised in hepatic actinomycosis.[w23]

Imaging

In the early stages of infection, imaging features are usually non-specific and non-diagnostic, and they may be similar to findings for other local inflammatory or neoplastic processes (especially tumours in the lung).[13] Cross sectional imaging with computed tomography or magnetic resonance imaging usually yields non-specific features of an abscess or phlegmon but does provide accurate anatomical localisation, which can aid tissue sampling (fig 1). Unlike most other infections, local or regional lymphadenopathy is rarely a feature. In the later stages of infection, there may be evidence of infiltration of surrounding tissues across tissue planes, with sinus tract formation that is characteristic of, but not specific to, actinomycosis.[22 23 24]

Histopathology

Demonstration of Gram positive filamentous organisms and sulphur granules on histological examination is strongly supportive of a diagnosis of actinomycosis (figs 2 and 3).

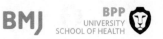

Differential diagnoses of actinomycosis

Type of actinomycosis	Differential diagnosis
Orocervicofacial[9]	Abscess by other typical bacteria, cyst, neoplasm, tuberculosis (scrofula), nocardiosis
Thoracic[19]	Tuberculosis, lymphoma, bronchogenic carcinoma, mesothelioma, blastomycosis, nocardiosis, histoplasmosis, cryptococcosis, pulmonary infarction, abscess or pneumonia by more typical pathogens
Abdominopelvic[3 16]	Intestinal tuberculosis, nocardiosis, tubo-ovarian or pelvic abscess, carcinoma, lymphoma, chronic appendicitis, regional enteritis, inflammatory bowel disease, diverticulitis, endometriosis, pelvic inflammatory disease
Central nervous system[13]	Infection or abscess by pyogenic bacteria, tuberculosis, nocardiosis, neoplasm, colloid or dermoid cysts, cholesteatoma, aneurysm of the basilar artery

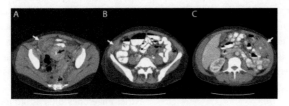

Fig 1 Axial computed tomograms with oral and intravenous contrast medium from the abdomen and pelvis of the same patient. (A) A low density collection with rim enhancement, consistent with an abscess, is seen in the right iliac fossa (white arrow); free fluid is seen in the presacral region of the pelvis (black asterisk); an intrauterine device is also present within the endometrial cavity of the uterus (black arrow). (B) Inflammatory thickening of the anterior abdominal wall musculature and underlying intraperitoneal fat is seen in the right iliac fossa (white arrow); compare this with normal appearances on the left. (C) A small rim enhancing collection is seen within the anterior abdominal wall musculature of the left upper quadrant consistent with another abscess (white arrow) and a bulky region of phlegmonous change in the underlying intraperitoneal fat (white asterisk). Although these features are non-specific, the constellation of inflammation and abscess formation across tissue planes in the presence of an intrauterine device is strongly suggestive of actinomycosis infection

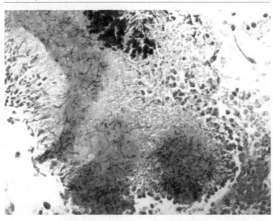

Fig 2 Gram positive filamentous actinomyces (Gram stain, original magnification ×40)

Sulphur granules are colonies of organisms that appear as round or oval basophilic masses with eosinophilic terminal "clubs" on staining with haematoxylin-eosin. Although the presence of sulphur granules is helpful in making the diagnosis, they are not always recovered in culture confirmed cases of actinomycosis.[3] In one series of 181 cases of actinomycosis, the average number per specimen examined was seven, but one to three granules were present in 56% of the cases, and only one granule was found in 26%. None was seen in seven cases in which actinomyces had been cultured.[10] Furthermore, granules are not specific to actinomycosis because they are seen in other diseases,

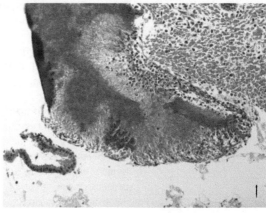

Fig 3 Sulphur granules showing dense aggregate of Gram positive filamentous non-spore forming actinomyces with adjacent neutrophilic cell infiltrate. The filaments are surrounded by eosinophilic proteinaceous material, which represents host reaction (Splendore-Hoeppli phenomenon) (haematoxylin-eosin stain, original magnification ×20)

including nocardiosis, chromomycosis, and botryomycosis.[3] Special stains including Gram, Gomori methanamine-silver, and Giemsa are needed to demonstrate the Gram positive filamentous branching bacteria at the periphery of the grains.[1] A species specific fluorescent antibody allows rapid identification by direct staining, even after fixation in formalin. One small study of cervicofacial actinomycosis showed good correlation between conventional staining and A israeli conjugate staining of tissue sections. This technique has the advantage of specificity and is useful in mixed infections.[w24]

Microbiology

Direct isolation of the organism from a clinical specimen or from sulphur granules is necessary for a definitive diagnosis. However, the failure rate of isolation is high (>50%) for various reasons, including previous antibiotic treatment, overgrowth of concomitant organisms, or inadequate methodology.[7] The most appropriate clinical specimens are samples of pus, tissue, or sulphur granules. Swabs are not ideal because, although they can be cultured, the initial sample cannot be analysed with microscopy—a Gram stain of the specimen is usually more sensitive than culture, particularly if the patient has received antibiotics.[1] Avoid antibiotic treatment before obtaining the specimen and transport it as quickly as possible to the laboratory.[9] Depending on the site of infection, tissue may be obtained via image guided (computed tomography or ultrasound) or direct surgical sampling.[25 w25-w27] Clinicians should tell the laboratory to expect the specimen and specifically request actinomycosis culture on the laboratory request form to ensure that prolonged culture on appropriate media is performed.

Actinomyces are slow growing organisms that can be cultured on selective agar medium at 37°C anaerobically for up to three weeks. In a general clinical microbiology laboratory, the organism is identified by colony morphology on agar and biochemical profiling.[1] Commercial biochemical kits have made identification easier and quicker, although one study reported the accuracy of kits to be poor (below 60%) compared with conventional biochemical tests.[26] Serological assays have been developed but sensitivity and specificity need to be improved before they become clinically useful.[1] New molecular genetic methods, such as polymerase chain reaction,[w28] 16s rRNA sequencing,[w28] fluorescence in situ hybridisation,[w28] and mass spectrometry,[w29] are available for more rapid and accurate identification in reference or research laboratories. The16s rRNA sequencing is currently the preferred method of detecting actinomyces in clinical material in UK reference laboratories.

How is actinomycosis managed?

Clinical experience has shown that actinomycosis can be cured by high doses of antibiotics, such as penicillin for six to 12 months.[1 9] However, the modern approach to treatment is more individualised, and the exact antibiotic regimen depends on the site of infection, severity of disease, and the patient's response to treatment. We would suggest discussing the patient with the microbiology or infectious diseases team to ensure that treatment is appropriate. Patients are regularly monitored to assess their clinical and radiological progress and ultimately to confirm resolution of the disease.

Which antibiotics can be used to treat actinomycosis?

Historically, patients with all forms of actinomycosis have been treated with high doses (18-24 million units a day) of intravenous penicillin G over two to six weeks, followed by oral penicillin V at a dose of 2-4 g/day for six to 12 months.[1 9] The risk of actinomyces developing penicillin resistance is low.[9] In vitro studies have reported that actinomyces are susceptible to a wide range of antimicrobial agents. A UK study of 87 clinical isolates of actinomyces showed that most were susceptible to β lactams (including benzylpenicillin, amoxicillin, ceftriaxone, meropenem, and piperacillin-tazobactam), doxycycline, clindamycin, erythromycin, and clarithromycin. Species identification was found to be crucial because of resistance to some antibiotics.[27] These findings were supported by another study in Denmark in 2009.[28] These studies also found that many species of actinomyces were susceptible to newer antimicrobial agents such as linezolid[27 28] and tigecycline,[28] whereas fluoroquinolones (such as ciprofloxacin and moxifloxacin) and tetracyclines performed poorly.[27 28] However, tetracyclines have been widely used clinically with success,[1 7] and although data on quinolones are limited, there have been anecdotal reports of cure with these antibiotics.[w30 w31]

Doxycycline, minocycline, clindamycin, and erythromycin are suitable for patients who are allergic to penicillin.[1 5 29 30 31] Erythromycin is a safe option for pregnant patients.[1]

Little clinical evidence is available on the newer β lactam agents except for reports of infections treated successfully with ceftriaxone,[w32] piperacillin-tazobactam,[w33] imipenem,[w34] and meropenem.[w35] Antibiotics with no in vitro activity against actinomyces include metronidazole, aminoglycosides, oxacillin, dicloxacillin, and cefalexin;

these antibiotics should not be used alone as therapeutic options.[w36]

What are the appropriate choices for initial antibiotic treatment?

The therapeutic regimen should take into account the site of infection and the other pathogens that may also be present. Although the role of these co-isolates in the pathogenesis of actinomycosis is unclear, many of the organisms are pathogens in their own right, so the initial phase of treatment should cover other bacteria found at the site of infection. A first line regimen might consist of a β lactam and a β lactamase inhibitor such as clavulanate or tazobactam, which offers additional cover against potential β lactamase producers such as S aureus, Gram negative anaerobes, and—in abdominal actinomycosis—Enterobacteriaceae.[9 27] In abdominal actinomycosis, a possible treatment of choice is a combination of amoxicillin and clavulanic acid with metronidazole (or clindamycin) for strict anaerobes plus an aminoglycoside, such gentamicin, for resistant Enterobacteriaceae. In such clinical settings piperacillin-tazobactam or a carbapenem (imipenem or meropenem) may be a suitable alternative.[27]

When should surgery be considered?

Although antibiotics are the cornerstone of treatment for actinomycosis, surgical resection of infected tissue may also be necessary in some cases, especially if extensive necrotic tissue, sinus tracts, or fistulas are present. It may also be needed if malignancy cannot be excluded or if large abscesses or empyemas cannot be drained by percutaneous aspiration.[9] The need for surgery must be assessed on an individual basis. Surgery may be a valid option for patients who do not respond to medical treatment. A retrospective analysis of patients with thoracic actinomycosis showed that surgery cleared the disease in five patients who responded unfavourably to initial antibiotics.[25] Surgery may also be used to control symptoms, as in the control of haemoptysis in thoracic actinomycosis.[w37]

What is the optimal duration of treatment?

The duration of antibiotic treatment will depend on the initial burden of disease, the performance of resectional surgery, and the patient's response to treatment.[9] The traditional recommendation of six to 12 months may not be needed for all patients. Several studies have reported using shorter courses of antibiotics for actinomycosis. Orocervicofacial disease has been cured after short courses of two to six weeks of antibiotics (oral and intravenous) combined with surgical drainage.[32]

Thoracic actinomycosis can also be treated with relatively brief courses of treatment. A survey described 19 patients in whom thoracic actinomycosis was cured with a median duration of six weeks of antibiotics (range, one week to six months). Surgical resection was performed in seven patients. Another study of 16 patients with thoracic actinomycosis reported cure with a median duration of two weeks of intravenous penicillin and three months of oral penicillin. Nine of these patients underwent surgical debulking.[32]

Studies have also shown that pelvic disease can be cured by shorter courses of antibiotics. One retrospective analysis demonstrated cure after surgical removal of the lesion and three months of antibiotics.[w38] Cure has also been reported after only one to two months of antibiotics.[w39 w40] If short

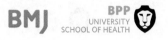

SOURCES AND SELECTION CRITERIA

We searched PubMed, Web of Science, and the Cochrane Library up to December 2010. We analysed randomised controlled trials, prospective analytical and retrospective studies, review articles, and case reports.

ADDITIONAL EDUCATIONAL RESOURCES

Resources for healthcare professionals

- Russo TA. Agents of actinomycosis. In: Mandell GL, Bennett JE, Dolin R, eds. *Principles and practice of infectious diseases*. 7th ed. Elsevier Churchill Livingstone, 2010:3209-19
- Smego RA Jr, Foglia G. Actinomycosis. *Clin Infect Dis* 1998;26:1255-61; quiz 62-3.
- Bonacho I, Pita S, Gomez-Besteiro MI. The importance of the removal of the intrauterine device in genital colonization by actinomyces. *Gynecol Obstet Invest* 2001;52:119-23

Resources for patients

- NHS choices (www.nhs.uk/conditions/Actinomycosis/Pages/Introduction.aspx)—Information on all types of actinomycoses; inludes video material
- Patient UK (www.patient.co.uk/doctor/Actinomycosis.htm)—Information on the causes, presentation, and management of actinomycosis

QUESTIONS FOR FUTURE RESEARCH

- What is the true burden of disease in different epidemiological settings?
- What are the exact associations between actinomyces and the coexisting bacteria with respect to the pathogenesis of disease, and what are the implications for treatment?
- What effect (if any) do various forms of immunosuppression have on the risk of actinomycosis?
- What are the comparative clinical efficacies of the different antimicrobial agents used in actinomycosis?
- Could treatment regimens be improved and, in particular, shortened?
- Can newer techniques (such as 16s rRNA sequencing) improve diagnosis and outcome in routine clinical practice?

TIPS FOR NON-SPECIALISTS

- If the patient is clinically stable, to ensure a definitive diagnosis avoid treating with antibiotics until a clinical specimen can be obtained
- If a sample of pus or sulphur granules is obtained from a sinus or abscess, ask specifically for actinomyces culture on the laboratory request form; avoid using a swab to obtain the sample
- Ensure the clinical specimen arrives quickly at the microbiology laboratory and warn the laboratory of its impending arrival
- Regular long term follow-up of the patient is important during extended antibiotic treatment to ascertain adherence and to assess for clearance of infection

term antibiotic treatment is attempted, the clinical and radiological response must be closely monitored.[32]

What is the treatment for immunocompromised patients?

Antibiotic regimens used to treat actinomycosis in immunocompetent patients are also suitable for immunocompromised patients.[1] However, there have been reports of refractory responses to treatment in certain settings, such as HIV, and it would be prudent to discuss the patient with a microbiologist or infectious diseases specialist.[W41]

What should happen to IUDs in pelvic or abdominal actinomycosis?

We recommend that IUDs are removed in patients with pelvic or abdominal actinomycosis. A randomised controlled trial showed that in addition to treatment with antibiotics, removal of the IUD was effective in eliminating genital actinomyces colonisation.[33] Furthermore, one report has recommended the removal of IUDs in patients with abdominal actinomycosis associated with an IUD.[W42]

What is the prognosis of actinomycosis?

Reports of mortality range from 0% to 28% depending on the site of infection, the time to diagnosis, and the time to the start of appropriate treatment, with the highest mortality seen in central nervous system disease.[2] It is therefore crucial to make an early and accurate diagnosis of actinomycosis.

Thanks to Suha Deen, consultant histopathologist, for providing the histopathology images and David Yu, radiology registrar, for sourcing the radiology images (both from Nottingham University Hospitals NHS Trust, UK).

Contributors: VKW helped design and draft the initial manuscripts. TDT helped in the design and co-wrote the final version. VCW helped on conception, provided final approval for submission, and is guarantor. All authors critically revised the manuscript.

Funding: No funding received.

Competing interests: All authors have completed the ICMJE uniform disclosure form at www.icmje.org/coi_disclosure.pdf (available on request from the corresponding author) and declare: no support from any organisation for the submitted work; no financial relationships with any organisations that might have an interest in the submitted work in the previous three years; no other relationships or activities that could appear to have influenced the submitted work.

Provenance and peer review: Not commissioned, externally peer reviewed.

1 Russo TA. Agents of actinomycosis. In: Mandell GL, Bennett JE, Dolin R, eds. *Principles and practice of infectious diseases* . 7th ed. Elsevier Churchill Livingstone, 2010:3209-19.
2 Acevedo F, Baudrand R, Letelier LM, Gaete P. Actinomycosis: a great pretender. Case reports of unusual presentations and a review of the literature. *Int J Infect Dis* 2008;12:358-62.
3 Smego RA Jr, Foglia G. Actinomycosis. *Clin Infect Dis* 1998;26:1255-61; quiz 62-3.
4 Schaal KP, Lee HJ. Actinomycete infections in humans—a review. *Gene* 1992;115:201-11.
5 Weese WC, Smith IM. A study of 57 cases of actinomycosis over a 36-year period. A diagnostic "failure" with good prognosis after treatment. *Arch Intern Med* 1975;135:1562-8.
6 Fiorino AS. Intrauterine contraceptive device-associated actinomycotic abscess and Actinomyces detection on cervical smear. *Obstet Gynecol* 1996;87:142-9.
7 Bennhoff DF. Actinomycosis: diagnostic and therapeutic considerations and a review of 32 cases. *Laryngoscope* 1984;94:1198-217.
8 Oostman O, Smego RA. Cervicofacial actinomycosis: diagnosis and management. *Curr Infect Dis Rep* 2005;7:170-4.
9 Brook I. Actinomycosis: diagnosis and management. *South Med J* 2008;101:1019-23.
10 Brown JR. Human actinomycosis. A study of 181 subjects. *Hum Pathol* 1973;4:319-30.
11 Pulverer G, Schutt-Gerowitt H, Schaal KP. Human cervicofacial actinomycoses: microbiological data for 1997 cases. *Clin Infect Dis* 2003;37:490-7.
12 Schaal KP, Beaman BL. Clinical significance of actinomycetes. In: Goodfellow M, Mordarski M, Williams ST, eds. *The biology of the Actinomycetes* . Academic Press, 1983:383-424.
13 Mabeza GF, Macfarlane J. Pulmonary actinomycosis. *Eur Respir J* 2003;21:545-51.
14 Kinnear WJ, MacFarlane JT. A survey of thoracic actinomycosis. *Respir Med* 1990;84:57-9.
15 Fowler RC, Simpkins KC. Abdominal actinomycosis: a report of three cases. *Clin Radiol* 1983;34:301-7.
16 Choi MM, Baek JH, Lee JN, Park S, Lee WS. Clinical features of abdominopelvic actinomycosis: report of twenty cases and literature review. *Yonsei Med J* 2009;50:555-9.
17 Agarwal K, Sharma U, Acharya V. Microbial and cytopathological study of intrauterine contraceptive device users. *Indian J Med Sci* 2004;58:394-9.
18 Cayley J, Fotherby K, Guillebaud J, Killick S, Kubba A, MacGregor A, et al. Recommendations for clinical practice: actinomyces like organisms and intrauterine contraceptives. The Clinical and Scientific Committee. *Br J Fam Plann* 1998;23:137-8.

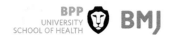

19 Smego RA Jr. Actinomycosis of the central nervous system. *Rev Infect Dis* 1987;9:855-65.

20 Lewis RP, Sutter VL, Finegold SM. Bone infections involving anaerobic bacteria. *Medicine (Baltimore)* 1978;57:279-305.

21 Felz MW, Smith MR. Disseminated actinomycosis: multisystem mimicry in primary care. *South Med J* 2003;96:294-9.

22 Ha HK, Lee HJ, Kim H, Ro HJ, Park YH, Cha SJ, et al. Abdominal actinomycosis: CT findings in 10 patients. *AJR Am J Roentgenol* 1993;161:791-4.

23 Kim TS, Han J, Koh WJ, Choi JC, Chung MJ, Lee JH, et al. Thoracic actinomycosis: CT features with histopathologic correlation. *AJR Am J Roentgenol* 2006;186:225-31.

24 Pickhardt PJ, Bhalla S. Unusual nonneoplastic peritoneal and subperitoneal conditions: CT findings. *Radiographics* 2005;25:719-30.

25 Song JU, Park HY, Jeon K, Um SW, Kwon OJ, Koh WJ. Treatment of thoracic actinomycosis: A retrospective analysis of 40 patients. *Ann Thorac Med* 2010;5:80-5.

26 Miller PH, Wiggs LS, Miller JM. Evaluation of API An-IDENT and RapID ANA II systems for identification of Actinomyces species from clinical specimens. *J Clin Microbiol* 1995;33:329-30.

27 Smith AJ, Hall V, Thakker B, Gemmell CG. Antimicrobial susceptibility testing of Actinomyces species with 12 antimicrobial agents. *J Antimicrob Chemother* 2005;56:407-9.

28 Hansen JM, Fjeldsoe-Nielsen H, Sulim S, Kemp M, Christensen JJ. Actinomyces species: a Danish survey on human infections and microbiological characteristics. *Open Microbiol J* 2009;3:113-20.

29 Fass RJ, Scholand JF, Hodges GR, Saslaw S. Clindamycin in the treatment of serious anaerobic infections. *Ann Intern Med* 1973;78:853-9.

30 Kolditz M, Bickhardt J, Matthiessen W, Holotiuk O, Hoffken G, Koschel D. Medical management of pulmonary actinomycosis: data from 49 consecutive cases. *J Antimicrob Chemother* 2009;63:839-41.

31 Martin MV. Antibiotic treatment of cervicofacial actinomycosis for patients allergic to penicillin: a clinical and in vitro study. *Br J Oral Maxillofac Surg* 1985;23:428-34.

32 Sudhakar SS, Ross JJ. Short-term treatment of actinomycosis: two cases and a review. *Clin Infect Dis* 2004;38:444-7.

33 Bonacho I, Pita S, Gomez-Besteiro MI. The importance of the removal of the intrauterine device in genital colonization by actinomyces. *Gynecol Obstet Invest* 2001;52:119-23.

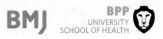

Cryptosporidiosis

A P Davies, clinical senior lecturer/honorary consultant microbiologist[1],
R M Chalmers, consultant clinical scientist and head of unit[2]

[1]School of Medicine, Swansea University, Swansea SA2 8PP

[2]UK Cryptosporidium Reference Unit, National Public Health Service for Wales, Swansea

Correspondence to: A P Davies
angharad.p.davies@swansea.ac.uk

Cite this as: BMJ 2009;339:b4168

DOI: 10.1136/bmj.b4168

http://www.bmj.com/content/339/bmj.b4168

Cryptosporidium is a protozoan parasite that has emerged as an important cause of diarrhoeal illness worldwide, particularly in young children and immunocompromised patients. In the UK *Cryptosporidium* is the commonest protozoal cause of acute gastroenteritis, with 3000-6000 laboratory confirmed cases annually, although this is almost certainly an underestimation of the disease burden. Two species, *Cryptosporidium hominis* and *Cryptosporidium parvum*, account for most of these laboratory-confirmed cases. Species distinction between *C hominis* and *C parvum* is quite recent and for several years both parasites were referred to as *C parvum* (sometimes genotypes 1 and 2). Large waterborne outbreaks highlight the parasite's clinical and economic importance.

The clinical problems associated with *Cryptosporidium* are increasingly becoming recognised internationally, and the parasite was included in the World Health Organization's Neglected Diseases Initiative 2004. These neglected diseases are defined as those that "exhibit a considerable and increasing global burden, and impair the ability of those infected to achieve their full potential, both developmentally and socio-economically".[1]

In this review, we assess the epidemiology, clinical presentation, diagnosis, and management of cryptosporidiosis, and consider its epidemiology.

Sources and selection criteria

We searched MEDLINE for authoritative articles and studies and by consulting the archived resources of the UK Cryptosporidium Reference Unit, Swansea, of which one of the authors (RMC) is the head. The Cochrane database contains a systematic review of treatment in the immunocompromised.[2]

Who gets cryptosporidiosis?

Anyone can be infected and become ill with *Cryptosporidium*. Cryptosporidiosis is commoner in young children, particularly in those under age 5 years, but the disease can also affect healthy people of any age. However,

most clinical problems are encountered in patients who are profoundly immunocompromised. Asymptomatic carriage of the organism is possible: a recent study of young children in day care nurseries found that three of 230 (1.3%, upper 95% CI 3.8%) were carrying the parasite without any symptoms.[3] Risk factors for the acquisition of *Cryptosporidium* identified from outbreaks and sporadic cases are listed in box 1.

How is cryptosporidiosis acquired?

Transmission is usually via the faeco-oral route. As well as person-to-person transmission of both *C parvum* and *C hominis*, particularly within households and nurseries, *C parvum* can also be acquired as a zoonosis, for example, during children's farm visits or exposure to animal dung during outdoor recreation. Oocysts, which are the transmissible form that contains infectious sporozoites, can survive for prolonged periods in damp soil and ingestion of very low numbers can cause disease.[w1 w2]

The largest outbreaks of cryptosporidiosis are associated with contamination of drinking water by sewage effluent or manure. Ordinary water disinfection processes do not kill *Cryptosporidium*, and filtering is required to remove the parasite. Improved quality of drinking water, particularly with the installation of filtration at previously unfiltered supplies, has reduced disease burden.[4 5] Nonetheless, there can still be a background risk in some mains water and many private water supplies.

Outbreaks of the disease associated with swimming pools are well recognised because oocysts are relatively resistant to chlorination, and pool water filtration is often inadequate. Patients with diarrhoeal illness should be advised not to go swimming, and in particular, patients with a confirmed diagnosis of cryptosporidiosis should be discouraged from using pools for two weeks after diarrhoea has stopped because oocysts can still be shed during this time.[6] Advice for patients diagnosed with cryptosporidiosis is outlined in box 2.

Food borne infection is probably less common but can be caused by contaminated fruit or vegetables, food washed in contaminated water, or inadequate pasteurisation of milk.

What are the clinical features of cryptosporidiosis?

Cryptosporidiosis presents as a gastroenteritis like syndrome. Symptoms indicate its pathogenesis[w3] with disease predominantly affecting the small bowel, with malabsorption, and some elements of inflammation. A 3-12 day dose dependent incubation period[7] precedes watery diarrhoea accompanied by abdominal cramps (in 96% of patients who present for consultation), vomiting (65%), mild fever (59%), and loss of appetite.[8] Symptoms can be prolonged, with a mean duration of 12.7 days, and can persist for up to a month.[8] The relapse of symptoms, indicating persistent infection, occurs in over a third of cases,[9] but after clearance of the parasite the epithelium recovers. In one study, 61 of 427 (14%) sporadic cases were hospitalised.[8] The differential diagnosis is usually of other causes of infectious gastroenteritis.

SUMMARY POINTS

- *Cryptosporidium* is a common cause of diarrhoea worldwide, and is the commonest protozoal cause of acute gastroenteritis in the UK
- In immunocompetent patients the illness is self-limiting but generally lasts one to two weeks and sometimes longer
- Laboratory diagnosis is required for confirmation
- Sources of infection include animals, as well as people, and the parasite is resistant to normal water disinfection
- In those with T-cell deficiencies the disease is chronic and protracted and may be severe, with complications including sclerosing cholangitis and rarely, biliary cirrhosis and pancreatitis. Specialist tests may be required
- Treatment options are limited. In the US nitazoxanide is licensed, and available by regular prescription, for disease in the immunocompetent, in whom it reduces the severity of symptoms, which may be prolonged. Nitazoxanide is available in the UK on a named-patient basis
- In England the Chief Medical Officer advises that patients whose T-cell function is compromised should boil all drinking water to reduce the risk of infection

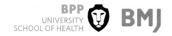

Types of specimens that can be examined for *Cryptosporidium*

	Appropriate patient group	Test and availability
Stool (most commonly examined specimen)	Any patient with community acquired or unexplained diarrhoea	Routine diagnostic tests available locally or specialist tests if negative and *Cryptosporidium* still suspected
Jejunal +/− gastric biopsy	Persistent idiopathic gastrointestinal symptoms in high risk groups	Specialist tests
Bile from endoscopic retrograde cholangio-pancreatography	If symptoms of cholangitis in high risk groups	Specialist tests
Sputum/ bronchoalveolar lavage	High risk patients with profound immunosuppression and unexplained respiratory symptoms	Specialist tests
Antral washout	High risk patients with profound immunosuppression and unexplained sinusitis	Specialist tests

---

BOX 1 RISK FACTORS FOR ACQUISITION OF *CRYPTOSPORIDIUM*

Drinking contaminated water

Travel to less industrialised countries

Use of swimming pools and water based recreation

Contact with animals in farms or petting zoos, especially young ruminants

Contact with animal dung, for example, during outdoor recreation

Contact with another person with diarrhoea, especially a child

Attendance at child care settings

Changing nappies or toileting young children (even those with no diarrhoea)

BOX 2 ADVICE FOR PATIENTS DIAGNOSED WITH CRYPTOSPORIDIOSIS

- Expect the diarrhoea to last longer than with some other causes of infectious gastroenteritis, and be prepared for the possibility that symptoms may relapse before the infection is completely cleared

- Observe stringent personal hygiene because the organism is highly infectious from person to person; wash hands carefully and do not share towels

- Avoid using swimming pools for two weeks after the diarrhoea has stopped

- Children should not attend nursery settings until 48 hours after diarrhoea has stopped

- Food handlers and those caring for vulnerable adults (such as patients in hospital and older people) should not attend work until 48 hours after diarrhoea has stopped

---

In the developing world, cryptosporidiosis is associated with substantial morbidity, and with children who are malnourished,[10] [11] [12] including those with apparently asymptomatic infection who may exhibit poor growth.[13]

Immunocompromised patients commonly experience chronic or intractable disease. Those patients most at risk are those with T-cell immune deficiency, including those with haematological malignancies (particularly children), patients with HIV infection with CD4 counts lower than 200 (and in particular those with counts below 50), and patients with primary T-cell deficiencies such as severe combined immunodeficiency and CD40 ligand deficiency (hyper IgM syndrome). In these immunocompromised patients the entire gastrointestinal tract can be affected, including the pancreatic duct and gall bladder. Complications include pancreato-biliary infection, which can lead to pancreatitis, sclerosing cholangitis, and rarely, subsequent biliary cirrhosis. Tracheo-bronchial involvement, though uncommon, can occur and sinusitis has been described.[14] Rarely, in advanced HIV, cryptosporidiosis is associated with pneumatosis cystoides intestinalis,[15] in which cysts containing gas occur in the gut wall, and can rupture, leading to pneumoretroperitoneum and pneumomediastinum.

There is also concern about cryptosporidiosis in bone marrow and solid-organ transplant patients. A review of the evidence regarding *Cryptosporidium* infection in immunocompromised patients found that the severe disease reported in those who had undergone bone-marrow transplant typically depended on the underlying diagnosis for which the transplant was performed.[15] Cryptosporidiosis in solid organ recipients and in patients with non-haematological malignancies has been described, but does not seem to be as problematic as it is in the highest risk groups.[15]

What are the long term effects of infection?

Little is known about the long term effects of *Cryptosporidium* infection. A case-control study found that infection with *C hominis* (but not *C parvum*) was associated with joint pain, eye pain, headaches, and fatigue during the two months after infection.[9] Seronegative reactive arthritis has been reported in adults[16] [17] and children[18] [19] including one report of Reiter's syndrome.[18] It has been suggested that *Cryptosporidium* infection may cause relapse of inflammatory bowel disease.[20] There are anecdotal reports of an association between *Cryptosporidium* and irritable bowel disease but this link, if it exists, is very unclear and requires further study.

How is infection with *Cryptosporidium* diagnosed?

Cryptosporidium causes a spectrum of disease from asymptomatic, through mild, to severe. Incidence of the disease is almost certainly underestimated[21] because a confirmed diagnosis can only be made after a stool sample is sent to the local microbiology laboratory. Although UK guidance states that all stool samples from community cases of diarrhoea should be tested for *Cryptosporidium*,[22] laboratories have varying criteria for selecting stools for testing.[23] Examination for *Cryptosporidium* may not necessarily be included in a request for "ova cysts and parasites" (as the methods of examination for the two tests differ). The usual methods of detecting *Cryptosporidium* oocysts in the stool are by acid-fast or auramine-phenol staining and microscopy, which often show the organisms in great numbers (figs 1 and 2) , or by antigen detection. Clinicians are advised to become familiar with local laboratory practice, and to specify *Cryptosporidium* on the request form to ensure appropriate testing is carried out.

More sensitive, specialist tests available in reference facilities include PCR, and for maximum sensitivity in exceptional circumstances, immunomagnetic separation with immunofluorescence microscopy, which can detect as few as two organisms per gram of stool.[w4]

In patients with profound T-cell immune deficiency, examination of small bowel or gastric biopsies can reveal the

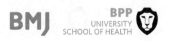

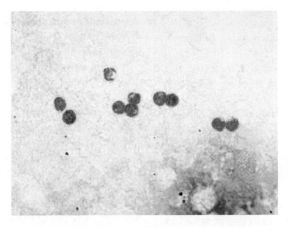

Fig 1 *Cryptosporidium parvum*: modified Ziehl-Neelson staining with ×100 objective. Courtesy of G Robinson, UK Cryptosporidium Reference Unit, Swansea

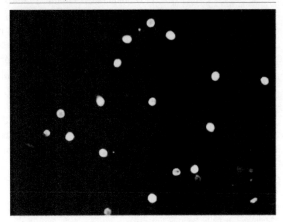

Fig 2 *Cryptosporidium parvum*: auramine phenol staining with ×50 objective. Courtesy of G Robinson, UK Cryptosporidium Reference Unit, Swansea

parasite or histopathological changes where the stool sample is negative. Other samples occasionally examined include bile, in cases of cholangitis, and sputum/bronchoalveolar lavage where pulmonary cryptosporidiosis is suspected. Possible specimen types are listed in the table.

How is cryptosporidiosis managed?

Immunocompetent patients

In immunocompetent patients, the disease, though unpleasant and debilitating, is self-limiting. Rehydration salts may be required. Patients and carers should be informed that symptoms may persist for longer than with other common causes of acute gastroenteritis, making the diagnosis helpful to the clinician. Cryptosporidiosis is highly infectious person-to-person, as large numbers of oocysts are excreted and the infectious dose is low (possibly in single figures[w1 w2]), so scrupulous personal hygiene is required. As with other causes of infectious gastroenteritis, UK guidance issued by a working group of the former Public Health Laboratory Advisory Committee on Gastrointestinal Infections[5] states that affected children should not attend day care centres until 48 hours after diarrhoea has stopped, and that food handlers and carers of highly susceptible patients should be excluded from work for the same period. Regulations for notifying infections vary among jurisdictions. In the UK, cryptosporidiosis is notifiable only where believed to be food borne or water borne. Elsewhere, for example, in the United States, it is a nationally notifiable disease.

Immunocompromised patients

In the high risk groups outlined earlier, infection can be severe and difficult to manage. Because treatment modalities are limited, prevention and risk reduction are the most important interventions. The Department of Health in England advises, on the basis of the Bouchier report,[24] that those with compromised T-cell function should boil all drinking water (including bottled water) to reduce the risk of infection.[25] Whether this permanent, blanket advice is still necessary and should be applied across the UK is currently under review.

The aim of treatment is symptomatic improvement, with complete clearance of the parasite being unlikely unless the underlying immune deficiency can be corrected.

Immune reconstitution

In patients with HIV, highly active antiretroviral therapy (HAART) is the treatment of choice. As well as improving the CD4 cell level and restoring a degree of immunity, protease inhibitors have reduced *Cryptosporidium* host cell invasion and parasite development in vitro, an effect enhanced with paromomycin.[w5] In other patients, improving immunity can also lead to improvement—for example, in a renal transplant patient, accidental reduction in immunosuppression was associated with parasite clearance and resolution of sclerosing cholangitis.[w6]

Specific therapy

Nitazoxanide (Alinia, Romark Laboratories) is approved by the United States Food and Drug Administration for use in immunocompetent patients older than 1 year and is available there by regular prescription. In the UK, nitazoxanide is not licensed but is available on a named patient basis. In a randomised placebo controlled trial of Zambian children with cryptosporidiosis, 100 mg nitazoxanide twice daily[26] resulted in statistically significant improvement in diarrhoea and parasite clearance amongst those who were HIV negative. In an HIV positive group, there was no benefit after the primary treatment course, but after a second course of therapy diarrhoea (but not parasite carriage) had resolved in most. A double blind placebo controlled study in Mexican HIV positive patients[27] used higher doses of nitazoxanide (500 or 1000 mg twice daily), and reported that parasite clearance was significantly better than placebo. Oocyst shedding and diarrhoea resolved in patients with CD4 greater than 50 but not in those with a lower CD4 count. Overall the data support the efficacy of nitazoxanide in immunocompetent patients, with some less conclusive evidence of benefit in immunosuppressed patients, although not, unfortunately, in the subgroup with the most advanced HIV disease. Nitazoxanide is well tolerated with a good safety profile.

All drugs that are currently available in the UK are of unproven benefit and unlicensed for the indication of cryptosporidiosis. Published trials are small and evidence is anecdotal and conflicting. Drugs that have been used to treat *Cryptosporidium* infection include the aminoglycoside paromomycin, and macrolides such as spiramycin, azithromycin, and clarithromycin, which all have anti-parasitic activity. A randomised double blind trial of paromomycin in 10 patients with AIDS and cryptosporidiosis found clinical and parasitological response reaching statistical significance.[28] Another small open uncontrolled prospective study of paromomycin in HIV positive patients with cryptosporidiosis found that most responded clinically

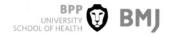

TIPS FOR NON-SPECIALISTS

- Consider cryptosporidiosis in any case of acute gastroenteritis, particularly in young children and especially if the symptoms are prolonged
- A request for "ova cysts and parasites" testing may not routinely include microscopy for *Crytosporidium* so specify on the request form if you suspect the diagnosis
- In immunocompetent patients no specific treatment is required
- If your patient with cryptosporidiosis is severely immunocompromised seek specialist advice

QUESTIONS FOR ONGOING AND FUTURE RESEARCH

- What is the true incidence of cryptosporidiosis in the community?
- Are there long term health effects of infection with *Cryptosporidium*, and if so what are they?
- What are the risk factors for cryptosporidiosis in the second half of the year?
- We are currently gathering evidence to discover whether we should be screening for *Cryptosporidium* carriage in high-risk patients such as those with primary immune deficiencies.

A PARENT'S PERSPECTIVE

Our son Sam got *Cryptosporidium* after visiting the sheep shed during lambing when he was of pre-school age, in a pushchair, but did not actively go into the pens. He got very ill, had a tummy ache, and lost weight. It was a very worrying time as the diagnosis took several weeks and the illness carried on and on.

A patient's perspective

The first inkling that something was wrong was when I woke in the night with intense cramping stomach pains. They came in waves over a couple of hours before the vomiting started. By morning I had vomited so much that it felt as though there was nothing left inside me, but I continued to retch on an empty stomach.

Around mid-morning the diarrhoea started. It was like nothing I had ever experienced before: the cramps would build and then the most awful, profuse, offensive, and watery diarrhoea would follow. It left me physically weak. I couldn't leave the bathroom, and certainly couldn't look after my children, not that I'd have wanted to in case they got it.

I could not face eating, but made myself sip water; however this often caused further episodes of vomiting and diarrhoea. I continued night and day like this for three days before finally I could venture out of the bedroom to take drinks and clear soup without immediately being ill again. It was a full ten days before I felt like I had enough energy to start eating normally or functioning. About two weeks after this I woke again in the night with stomach cramps, no way near as severe as the first attack, but it filled me with dread as to what was going to follow. The diarrhoea only lasted 24 hours this time, there was no vomiting, and then all my symptoms resolved.

I have not had cryptosporidiosis since, but it is an episode of illness I will never forget, and a disease I have the greatest respect for.

ADDITIONAL EDUCATIONAL RESOURCES

Resources for healthcare professionals

- Health Protection Agency (www.hpa.org.uk/infections/topics_az/crypto/menu.htm)—Epidemiological data, general information and guidelines
- Drinking Water Inspectorate (www.dwi.gov.uk/consumer/consumer/crypto.htm)—Wwebpage about cryptosporidiosis in water supplies
- Chartered Institute of Environmental Health (www.cieh.org/policy/cryptosporidium.html)—Comprehensive listings of UK guidance and links to other relevant sites

Resources for patients

- Association of Medical Microbiologists (www.amm.co.uk/files/factsabout/fa_crypto.htm)—Fact sheet for patients
- Institute of Child Health/Great Ormond Street (www.ich.ucl.ac.uk/factsheets/families/F000291)—Factsheet: *Reducing Exposure to Cryptosporidial Infection—Advice for Families with an Immuno-compromised Child*

What else is known about the epidemiology of cryptosporidiosis?

Of the two species accounting for most disease in humans, *C hominis* seems to be largely host adapted to humans while *C parvum* can result in infection in both humans and animals. Less commonly, other species such as *C meleagridis*, *C canis*, and *C felis*, and unusual genotypes have also been reported in patients with diarrhoea but their acquisition is not fully understood.[31] Interestingly, a recent study of young children in day care centres found that unusual genotypes were found proportionately much more frequently in asymptomatic carriers than in patients with symptomatic disease, raising the possibility that some genotypes may be commoner than previously thought and possibly have lower pathogenicity.[2]

In the UK, *C parvum* infections peak in spring and *C hominis* peaks in late summer and autumn. There has been a reduction in the number of cases in the first half of the year, but the number of cases in the second part of the year remains high, with the risk factors not clearly identified.

Risk factors for acquisition of *C hominis* and *C parvum* also differ. Infections associated with foreign travel, in children under one year and in adults, particularly girls and women aged 15 to 44 years, tend to be caused by *C hominis*.[31] *C hominis* is also associated with changing children's nappies (whether or not the child was symptomatic) or swimming in a toddler pool, while *C parvum* is associated with farm animal contact.[8]

Thus, although routine diagnosis outside a reference laboratory is to genus level only, typing to species level yields useful epidemiological information that may shed light on likely sources and routes of transmission.

Contributors: APD and RMC contributed equally to this work. Both authors are responsible for the overall content as guarantors.

Competing interests: None declared.

Provenance and peer review: Not commissioned, externally peer reviewed.

1 Savioli L, Smith H, Thompson A. Giardia and Cryptosporidium join the 'Neglected Diseases Initiative'. *Trends Parasitol* 2006;22:203-8.
2 Abubakar I, Aliyu S, Hunter P. Prevention and treatment of cryptosporidiosis in immunocompromised patients. *Cochrane Database Syst Rev* 2007;24(1):CD004932.
3 Davies AP, Campbell B, Evans MR, Bone A, Roche A, Chalmers RM. Asymptomatic carriage of protozoan parasites inchildren in day care centres in the United Kingdom. *Pediatr Infect Dis J* 2009;28:838-40.
4 Lake IR, Nichols G, Bentham G, Harrison FC, Hunter PR, Kovats SR. Cryptosporidiosis decline after regulation, England and Wales, 1989-2005. *Emerg Infect Dis* 2007;13:623-5.
5 Sopwith W, Osborn K, Chalmers R, Regan M. The changing epidemiology of cryptosporidiosis in North West England. *Epidemiol Infect* 2005;133:785-93.
6 Working Group of the former PHLS Advisory Committee on Gastrointestinal Infections.Preventing person-to-person spread following gastrointestinal infections: guidelines for public health physicians and environmental health officers. *Commun Dis Public Health* 2004;7:362-84.
7 Chappell CL, Okhuysen PC, Sterling CR, Wang C, Jakubowski W, Dupont HL. Infectivity of Cryptosporidium parvum in healthy adults with pre-existing anti-C. parvum serum immunoglobulin G. *Am J Trop Med Hyg* 1999;60:157-64.
8 Hunter PR, Hughes S, Woodhouse S, Syed O, Verlander NQ, Chalmers RM, et al. Sporadic cryptosporidiosis case-control study with genotyping. *Emerg Infect Dis* 2004;10:1241-9.
9 Hunter PR, Hughes S, Woodhouse S, Raj N, Syed Q, Chalmers RM, et al. Health sequelae of human cryptosporidiosis in immunocompetent patients. *Clin Infect Dis* 2004;39:504-10.
10 Sallon S, Deckelbaum RJ, Schmid II, Harlap S, Baras M, Spira DT. Cryptosporidium, malnutrition, and chronic diarrhea in children. *Am J Dis Child* 1988;142:312-5.
11 Sarabia-Arce S, Salazar-Lindo E, Gilman RH, Naranjo J, Miranda E. Case-control study of Cryptosporidium parvum infection in Peruvian children hospitalized for diarrhea: possible association with malnutrition and nosocomial infection. *Pediatr Infect Dis J* 1990;9:627-31.

but that continuous maintenance therapy was required to prevent relapse.[29] The largest prospective, double blind, placebo controlled trial included 35 adults who were HIV positive.[30] Paromomycin was not more effective than placebo but the study lacked power to conclusively refute its usefulness. There are anecdotal reports of both responses[w7,w8,w9] and failures[w10] with azithromycin. Case reports[w11 w12] and one uncontrolled series of patients with AIDS[w13] describe success with azithromycin and paromomycin combination treatments.

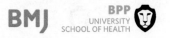

12 Lima AA, Fang G, Schorling JB, De Albuquerque L, Mcauliffe JF, Mota S, et al. Persistent diarrhea in Northeast Brazil: etiologies and interactions with malnutrition. *Acta Paediatr* 1992;81:39-44.

13 Checkley W, Gilman RH, Epstein LD, Suarez M, Diaz JF, Cabrera L, et al. Asymptomatic and symptomatic cryptosporidiosis: their acute effect on weight gain in Peruvian children. *Am Journal of Epidemiol* 1997;145:156-3.

14 Dunand VA, Hammer SM, Rossi R, Poulin M, Albrecht MA, Doweiko JP, et al. Parasitic sinusitis and otitis in patients infected with human immunodeficiency virus: report of five cases and review. *Clin Infect Dis* 1997;25:267-72.

15 Hunter PR, Nichols G. Epidemiology and clinical features of cryptosporidium infection in immunocompromised patients. *Clin Micro Rev* 2002;15:145-54.

16 Hay EM, Winfield J, McKendrick MW. Reactive arthritis associated with Cryptosporidium enteritis. *BMJ* 1987;295:248.

17 Ozgul A, Tanyuksel M, Yazicioglu K, Arpacioglu O. Sacroiliitis associated with Cryptosporidium parvum in an HLA-B27-negative patient. *Rheumatology* 1999;38:288-9.

18 Shepherd RC, Smail PJ, Sinha GP. Reactive arthritis complicating cryptosporidial infection. *Arc Dis Child* 1989;64:743-4.

19 Cron RQ, Sherry DD. Reiter's syndrome associated with cryptosporidial gastroenteritis. *J Rheumatol* 1995;22:1962-3.

20 Manthey MW, Ross AB, Soergel KH. Cryptosporidiosis and inflammatory bowel disease. Experience from the Milwaukee outbreak. *Dig Dis Sci* 1997;42:1580-6.

21 Adak GK, Long SM, O'Brien SJ. Trends in indigenous foodborne disease and deaths, England and Wales: 1992-2000. *Gut* 2002;51:832-41.

22 Health Protection Agency. *Investigation of specimens other than blood for parasites* . National Standard Method BSOP 31. Health Protection Agency, 2007.

23 Chalmers RM, Hughes S, Thomas AL, Woodhouse S, Thomas PD, Hunter P. Laboratory ascertainment of Cryptosporidium and local authority policies for investigating sporadic cases of cryptosporidiosis in two regions of the United Kingdom. *Commun Dis Public Health* 2002;5:114-8.

24 Expert Group chaired by Bouchier I. *Cryptosporidium in water supplies; Third report of the group of experts.* London: Department of the Environment, Transport and the Regions, Department of Health, 1998:1-171.

25 CMO Update 23. Cryptosporidium in water: advice to the immunocompromised. A communication to all doctors from the Chief Medical Officer (August 1999).

26 Amadi B, Mwiya M, Musuku J, Watuka A, Sianongo S, Ayoub A, et al. Effect of nitazoxanide on morbidity and mortality in Zambian children with cryptosporidiosis: a randomised controlled trial. *Lancet* 2002;360:1375-80.

27 Rossignol JF, Hidalgo H, Feregrino M, Higuera F, Gomez WH, Romero JL, et al. A double 'blind' placebo-controlled study of nitazoxanide in the treatment of cryptosporidial diarrhoea in AIDS patients in Mexico. *Trans R Soc Trop Med Hyg* 1998;92:663-6.

28 White AC Jr, Chappell CL, Hayat CS, Kimball KT, Flanigan TP, Goodgame RW. Paromomycin for cryptosporidiosis in AIDS: a prospective, double-blind trial. *J Infect Dis* 1994;170:419-24.

29 Bissuel F, Cotte L, Rabodonirina M, Rougier P, Piens MA, Trepo C. Paromomycin: an effective treatment for cryptosporidial diarrhea in patients with AIDS. *Clin Infect Dis* 1994;18:447-9.

30 Hewitt RG, Yiannoutsos CT, Higgs ES, Carey JT, Geiseler PJ, Soave R, et al for the AIDS Clinical Trials Group. Paromomycin: no more effective than placebo for treatment of cryptosporidiosis in patients with advanced human immunodeficiency virus infection. *Clin Infect Dis* 2000;31:1084-92.

31 Chalmers RM, Elwin K, Thomas AL, Guy EC, Mason B. Long-term Cryptosporidium typing reveals the aetiology and species-specific epidemiology of human cryptosporidiosis in England and Wales, 2000 to 2003. *Euro surveill* 2009;14:pii 19086.

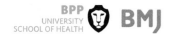

The prevention and management of rabies

Natasha S Crowcroft, chief, infectious diseases[1], Nisha Thampi, medical director[2]

[1]Public Health Ontario, 480 University Avenue, Suite 300, Toronto, ON, M5G 1V2, Canada

[2]Infection Prevention & Control, Division of Infectious Diseases, Children's Hospital of Eastern Ontario, Canada

Correspondence to: N S Crowcroft natasha.crowcroft@oahpp.ca

Cite this as: BMJ 2015;350:g7827

DOI: 10.1136/bmj.g7827

http://www.bmj.com/content/350/bmj.g7827

Rabies is a lyssavirus infection resulting in acute encephalitis or meningoencephalitis that is virtually always fatal. The disease can be caused by several different rabies and rabies-like viruses (box 1). Rabies is a neglected tropical disease that predominantly affects the most vulnerable humans—children living in the most disadvantaged areas of the poorest countries.[1] Many countries have successfully reduced the impact of the disease by tackling the gap between public and animal health through a concerted "one health" approach.[2]

Clinicians worldwide need to be aware of rabies and vigilant about the possible exposure of patients to infection because timely prevention is life saving. The purpose of the review is to give an overview of rabies prevention and the management of patients who may have been exposed to infection or are suspected of having rabies.

What is the global burden of rabies?

Countries predominantly affected by rabies often have poor diagnostic and reporting capacities, leading to a lack of accurate data and considerable uncertainty around estimates of global burden.[3] Efforts to improve data quality have been hampered by duplicative reporting systems requirements to different agencies representing animal or human health. In 2011 the World Health Organization reporting database Rabnet closed, as limited data and under-reporting contributed to a lack of priority for this disease.[3]

In the absence of high quality reporting, estimates of global burden in 2010 ranged from 26 400 to 61 000 deaths, depending on the method applied. Considerable geographical variation exists worldwide, with 95% of rabies cases in humans occurring in Africa and Asia; 84% of these in rural areas.[2] Dogs are the source of infection in more than 99% of cases in humans.

The global economic burden of rabies has been estimated at $6bn (£3.8bn; €5bn), comprising the cost of both disease in humans, domestic animals, and wildlife and prevention through control measures in animals and post-exposure prophylaxis in humans.[2] From a health policy maker perspective, control of canine rabies is highly cost effective and even cost saving.[4] Post-exposure prophylaxis is also cost effective[5] but expensive for individuals and does not contribute to public health measures to interrupt transmission. While post-exposure prophylaxis is usually publicly funded in developed settings, it may be unaffordable for individuals in the highest risk areas, and help may be sought from traditional healers.[6] In India, the

country with the highest number of deaths from rabies, only one in six patients receives appropriate post-exposure prophylaxis.[2]

In areas where canine rabies is eliminated, such as North America, the costs of post-exposure prophylaxis have not diminished because rabies continues to circulate in wildlife.[7] For countries with good control programs, a challenge is to continue to be vigilant and to bear the costs of post-exposure prophylaxis given recurrent importations from neighboring countries with poor control, as seen recently in Greece.[8]

What are the trends in global rabies control and elimination?

Although there is uncertainty about, and under-reporting of, rabies, estimates are that the global burden of the disease decreased from 3234 to 1462 disability adjusted life years between 1990 and 2010.[9]

Vaccination of dogs is the key to primary prevention in humans. This is feasible even in the poorest parts of the world.[10] Success relies on concerted multidisciplinary partnerships involving governments, animal and human health authorities, and a national reference laboratory to support diagnosis and surveillance.

Since rabies can be eliminated through vaccination of dogs, why do so many countries continue to have challenges in disease control? One reason is lack of communication between those responsible for human and animal health, including physicians and veterinarians.[11]

Terrestrial rabies has the potential to be eliminated, but this is unlikely to happen to bat rabies, which accounts for a small proportion of cases in humans each year. Bats are an essential part of the ecosystem and protected by law in many countries. Rabies vaccination is effective in bats, but there is no means of delivering it.

Who is at risk?

Those living in rabies endemic countries, without control measures in dogs and wildlife and access to post-exposure prophylaxis, are at greatest risk. Half of the human population worldwide lives in countries endemic for canine rabies (fig 1).[2] Children are especially at risk because they are more likely to approach animals without caution, including apparently tame wild animals, and therefore to be attacked and bitten, especially on the arms and face. In rabies-free countries, all cases of terrestrial rabies are linked with importations (rabies-like viruses in bats do not affect a country's rabies-free status). For example, since 1946, 25 cases of human terrestrial rabies have been reported in the United Kingdom, associated with exposures to rabid dogs in countries such as the Philippines, Nigeria, India, and South Africa.[12] Travelers and residents in rabies endemic countries should avoid contact with free-roaming animals, especially dogs.

Vampire bats have been associated with several rabies outbreaks in South America. Bats carry rabies-like viruses (rabies related lyssaviruses) even in terrestrial rabies-free countries in Europe and Australia.[2][13] In 2002, a patient developed rabies after exposure to a bat, the only

THE BOTTOM LINE

- Rabies remains a fatal disease in the majority of patients once symptoms develop
- Treatment is supportive; protocols for curative therapy currently remain experimental
- Given the extremely high mortality, prevention is of the utmost importance
- Post-exposure prophylaxis through vaccine and immunoglobulin given soon after exposure to rabies virus is highly effective in preventing rabies
- Rabies elimination requires concerted action by animal and human health authorities, focused on control of rabies in dogs and wild animals and timely prophylaxis for exposed people

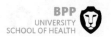

BOX 1 RABIES AND RABIES-LIKE VIRUSES

- *Rabies virus*—various strains found in terrestrial mammals worldwide (except for Australia, Antarctica, some islands), as well as bats in the Americas
- *Australian bat lyssavirus*—bats in Australia and perhaps several nearby islands
- *European bat lyssavirus types 1 and 2, Bokeloh bat lyssavirus, West Caucasian bat virus*—bats in various parts of Europe
- *Khujand virus, Aravan virus, Irkut virus*—bats in Asia
- *Duvenhage virus, Lagos bat virus, Shimoni bat virus, Mokola virus, Ikoma lyssavirus*—bats or unknown host, Africa

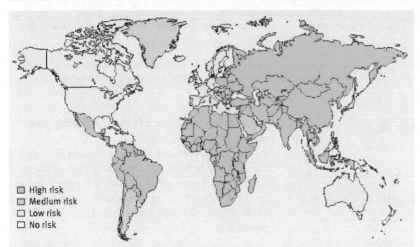

☐ High risk
☐ Medium risk
☐ Low risk
☐ No risk

In countries of categories I, II, and III, contacts with suspect rabid animals, including bats, should be followed by rabies post-exposure prophylaxis
High risk - Pre-exposure immunization recommended for travelers/people likely to come into contact with domestic animals, particularly dogs and other rabies vectors
Medium risk - Pre-exposure immunization recommended for travelers/people likely to come into contact with bats and other wildlife
Low risk - Pre-exposure immunization recommended for people likely to come into contact with bats
No risk - no risk at all

Fig 1 Map of rabies endemic areas

Risk of exposure to rabies
Risk that animal has rabies; depends on level of rabies control in the country, species (dogs are high risk), vaccination status of animal, local epidemiology
Or risk that rabies was cause of death in transplant donor; overall risk is very low

Risk of introduction of virus into body
Type of exposure - increasing risk from lick to scratch through to bite
Location of injury - bites to face are highest risk
Or type of transplantation - tissue and solid organ transplantation are documented sources of rabies

Risk of virus entering nerves, leading to rabies infection
Reduced by:
Post-exposure prophylaxis:
1. washing of wound
2. vaccine
3. rabies immunoglobulin
And/or pre-exposure vaccination

Fig 2 Components involved in risk of acquiring rabies

case acquired that way in the United Kingdom in over a century.[14] In Canada, six of eight cases identified nationally since 1970 have been attributed to infections with rabies strains associated with bats.[15] Although bats may be more important as reservoirs of rabies-like viruses than sources of infection in humans, people need to be aware of the risk of acquiring rabies from bats and seek immediate medical attention should they or their family members have contact.

How is rabies transmitted?

Lyssaviruses cannot cross intact skin. Rabies gets into the body through wounds or direct exposure of mucous membranes, usually as a result of bites from infected animals, or through transplantation of tissues or organs from someone who died from rabies (fig 2). Humans are an end host; anecdotal cases of transmission from human to human have not been confirmed outside of transplantation,[16] including transmission from patients to healthcare workers.

The incubation period is variable, with a mean incubation time in one study of 273.6 days (median 80 days, range 12 days to 10 years).[17] The longer incubation periods emphasize that post-exposure prophylaxis is always indicated even if exposure occurred months or years earlier, provided neurological symptoms have not developed.

Can it be prevented?

Rabies vaccination has been available for more than 125 years.[18] Several modern cell culture and embryonated egg-based rabies vaccines (CCEEVs) containing inactivated rabies virus are available. Older nerve tissue vaccines should no longer be used as they may induce severe adverse reactions and are less effective than CCEEVs. Those who begin post-exposure prophylaxis with one of these older vaccines should restart the series with CCEEVs.[2]

Pre-exposure vaccination

Pre-exposure vaccination is strongly recommended for anyone who is at "continuous frequent or increased risk for exposure to the rabies virus."[2] It is recommended that laboratory staff, veterinarians, and anyone who works with animals and wildlife receive pre-exposure prophylaxis to reduce their occupational risk of infection.[19] [20] It should also be an important prevention strategy in other high risk groups, including infants and children in areas with a high incidence of canine rabies,[21] and where access to immediate care or rabies immunoglobulin is limited.

WHO recognizes two pre-exposure vaccination schedules; one administered intramuscularly and the other intradermally (box 2). Periodic boosters for immunized people are not usually recommended, apart from some workers at continual risk who should undergo serological monitoring and receive a booster if and when required. In the event of an exposure to rabies, post-exposure prophylaxis is still required for those who have received pre-exposure vaccination.

Routes for administering vaccines

In the WHO recommended schedules, the vaccines for both pre-exposure and post-exposure immunization can be administered by two routes: intramuscular and intradermal. The intramuscular route is universally recommended and most commonly used where resources are not a problem. The intradermal route has the advantages of being dose sparing, resulting in equivalent protection at up to 60-80% of the cost of the intramuscular route, and requiring a single visit for post-exposure prophylaxis in people with documented previous complete pre-exposure or post-exposure prophylaxis. The reduced costs increase the likelihood that patients will complete post-exposure prophylaxis. Intradermal immunization against rabies is used mainly in countries where WHO recommended vaccines have regulatory approval for this route of use.

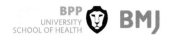

Table 1 Recommended post-exposure regimens for rabies. Adapted from World Health Organization[2]

Route	Schedule (day 0 is date of first dose)
For non-immunized or incompletely immunized people	
Intramuscular:	
5 dose Essen regimen	One intramuscular dose on each of days 0, 3, 7, 14, and 28 plus rabies immunoglobulin for category III exposures; in immunocompetent people, a reduced course with four vaccine doses on days 0, 3, 7, and 14 may be considered, provided they receive wound care plus rabies immunoglobulin for both categories II and III exposures and a WHO prequalified rabies vaccine is used
4 dose Zagreb regimen	Two doses of vaccine on day 0, one dose on days 7 and 21
Intradermal*:	
Thai Red Cross regimen	Two intradermal doses of 0.1 mL vaccine at two different sites on days 0, 3, 7, and 28
For people with documented previous complete pre-exposure or post-exposure prophylaxis with rabies CCEEVs†	
Intramuscular	One intramuscular dose at one site on both days 0 and 3 (no rabies immunoglobulin required)‡
Intradermal	"One visit four-site" intradermal regimen. Four injections of 0.1 mL equally distributed over left and right deltoids, thigh, or suprascapular areas at one visit

CCEEVs=cell culture and embryonated egg-based rabies vaccines.

*WHO states that this regimen can be used for people with category II or III exposure in countries in which the intradermal route has been endorsed by the national health authorities.

†People with category III exposures who have received complete pre-exposure or post-exposure prophylaxis with a vaccine of unproved potency should be managed as if unvaccinated and receive a full post-exposure vaccination course, including rabies immunoglobulin.

‡This regimen can also be given to people vaccinated against rabies who have detectable rabies virus neutralizing antibody.

BOX 2 SCHEDULE FOR PRE-EXPOSURE VACCINATION (DAY 0 IS DATE OF FIRST DOSE)

- Intramuscular—one dose on each of days 0, 7, and 21 or 28*
- Intradermal—one injection on each of days 0, 7, and 21 or 28†

*WHO recommends following the schedule as closely as possible. The series need not be restarted if doses are not given exactly to schedule

†Vials should be used within six hours of opening. To maximize cost savings, sessions should involve enough people to avoid vaccine wastage

---

BOX 3 EXAMPLES OF NATIONAL SOURCES OF ADVICE ON RABIES DIAGNOSIS, PREVENTION, AND POST-EXPOSURE PROPHYLAXIS

Australia—Australian immunization handbook

- www.health.gov.au/internet/immunise/publishing.nsf/Content/handbook10-4-16
- www.health.gov.au/internet/main/publishing.nsf/Content/cdna-song-abvl-rabies.htm

Bangladesh—national guideline for rabies prophylaxis and intradermal application of cell culture rabies vaccines

- www.dghs.gov.bd/bn/licts_file/images/Guideline/2010_National_Guideline_of_ID_PET_Final_Jun2010.pdf

Canada—Canadian immunization guide

- www.phac-aspc.gc.ca/publicat/cig-gci/p04-rabi-rage-eng.php

India—national guidelines for rabies prophylaxis and intradermal administration of cell culture rabies vaccines

- www.ncdc.gov.in/Rabies_Guidelines.pdf

New Zealand—communicable disease control manual

- www.health.govt.nz/system/files/documents/publications/cd-manual-rabies-may2012.pdf

United Kingdom—immunization against infectious diseases (the green book)

- www.gov.uk/government/publications/rabies-the-green-book-chapter-27

United States—Advisory Committee on Immunization Practices

- www.cdc.gov/mmwr/preview/mmwrhtml/rr5902a1.htm#tab3

Disadvantages include the additional training required to ensure that the vaccine is administered correctly, and safety concerns about multi-use vials; the intradermal route is not recommended for pre-exposure prophylaxis in immunocompromised patients or those taking chloroquine for malaria treatment or prophylaxis.[2] [22]

Greater awareness of the risks of undiagnosed encephalitis is needed in the context of organ transplant related rabies. Those who die of encephalitis of unknown cause ideally should be excluded from being donors.[23] Antemortem diagnostic tests for rabies are not sufficiently reliable for screening to exclude rabies, nor is relying on a negative report of potential exposure.[24] [25]

What measures should be taken after a possible rabies exposure (such as dog bite)?

Post-exposure prophylaxis should be initiated immediately after exposure is suspected, especially if an unprovoked animal bites. Several different WHO approved schedules have been adopted for local use (table 1 and box 2); all include wound cleaning, followed by active and passive immunization.

Local recommendations should be followed since these are relevant to the approved vaccines and rabies immunoglobulin available in the vicinity. Expert advice is available in many countries through public health departments and national immunization guides (box 3). Post-exposure prophylaxis is highly effective in preventing the virus from reaching the nervous system. Few failures have been noted and most deviated from WHO recommended protocols.[26] [27] Failures among those with complete pre-exposure immunization are even rarer if post-exposure immunization is given as per WHO protocols, with survival following documented exposure 20 years after the completion of pre-exposure immunisation.[28] Post-exposure prophylaxis is considered futile when administered after the onset of clinical symptoms.

Step 1: wound care

Immediate wound cleaning greatly decreases the risk of developing rabies. Recommended first aid for bite wounds and scratches includes thorough flushing with soap and water, detergent, povidone iodine, or other virucidal substances. Care should be taken to avoid contamination or enlargement of the wound. A bleeding wound is a source of high risk infection. Rabies immunoglobulin must be infiltrated into the wound. Deferred surgical closure of the wound has been recommended, given case reports of post-exposure prophylaxis failures associated with primary repair.[27]

Step 2: vaccination

The decision on whether to initiate vaccination is sometimes difficult to make and may require expert advice (fig 2). A risk assessment should be guided by:

Location (country) of the potential rabies exposure—this helps to determine the likelihood of the animal being rabid. Post-exposure immunization may not be warranted if exposure occurred in a rabies-free country or region

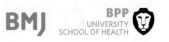

Table 2 Decision aid for post-exposure prophylaxis according to type of exposure. Adapted from World Health Organization[2]

Category of exposure	Type of exposure to domestic or wild* animal suspected or confirmed to be rabid, or animal unavailable for testing	Recommended post-exposure prophylaxis
I	Touching or feeding animals; licks on intact skin; contact of intact skin with secretions or excretions of rabid animal or human case	None, if reliable case history is available
II	Nibbling of uncovered skin; minor scratches or abrasions without bleeding	Administer vaccine immediately† stop treatment if animal remains healthy throughout an observation period of 10 days‡ or is proved to be negative for rabies by reliable laboratory using appropriate diagnostic techniques
III	Single or multiple transdermal bites§ or scratches, licks on broken skin; contamination of mucous membrane with saliva (that is, licks) exposure to bats¶	Administer rabies vaccine immediately, and rabies immunoglobulin, preferably as soon as possible after initiation of post-exposure prophylaxis. Rabies immunoglobulin can be injected up to seven days after first vaccine dose has been administered. Stop treatment if animal remains healthy throughout an observation period of 10 days (does not apply to bats) or is proved to be negative for rabies by a reliable laboratory using appropriate diagnostic techniques

*Post-exposure prophylaxis not routinely required for exposure to rodents, rabbits, or hares.

†Treatment may be delayed if an apparently healthy dog or cat is from a low risk area and placed under observation.

‡Applies to dogs and cats only. Except for threatened or endangered species, other domestic and wild animals suspected of being rabid should be euthanized and their tissues examined for the presence of rabies antigen by appropriate laboratory techniques.

§Bites especially on the head, neck, face, hands, and genitals are category III exposures because of the rich innervation of these areas.

¶Post-exposure prophylaxis should be considered when contact between a human and a bat has occurred, unless the exposed person can rule out a bite or scratch or exposure of a mucous membrane.

BOX 4 STANDARD CASE DEFINITION FOR RABIES IN HUMANS, ADAPTED FROM THE WORLD HEALTH ORGANIZATION[2]

Clinical case

Patients presenting with an acute neurological syndrome (that is, encephalitis) dominated by forms of hyperactivity (that is, furious rabies) or paralytic syndromes (that is, dumb rabies) progressing towards coma and death, usually by cardiac or respiratory failure, typically within 7-10 days after the first sign, if no intensive care is instituted.

One or more of the following laboratory criteria should be used to confirm a clinical case:

- Presence of viral antigens
- Isolation of virus in cell culture or in laboratory animals
- Presence of viral specific antibodies in the cerebrospinal fluid or in the serum of an unvaccinated person
- Presence of viral nucleic acids detected by molecular methods in samples (for example, brain biopsy sample, skin, saliva, concentrated urine) collected post mortem or when the patient is alive

---

Severity of exposure (table 2)

Clinical features of the animal

Vaccination status of the animal and its availability for observation or testing (usually only applies to dogs, cats, and ferrets)

Species of animal (if known).

The decision about whether to initiate vaccination should be made quickly so that post-exposure vaccination can be started immediately and continued while the animal is being observed or pending the results of laboratory tests. Superficial scratches and bites, particularly by bats, should be taken seriously, as the bat rabies virus has been shown to replicate in epithelial cells.[29] Even in the absence of a history of animal bites, the discovery of a bat in a room with a young person who cannot reliably report a bite, should raise concerns, especially when the person was sleeping. Assessment is required to rule out possible contact. Nevertheless, the likelihood of a case of human rabies after bat exposure without a bite or other close contact (for example, a bat flying into a room, observed by one or more adults, and safely removed or leaves without any direct contact) is extremely low.[7]

If the animal in question is a dog, cat, or ferret and can be observed for 10 days, post-exposure vaccination may be started and discontinued if the animal remains well at the end of the observation period. While most countries use a five dose schedule, several have now adopted a WHO recommended four dose schedule, with vaccine administered intramuscularly at 0.1 mL on days 0, 3, 7, and 14 (table 1). With this reduced schedule, rabies immunoglobulin is recommended for category II as well as category III exposures. If someone is immunocompromised, a fifth dose at day 28 is still recommended.[30] Minor reactions at local injection site are common and more likely to occur after an intradermal vaccine, whereas serious adverse events, including Guillain-Barré syndrome and allergic reactions are rare.[31]

Specialized advice is needed for immunocompromised patients. They may need additional monitoring to assess whether an adequate immune response has been mounted after vaccination and whether additional boosters are indicated.

Vaccinated people only require two boosters, given intramuscularly on days 0 and 3, or intradermally in four doses at a single visit (table 1); no rabies immunoglobulin is required.[2]

Step 3: rabies immunoglobulin

Several different rabies immunoglobulin products are available but access to them is limited by global shortages and high cost.[32] [33] Rabies immunoglobulin provides passive antibodies at the site of exposure. It is given once, as soon as possible, and within seven days after the first vaccine dose, before patients develop an active immune response.[2] The recommended total dose is 20 IU/kg. As far as possible, all of the dose should be administered locally around the wound.

What are the symptoms of rabies?

Clinicians suspecting rabies should immediately contact public health authorities and the relevant reference laboratory for advice.

The incubation period after a bite may be as short as a few days or as long as years, and depends on the animal, viral inoculums, and location of the bite.[34] However, most cases present within the first two months after inoculation.

Prodromal symptoms are often non-specific, resembling systemic viral infections, although there may be initial neuropathic pain at the site of the bite or weakness of the affected limb. Signs suggestive of rabies include intense pruritus, beginning at the site of the bite and progressing to involve the limb or side of the face, and myoedema, a mounding of the muscle elicited by being struck with a reflex hammer and that resolves within seconds.[35][36]

Prodromal symptoms are quickly followed by the acute neurological phase, when the virus manifests itself in the central nervous system. This phase is referred to as paralytic or furious rabies (box 4), and progression towards coma and death occurs within one to two weeks from the onset of neurological dysfunction.[37] Furious rabies, which affects two thirds of patients, is characterized by persistent fever, agitation, confusion, and seizures, and it is distinguished from other forms of encephalitis by the presence of hydrophobia, aerophobia, hypersalivation, and dysphagia.[37] Patients with paralytic rabies do not present with the cardinal symptoms seen in those with the furious form and may have early features such as piloerection and fasciculations. They may also present with an ascending paralysis or symmetric quadriparesis; however, they can be distinguished from Guillain-Barré syndrome by the presence of persistent fever, an intact sensation except at the bite site, myoedema, and bladder dysfunction. Other manifestations are also being increasingly recognized, especially among patients with bat related rabies, including tremor, myoclonus, and cranial nerve, motor, or sensory deficits, which may contribute to under-reporting.[35][38]

The diagnosis is made clinically and confirmed by nuchal skin biopsy, with viral antigens or RNA detected at the base of hair follicles containing peripheral nerves, saliva, or brain tissue, the last submitted post mortem.[2] Neutralizing antibodies in the serum may be detected seven or eight days after the onset of clinical symptoms, although they may not develop at all,[38] and are occasionally found in cerebrospinal fluid.

Are any treatments available for rabies?

Death is almost always inevitable in unimmunized patients; only supportive measures are recommended after the onset of neurological signs and symptoms. The "Milwaukee protocol" is a controversial intensive care strategy that was developed for a patient who survived a bat bite despite not having received post-exposure prophylaxis and presenting with encephalitis.[39] Numerous patients have subsequently failed this experimental protocol, which involves antiviral therapy and induction of a therapeutic coma to maintain a burst suppression pattern on the electroencephalogram.[40] Suggested favorable factors for initiation of aggressive treatment include young age and normal immune status, receipt of rabies vaccine before the onset of neurological illness, mild neurological disease at the time of presentation, presence of anti-rabies virus neutralizing antibodies in the serum and cerebrospinal fluid early in the course of illness, and infection by a bat rabies variant, which may be associated with paralytic rabies and thus detectable serum antibodies.[38]

For patients admitted to hospital with rabies encephalitis, palliative measures include sedation and physical and emotional support, as such patients tend to be severely agitated and anxious. A private room is recommended to provide these measures; however, additional barrier precautions are not required as the virus is transmitted through a break in skin and not through inhaled droplets or contact with blood or faeces. Hospital contacts of patients with rabies do not require post-exposure prophylaxis unless they are bitten or their mucous membranes or any open wounds come into contact with the saliva, cerebrospinal fluid, or brain tissue of affected patients.[2]

Are any new treatment or prevention strategies on the horizon?

Antiviral drugs with in vitro activity against rabies virus include ribavirin and interferon-alpha, but they have shown limited activity in the setting of infection; other antiviral treatments for rabies are not on the near horizon. To tackle the global shortage of rabies immunoglobulin, clinical trials are under way to evaluate a human monoclonal antibody and a cocktail of humanized mouse monoclonal antibody.[2] New vaccines, including a less expensive vaccine for post-exposure prophylaxis, new delivery systems for intradermal vaccines, and dose sparing adjuvants for humans are early in development.[1][22]

Priorities for research include multi-level and multi-sectoral population and public health research into interventions aimed at policy makers, health systems, animal health, and the public for achieving elimination of rabies in dogs and optimizing delivery of pre-exposure prophylaxis and post-exposure prophylaxis to humans.[11]

What is the advice for travelers to rabies endemic countries?

Travelers to areas where rabies is enzootic should be aware of the risks and whether appropriate post-exposure prophylaxis will be available at their destination.[41] In a review of recent cases, immigrants who had traveled home to visit family and friends, including for short trips, seemed to be at higher risk, with delays in post-exposure prophylaxis.[17] Pre-exposure vaccination should be considered by travelers to endemic areas who are likely to come in contact with animals, or short term travelers making repeated visits. Short term travelers to rabies endemic countries with ready access to medical care while traveling may choose not to have pre-exposure vaccination as the risk is lower, immunization is expensive, and pre-exposure vaccination is often not publicly funded or covered by health insurance. Such people need to be fully informed about what to do in case of potential exposure to rabies during their trip.

When travelers to endemic countries seek advice too late to complete a course of post-exposure prophylaxis, they need to be aware that full post-exposure vaccination must be sought in case of a high likelihood of exposure to rabies. Options to be considered include the intradermal single visit regimen, if available; traveling with an incomplete series to be completed on return; or completing the series on arrival at the destination.

We thank PHO Library Services and Allison Crehore for help with the literature review, Winsley Rose for advice on treatment of patients, Kwame McKenzie for assistance with reviewing drafts, and the reviewers for their expert comments. This article is dedicated to the memory of Declan McKeever.

Contributors: NSC conducted the literature search and wrote the article. NT contributed to the section on rabies treatment and clinical parts of the article. Both authors contributed to the final draft for submission and are the guarantors.

Competing interests: We have read and understood the BMJ policy on declaration of interests and declare the following interests: none.

SOURCES AND SELECTION CRITERIA

In a non-systematic review of literature, we built on an existing collection of literature on rabies that had been accumulated since 2000. We searched PubMed using MeSH term "rabies", limited to studies in English in humans conducted in the past five years. From that search we reviewed 846 abstracts for relevance and reviewed relevant papers in full, as well as reviewing bibliographies to identify further papers and searching key sources of grey literature, including the World Health Organization and national health authorities. The final list of references was also influenced by the scope and format of the article.

ADDITIONAL EDUCATIONAL RESOURCES

Resources for healthcare professionals

- World Health Organization (www.who.int/mediacentre/factsheets/fs099/en/)—provides a range of information and data on rabies
- Mission Rabies (www.missionrabies.com/)—a charity aiming to eliminate rabies through vaccination of dogs
- US Centers for Disease Control and Prevention (www.cdc.gov/rabies/)—contains excellent resources on rabies
- European Centre for Disease Control (www.ecdc.europa.eu/en/healthtopics/rabies/Pages/index.aspx)—has good information on rabies in Europe.

Resources for the public

- Disease Daily (http://healthmap.org/site/diseasedaily)—contains information about infectious diseases written by health professionals for the public
- National Health Service UK (www.nhs.uk/conditions/rabies/Pages/Introduction.aspx)—a certified source of reliable information about rabies written for the public

Provenance and peer review: Commissioned; externally peer reviewed.

1. Wunner WH, Briggs DJ. Rabies in the 21 century. *PLoS Negl Trop Dis* 2010;4:e591.
2. World Health Organization. WHO expert consultation on rabies: second report. WHO Press, 2013.
3. Nel LH. Discrepancies in data reporting for rabies, Africa. *Emerg Infect Dis* 2013;19:529-33.
4. Fitzpatrick MC, Hampson K, Cleaveland S, Mzimbiri I, Lankester F, Lembo T, et al. Cost-effectiveness of canine vaccination to prevent human rabies in rural Tanzania. *Ann Intern Med* 2014;160:91-100.
5. Shim E, Hampson K, Cleaveland S, Galvani AP. Evaluating the cost-effectiveness of rabies post-exposure prophylaxis: a case study in Tanzania. *Vaccine* 2009;27:7167-72.
6. Rumana R, Sayeed AA, Basher A, Islam Z, Rahman MR, Faiz MA.. Perceptions and treatment seeking behavior for dog bites in rural Bangladesh. *Southeast Asian J Trop Med Public Health* 2013;44:244-8.
7. De Serres G, Skowronski DM, Mimault P, Ouakki M, Maranda-Aubut R, Duval B. Bats in the bedroom, bats in the belfry: reanalysis of the rationale for rabies postexposure prophylaxis. *Clin Infect Dis* 2009;48:1493-9.
8. Tsiodras S, Dougas G, Baka A, Billinis C, Doudounakis S, Balaska A, et al. Re-emergence of animal rabies in northern Greece and subsequent human exposure, October 2012-March 2013. *Euro Surveill* 2013;18:20474.
9. Murray CJ, Vos T, Lozano R, Naghavi M, Flaxman AD, Michaud C, et al. Disability-adjusted life years (DALYs) for 291 diseases and injuries in 21 regions, 1990-2010: a systematic analysis for the Global Burden of Disease Study 2010. *Lancet* 2012;380:2197-223.
10. Lembo T, Hampson K, Kaare MT, Ernest E, Knobel D, Kazwala RR, et al. The feasibility of canine rabies elimination in Africa: dispelling doubts with data. *PLoS Negl Trop Dis* 2010;4:e626.
11. Zinsstag J. Towards a science of rabies elimination. *Infect Dis Poverty* 2013;2:22.
12. Public Health England. Rabies. 2013. www.hpa.org.uk/Topics/InfectiousDiseases/InfectionsAZ/Rabies/GeneralInformation/.
13. Vigilato MA, Cosivi O, Knöbl T, Clavijo A, Silva HM. Rabies update for Latin America and the Caribbean. *Emerg Infect Dis* 2013;19:678-9.
14. Public Health Laboratory Service. Fatal infection with European bat lyssavirus rabies-related virus in Scotland. *Commun Dis Rep CDR Wkly* 2002;12(48). www.hpa.org.uk/cdr/archives/2002/cdr4802.pdf.
15. Johnstone J, Saxinger L, McDermid R, Bagshaw S, Resch L, Lee B, et al. Human rabies-Alberta, Canada, 2007. *MMWR Morb Mortal Wkly Rep* 2008;57:197-200.
16. Helmick CG, Tauxe RV, Vernon AA. Is there a risk to contacts of patients with rabies? *Rev Infect Dis* 1987;9:511-8.
17. Carrara P, Parola P, Brouqui P, Gautret P. Imported human rabies cases worldwide, 1990-2012. *PLoS Negl Trop Dis* 2013;7:e2209.
18. Bourhy H, Dautry-Varsat A, Hotez PJ, Salomon J. Rabies, still neglected after 125 years of vaccination. *PLoS Neglect Trop Dis* 2010;4:e839.
19. Centers for Disease Control and Prevention. Rabies in a laboratory worker-New York. *MMWR Morb Mortal Wkly Rep* 1977;26:183-4.
20. Winkler WG, Fashinell TR, Leffingwell L, Howard P, Conomy P. Airborne rabies transmission in a laboratory worker. *JAMA* 1973;226:1219-21.
21. Both L, Banyard AC, van Dolleweerd C, Horton DL, Ma JK, Fooks AR. Passive immunity in the prevention of rabies. *Lancet Infect Dis* 2012;12:397-407.
22. Madhusudana SN, Mani RS. Intradermal vaccination for rabies prophylaxis: conceptualization, evolution, present status and future. *Expert Rev Vaccines* 2014;13:641-55.
23. Kaul DR. Donor-derived infections with central nervous system pathogens after solid organ transplantation. *JAMA* 2013;310:378-9.
24. Bronnert J, Wilde H, Tepsumethanon V, Lumlertdacha B, Hemachudha T. Organ transplantations and rabies transmission. *J Travel Med* 2007;14:177-80.
25. Vora NM, Basavaraju SV, Feldman KA, Paddock CD, Orciari L, Gitterman S, et al. Raccoon rabies virus variant transmission through solid organ transplantation. *JAMA* 2013;310:398-407.
26. Wilde H. Failures of post-exposure rabies prophylaxis. *Vaccine* 2007;25:7605-9.
27. Wilde H, Sirikawin S, Sabcharoen A, Kingnate D, Tantawichien T, Harischandra PA, et al. Failure of postexposure treatment of rabies in children. *Clin Infect Dis* 1996;22:228-32.
28. Maier T, Schwarting A, Mauer D, Ross RS, Martens A, Kliem V, et al. Management and outcomes after multiple corneal and solid organ transplantations from a donor infected with rabies virus. *Clin Infect Dis* 2010;50:1112-9.
29. Morimoto K, Patel M, Corisdeo S, Hooper DC, Fu ZF, Rupprecht CE, et al. Characterization of a unique variant of bat rabies virus responsible for newly emerging human cases in North America. *Proc Natl Acad Sci U S A* 1996;93:5653-8.
30. Rupprecht CE, Briggs D, Brown CM, Franka R, Katz SL, Kerr HD, et al. Use of a reduced (4-dose) vaccine schedule for postexposure prophylaxis to prevent human rabies: recommendations of the advisory committee on immunization practices. *MMWR Recomm Rep* 2010;59(RR-2):1-9.
31. Bernard KW, Smith PW, Kader FJ, Moran MJ. Neuroparalytic illness and human diploid cell rabies vaccine. *JAMA* 1982;248:3136-8.
32. Knobel DL, Cleaveland S, Coleman PG, Fèvre EM, Meltzer MI, Miranda ME, et al. Re-evaluating the burden of rabies in Africa and Asia. *Bull World Health Organ* 2005;83:360-8.
33. Sudarshan MK, Mahendra BJ, Madhusudana SN, Ashwoath Narayana DH, Rahman A, Rao NS, et al. An epidemiological study of animal bites in India: results of a WHO sponsored national multi-centric rabies survey. *J Commun Dis* 2006;38:32-9.
34. Smith JS, Fishbein DB, Rupprecht CE, Clark K. Unexplained rabies in three immigrants in the United States. A virologic investigation. *N Engl J Med* 1991;324:205-11.
35. Hemachudha T, Laothamatas J, Rupprecht CE. Human rabies: a disease of complex neuropathogenetic mechanisms and diagnostic challenges. *Lancet Neurol* 2002;1:101-9.
36. Hemachudha T, Phanthumchinda K, Phanuphak P, Manutsathit S. Myoedema as a clinical sign in paralytic rabies. *Lancet* 1987;1:1210.
37. Noah DL, Drenzek CL, Smith JS, Krebs JW, Orciari L, Shaddock J, et al. Epidemiology of human rabies in the United States, 1980 to 1996. *Ann Intern Med* 1998;128:922-30.
38. Udow SJ, Marrie RA, Jackson AC. Clinical features of dog- and bat-acquired rabies in humans. *Clin Infect Dis* 2013;57:689-96.
39. Willoughby RE Jr, Tieves KS, Hoffman GM, Ghanayem NS, Amlie-Lefond CM, Schwabe MJ, et al. Survival after treatment of rabies with induction of coma. *N Engl J Med* 2005;352:2508-14.
40. Jackson AC. Current and future approaches to the therapy of human rabies. *Antiviral Res* 2013;99:61-7.
41. Jentes ES, Blanton JD, Johnson KJ, Petersen BW, Lamias MJ, Robertson K et al. The global availability of rabies immune globulin and rabies vaccine in clinics providing indirect care to travelers. *J Travel Med* 2014;21:62-6.

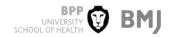

Diagnosis and management of schistosomiasis

Darren J Gray, research fellow[1], visiting scientist[2], Allen G Ross, professor and chair of public health[1], director, population health research[3], Yue-Sheng Li, senior research fellow[2], honorary director[4], Donald P McManus, laboratory head and National Health and Medical Research Council (Australia) senior principal research fellow[2]

[1]Griffith Health Institute, Griffith University, Brisbane, Australia

[2]Molecular Parasitology Laboratory, Infectious Diseases Division, Queensland Institute of Medical Research, Herston, Brisbane, Queensland, Australia

[3]School of Public Health, Griffith University, Meadowbrook, Australia

[4]Hunan Institute of Parasitic Diseases, World Health Organization Collaborating Centre for Research and Control of Schistosomiasis in Lake Region, Yueyang, People's Republic of China

Correspondence to: D P McManus Don.McManus@qimr.edu.au

Cite this as: BMJ 2011;342:d2651

DOI: 10.1136/bmj.d2651

http://www.bmj.com/content/349/bmj.g4929

Schistosomiasis, or bilharzia, is a common intravascular infection caused by parasitic Schistosoma trematode worms.[1][2] A systematic review and meta-analysis published in 2006 estimated that more than 200 million people are infected across Africa, Asia, and South America, and close to 800 million are at risk of infection.[3] Meta-analyses have estimated that the current disease burden may exceed 70 million disability adjusted life years.[4][5] The disease is also associated with anaemia, chronic pain, diarrhoea, exercise intolerance, and undernutrition, and female urogenital schistosomiasis may be a risk factor for HIV infection.[4][w1][5] Figure 1 shows the proposed pathway of schistosomiasis associated disease and disability derived from meta-analyses of disability-related outcomes.[4]

Schistosome transmission requires contamination of water by faeces or urine containing eggs, a specific freshwater snail as intermediate host, and human contact with water inhabited by the intermediate host snail.[1][2] Schistosomiasis transmission is highly dependent on environmental conditions, particularly those affecting the snail host. Climate change will alter aquatic environments and subsequently the transmission and distribution of waterborne diseases.[6][w2]

In this review, we introduce the schistosome parasites and describe the pathophysiology and the clinical disease they cause. We discuss current diagnostic tools and the management of schistosomiasis, based on evidence from studies of both high and lower quality as well as information from current international guidelines.

SUMMARY POINTS

- Schistosomiasis, or bilharzia, is a common intravascular infection caused by parasitic Schistosoma trematode worms
- It is prevalent in Africa, the Middle East, South America, and Asia
- Acute schistosomiasis, or Katayama syndrome, can present as fever, malaise, myalgia, fatigue, non-productive cough, diarrhoea (with or without blood), haematuria (S haematobium), and right upper quadrant pain
- Chronic and advanced disease results from the host's immune response to schistosome eggs deposited in tissues and the granulomatous reaction evoked by the antigens they secrete
- S mansoni, S japonicum, S intercalatum, and S mekongi cause intestinal disease; S haematobium causes urinary disease
- Neuroschistosomiasis is arguably the most severe clinical syndrome associated with schistosome infection
- Microscopic examination of excreta (stool, urine) is the gold standard diagnostic test but requires the adult worms to be producing eggs; serological tests can diagnose less advanced infections
- Praziquantel 60 mg/kg in three doses over one day (S japonicum and S.mekongi); and 40 mg/kg in doses over one day (S mansoni, S haematobium, S intercalatum) remains the treatment of choice although others are being investigated
- Preventive chemotherapy is with a single oral dose of praziquantel 40 mg/kg

Where and how is schistosomiasis acquired?

The global distribution of schistosomiasis is shown in figure 2, which is based on WHO statistics.[1] The majority of infections with Schistosoma haematobium, Schistosoma mansoni and Schistosoma intercalatum are found in sub-Saharan Africa.[1] S mansoni remains endemic in parts of Brazil, Venezuela, and the Caribbean. Schistosoma japonicum infection occurs in the People's Republic of China, the Philippines, and small pockets in Indonesia, despite substantial and largely successful control measures.[1][2] Schistosoma mekongi is found along the Mekong River in Cambodia and Lao People's Democratic Republic (Laos).[1][2][7] Infection is usually acquired through activities such as swimming, bathing, fishing, farming, and washing clothes. Important transmission sites include Lake Malawi and Lake Victoria in Africa, the Poyang and Dongting Lakes in China, and along the Mekong River in Laos. The life cycle of the schistosome is depicted in figure 3. Intermediate snail hosts are more likely to inhabit still to moderately flowing fresh water and infection increases exponentially with length of time in contact with water, peaking at 30 minutes.[w3]

What are the clinical features of schistosomiasis?

Schistosomiasis progresses in three distinct phases: acute, chronic, and advanced disease.

Early manifestations

Rash

A maculopapular eruption, comprising discrete erythematous raised lesions that vary in size from 1 cm to 3 cm, may arise at the site of percutaneous penetration by schistosome cercariae. (fig 4) Migrants or tourists infected for the first time may develop a skin reaction within a few hours, although a rash may appear up to a week later. This is less severe than, although similar to, "swimmers itch", which is not a sequela of acute schistosomiasis but rather an immune reaction that develops in sensitised people when they are reinfected by species of schistosomes that do not colonise humans.[1][2]

Acute schistosomiasis (Katayama syndrome)

The symptoms of acute schistosomiasis are mediated by the immune complex[w4-w7] and usually begin with the deposition of schistosome eggs into host tissues. Symptoms may include fever, malaise, myalgia, fatigue, non-productive cough, diarrhoea (with or without the presence of blood), haematuria (S haematobium), and right upper quadrant pain. Acute schistosomiasis is seen in people who are infected for the first time when travelling to endemic areas. In the case of S japonicum it is also associated with either a superinfection or a hypersensitivity reaction in

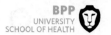

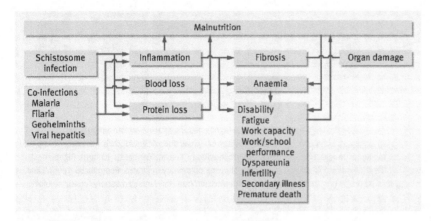

Fig 1 Proposed pathways of schistosomiasis associated disease and disability. Adapted from King et al[4] with permission from Elsevier

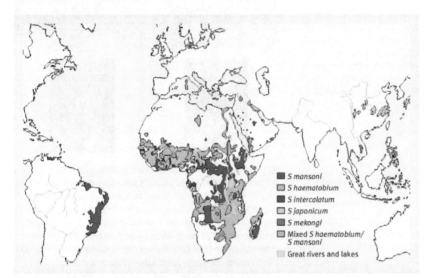

Fig 2 Global distribution of schistosomiasis. Adapted from Gryseels et al[2] with permission from Elsevier.

previously infected people.[8] Differential diagnoses include gastroenteritis, hepatitis A, B, and C, HIV, salmonellosis, and urinary tract infection.[8]

Chronic and advanced disease

Mature, patent, schistosome infections are associated with a chronic local inflammatory response to schistosome eggs trapped in host tissues, which may lead to inflammatory and obstructive disease in the urinary system (*S haematobium*) or intestinal disease, hepatosplenic inflammation, and liver fibrosis (*S mansoni, S intercalatum, S japonicum and S mekongi*).[1] [2] Immunopathological studies have shown that schistosomiasis results from the host's immune response to schistosome eggs (fig 5) and the granulomatous reaction evoked by the antigens they secrete.[1] [2] [9] [10] Granulomas, which develop at the sites of maximal accumulation of eggs, destroy the eggs but result in fibrosis in host tissues.[1] [2] [w8-w12] Granuloma formation and the local inflammatory response mediated by CD4+ T-helper-2 lymphocytes help facilitate the passage of eggs into the lumen of the gut or urinary tract.[w13]

Gastrointestinal and liver disease

Eggs retained in the gut wall induce inflammation, hyperplasia, ulceration, micro-abscess formation, and polyposis. Symptoms of gastrointestinal disease include colicky hypogastric pain or pain in the left iliac fossa, diarrhoea (particularly in children) that may alternate with constipation, and haematochezia (blood in the faeces). Severe chronic intestinal disease may result in colonic or

rectal stenosis. Colonic polyposis may manifest as a protein losing enteropathy. An inflammatory mass in the colon may even mimic cancer.[1] [2]

Eggs of *S mansoni* and *S japonicum* embolise to the liver, where the granulomatous inflammatory response induces presinusoidal inflammation and periportal or clay-pipe-stem fibrosis,[1] [2] which population studies have shown are associated with sustained heavy infection and can take many years to develop.[1] [2] [w14-w19] Hepatomegaly, secondary to granulomatous inflammation, occurs early in the evolution of chronic disease. Periportal collagen deposits lead to the progressive obstruction of blood flow, portal hypertension, and ultimately varices, variceal bleeding, splenomegaly, and hypersplenism.[1] Periportal fibrosis can be seen on ultrasonography, computed tomography, or magnetic resonance imaging and is characteristic of schistosomiasis.

Genitourinary disease

Urinary tract disease develops after infection with *S haematobium* and granulomatous inflammation in response to deposition of eggs in tissues.[1] [2] [w10] Haematuria, appearing 10-12 weeks after infection, is the first sign of established disease (fig 4). Dysuria and haematuria occur in early and late disease. Late disease manifestations also include proteinuria (often nephrotic syndrome), bladder calcification, ureteric obstruction, secondary bacterial infection in the urinary tract, renal colic, hydronephrosis, and renal failure.[1] [2] [w10] Structural abnormalities of the urinary tract may occur in children.[1] [2] [w20] Cystoscopy may reveal characteristic "sandy patches," which are areas of roughened bladder mucosa surrounding egg deposits.[1] [2] Epidemiological studies have associated chronic urinary schistosomiasis with squamous cell carcinoma of the bladder in Egypt and other parts of Africa.[w21-w25] In Egypt, the incidence of bladder cancer has decreased in line with decreasing prevalence of schistosomiasis over the past few decades.[w26] [w27] [1] [2] *S haematobium* bladder squamous cell carcinomas tend to be well differentiated and metastasise locally.[w21-w27] Nitrosamines, β-glucuronidase, and inflammatory gene damage have been proposed as possible carcinogenic factors.[1] [2] [w25] However, another explanation is that schistosomiasis lesions intensify the exposure of the bladder epithelium to mutagenetic substrates from tobacco or chemicals.[1] [w22] *S haematobium* causes genital disease in about a third of infected women.[2] Vulval schistosomiasis may also facilitate the transmission of HIV, according to clinical findings; pathophysiological and immunological data, and epidemiological surveillance information.[1] [2] [w24] [w28] [w29]

Additional morbidity associated with schistosomiasis

Neuroschistosomiasis (fig 6, box 1) is arguably the most severe clinical outcome associated with schistosome infection and includes signs and symptoms of increased intracranial pressure, myelopathy, and radiculopathy.[1] [2] [11] [12] [w30] Case studies suggest that neurological complications early in the course of infection are due to egg deposition following aberrant migration of adult worms to the brain or spinal cord. The mass effect of thousands of eggs and large granulomas in the brain or spinal cord underpin neuroschistosomiasis. Complications of cerebral disease include encephalopathy with headache, visual impairment, delirium, seizures, motor deficit, and ataxia; spinal symptoms comprise lumbar pain, lower limb radicular pain, muscle weakness, sensory loss, and bladder dysfunction.[11]

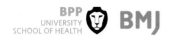

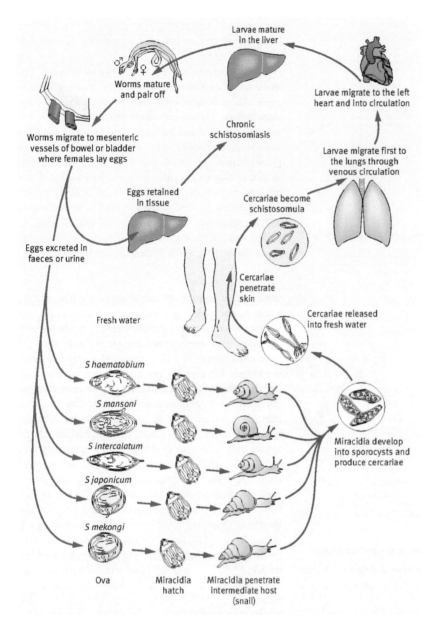

Fig 3 Schistosome lifecycle. Freshwater molluscs act as intermediate hosts and higher order vertebrates as definitive hosts. Adult male and female worm pairs (slender female schistosome lies within the ventral gynaecophoric canal of the male) produce numerous eggs, most of which are deposited in the capillaries and tissues of the parasitised target organ and some of which are excreted via the urine or faeces. The shape of the eggs and the location of their excretion differentiate the various species. S haematobium inhabits the urinary system and the sacral and pelvic vessels, while intestinal schistosomes inhabit the intestinal mucosa. Some eggs are carried downstream in the portal circulation and, in the case of an S mansoni or S japonicum infection, are trapped in the liver. Once excreted, an ovum hatches in contact with fresh water and a free living motile miracidium is released to infect the specific freshwater snail intermediate host—with S mansoni this is generally Biomphalaria glabrata (Americas) or B pfeifferi (Africa). After about 30 days infected snails release free swimming cercariae in response to sunlight. These can penetrate the skin of the mammalian host within 12-24 hours, invade the lymphatic system, and enter the circulation via the lungs as maturing schistosomula.

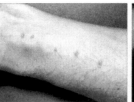 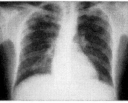

Fig 4 Clinical manifestations of acute schistosomiasis. Left: maculopapular rash (www.dpd.cdc.gov/dpdx/HTML/ImageLibrary/A-F/ CercarialDermatitis/body_CercarialDermatitis_il2.htm). Right: chest radiograph showing pulmonary infiltrates. Reproduced from McManus et al[13] with permission from the American Society for Microbiology.

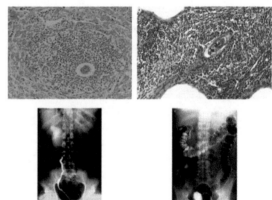

Fig 5 Chronic/advanced schistosomiasis pathology. (A) Characteristic perioval granuloma formed around S japonicum egg in mouse liver. (B) Granuloma formed around an S mansoni egg in human lung tissue. (C) Retrograde pyelogram showing right sided ureteric stricture due to infection with S haematobium. (D) Double contrast barium enema of a patient infected with S mansoni. The right side of the transverse colon (left of image) has a normal smooth mucosal lining. The left transverse colon, splenic flexure, and descending colon have a fine irregular granular mucosal surface, owing to numerous small lesions caused by deposition of schistosome eggs. The lesions result in inflammation and erosion of the mucosa. Reprinted from McManus et al[13]with permission from the American Society for Microbiology. Courtesy of the Wellcome Trust.

[12] Myelopathy (acute transverse myelitis and subacute myeloradiculopathy) of the lumbosacral region is the most commonly reported neurological manifestation of both S mansoni and S haematobium infection, whereas acute encephalitis of the cortex, subcortical white matter, basal ganglia, or internal capsule is reportedly typical of S japonicum.[11] [12]

Population studies of children have shown that schistosome infection can cause growth retardation and anaemia, as well as possible cognitive and memory impairment, which limits their potential.[1] [2] [13] Randomised controlled trials have shown that successful treatment

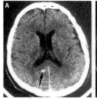 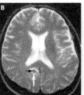 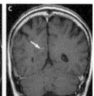

Fig 6 Pathology in neuroschistosomiasis. (A) Unenhanced axial CT scan shows small, oval, hyperdense lesion (black arrow) in the paraventricular zone, dorsal of the right posterior horn. (B) Axial T2-weighted (2437/90/1 [repetition time/echo time/excitations]) MRI shows hypointense lesion (white arrow) with small centrally located area of intermediate signal (black arrow). (C) Coronal contrast-enhanced T1-weighted (600/15/2) MRI shows oval lesion of intermediate signal (arrow) with ring-like and septum-like contrast enhancement. Reprinted from McManus et al[13]with permission from the American Society for Microbiology. Courtesy of the Wellcome Trust.

in children leads to appreciable but incomplete catch-up growth and improvement in haemoglobin levels.[1] [2] [13] [w26-w31] Schistosome infection seems to adversely affect maternal health and the unborn foetus. Chronic infection with S mansoni and (rarely) S haematobium, but not S japonicum, may cause pulmonary hypertension, cor pulmonale, glomerulonephritis, or transverse myelitis.[w31-w36]

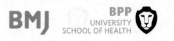

BOX 1 NEUROSCHISTOSOMIASIS

Diagnosis

- The finding of eggs in the stool or positive serology provides supportive but not direct evidence of schistosomal involvement in the central nervous system. A positive diagnostic finding coupled with neuroimaging and neurological symptoms should place neuroschistosomiasis high on the list of differentials. A definitive diagnosis can only be ascertained with histopathological study at biopsy or at necropsy, showing schistosome eggs and granulomas.

Signs and symptoms

- Focal or generalised epilepsy (S japonicum)
- Transverse myelitis (S mansoni and S haematobium)
- Nystagmus
- Speech disturbances
- Motor weakness (hemiplegia, paraplegia, or quadriplegia)
- Papilloedema
- Lumbar pain and lower limb radicular pain (S mansoni and S haematobium)
- Sensory loss (T12 to L1)
- Bladder dysfunction

Neuro-imaging

- Computerised tomography
- Magnetic resonance imaging
- Myelography

Management

- Consult with a neurologist and an infectious disease physician
- Treatment with corticosteroids and anticonvulsants within two months of infection
- Praziquantel chemotherapy two months after known water contact

---

BOX 2 KEY INDICATORS FOR POSITIVE DIAGNOSIS OF SCHISTOSOMIASIS

Medical history

- Have you travelled to or emigrated from an endemic country recently? If so from where?
- Have you been in contact with a freshwater source (such as lakes, rivers, or streams)?
- (Patients returning/emigrating from Africa or the Middle East may have either intestinal or urinary schistosomiasis and those from Asia or South America may have intestinal schistosomiasis)

Physical examination

- An urticarial rash (maculopapular lesions) may be present where the cercariae penetrated the skin (discrete erythematous raised lesions that vary in size from 1-3 cm)
- On palpation of the abdomen, hepatomegaly (tender left lobe) and in about a third of patients splenomegaly may be detected
- Auscultation of the lungs frequently detects dry or moist rales during the acute phase
- Generalised lymphadenopathy may be present

Laboratory investigations

- Stool/urine examination for schistosome eggs
- Full blood count: eosinophilia (>80% of patients) with acute infections; anaemia and thrombocytopenia may be present in chronic and advanced schistosomiasis
- Coagulation profile: prolonged prothrombin time, indicated by an increased international normalised ratio, may be evident in chronic and advanced cases
- Urea, electrolytes, and liver function: raised urea and creatinine may be evident; and hyperglobulinaemia and hypoalbuminaemia may be present in chronic and advanced schistosomiasis
- Serology: may be diagnostic in patients in whom no eggs are present, such as those with Katayama syndrome
- Rectal or bladder biopsy for the identification of eggs may be performed if stool or urine are egg-negative but schistosomiasis is still suspected

Radiology

- Chest radiograph: pulmonary infiltrates are common in acute cases (Katayama syndrome)
- Abdominal ultrasound: can establish extent of liver and spleen pathology in intestinal schistosomiasis
- Pelvic ultrasound: can establish extent of bladder, ureteral, and renal pathology in urinary schistosomiasis

---

How is schistosomiasis diagnosed?

Box 2 outlines the approach to making a positive diagnosis of schistosomiasis including important questions to ask on medical history, specific signs to look for on physical examination, and relevant supportive laboratory and radiological investigations that should be undertaken. Figure 7 presents an algorithm for diagnosis and management. Microscopic examination of excreta (stool, urine) remains the gold standard test for diagnosis of schistosomiasis albeit with some limitations.[1] Schistosome eggs are easy to detect and identify on microscopy owing to their characteristic size and shape with a lateral or terminal spine (fig 8). Wait at least two months after the last known freshwater contact before looking for eggs, as a patent infection takes this long to start producing eggs.[1] [2W37-W42]

S mansoni, S japonicum, S mekongi, and S intercalatum (intestinal schistosomiasis) are diagnosed by observing even a single egg in thick smears of stool specimens (2-10 mg) with or without suspension in saline. The extent to which eggs are shed varies and as many as three specimens may be needed to make a diagnosis in some patients. Formalin based techniques for sedimentation and concentration may increase the diagnostic yield[1] in patients with a light infection, such as returned travellers.[W43] The rapid, simple, and inexpensive Kato-Katz thick smear stool examination—recommended by WHO for intestinal schistosomiasis when the intensity of infection is high— is widely used in field studies, and requires 40-50 mg of faeces.[14] It has specificity of 100% but its sensitivity varies with prevalence and intensity of infection, as well as with the number of stool specimens collected and slides prepared for microscopy.[W44-W47] For example, one diagnostic study[W44] showed that the sensitivity increased from 85% for one stool to 100% for four stools, while another[W45] showed that the sensitivity increased from 70% for one smear to 92% for four smears. Several population based studies have shown that mean egg burdens correlate with the mean severity of disease.[1] [2] [W46] [W47] However, it is not necessary to quantify the egg burden in order to provide clinical care.

S haematobium eggs are released in urine and are detected by microscopy in a urine sample concentrated by sedimentation, centrifugation, or filtration and forced over a paper or nitrocellulose filter.[1] [2] A urine sample is ideally collected between 10 am and 2 pm to coincide with the maximum excretion of eggs. Self reported blood in the urine and microhaematuria on reagent strips indicates potential infection in those living in endemic areas.[W48-W50]

Specific and highly sensitive PCR based assays have been developed for the detection of schistosome DNA in faeces or sera and plasma.[15] [16] [17] This approach has the potential to provide a test for diagnosing schistosomiasis in all phases of clinical disease, including the capacity to diagnose Katayama syndrome and active disease, and for the evaluation of treatment. The miracidium hatching test has been used by public health workers in China to rule out S japonicum infection.[2W51] Eggs are concentrated by placing faeces in a nylon tissue bag suspended in distilled water. Miracidia that hatch are visualised macroscopically, and their presence is diagnostic of infection.

A biopsy of bladder or rectal mucosa may be considered for diagnosis in patients with a typical clinical presentation of schistosomiasis but with no eggs detectable in urine or faeces.[2]

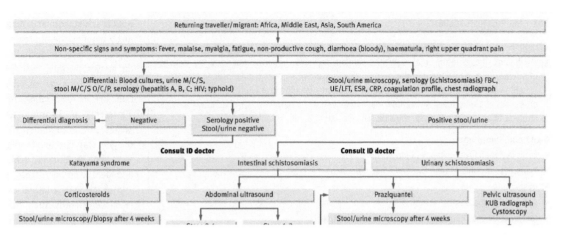

Fig 7 Diagnostic and treatment algorithm. M/C/S=microscopy/culture/sensitivity; O/C/P=ova/cysts/parasites; FBC=full blood count; UE/LFT=urea, electrolytes, and liver function test; ESR=erythrocyte sedimentation rate; CRP=C-reactive protein; ID doctor=infectious diseases doctor; KUB=kidney, ureter, and bladder; SCC=squamous cell carcinoma.

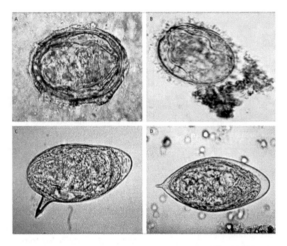

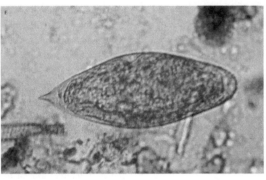

Fig 8 Schistosome eggs from species (A) *S japonicum*, (B) *S mekongi*, (C) *S mansoni*, (D) *S haematobium*,(E) *S intercalatum*. Courtesy of the Centers for Disease Control and Prevention, (A, C, D, and E) and www.dpd.cdc.gov/dpdx/HTML/ImageLibrary/Schistosomiasis_il.htm (B). Reproduced from Ross et al[8] with permission from Elsevier.

Indirect methods for diagnosing schistosome infection using clinical, subclinical, or biochemical morbidity markers are not specific given the generalised presentation of schistosomiasis. Current indirect methods include the use of clinical assessment of the patient coupled with ultrasound, liver biopsy, and subsequent histological examination and the measurement of biochemical markers.[1][2] Case studies have suggested that additional supportive laboratory evidence of schistosomiasis might include evidence of peripheral blood eosinophilia, anaemia (iron deficiency anaemia, anaemia of chronic disease, or macrocytic anaemia),

hypoalbuminaemia, raised concentrations of urea and creatinine, and hypergammaglobulinaemia.[1][2] Splenomegaly develops in some patients with pancytopenia.[1] Biochemical markers of liver fibrosis (pro-collagen peptides type III and IV, the P1 fragment of laminin, hyaluronic acid, fibrosin, tumour necrosis factor αR-II, and sICAM-1) measured in serum have potential to provide a highly sensitive and cost-effective method for assessment of schistosome induced fibrosis.[18][W55-W54] A biopsy of the liver may be necessary in some patients with co-infection (eg with hepatitis virus).[1] Liver involvement in patients with schistosomiasis may be suggested by the characteristic appearance of the organ on abdominal imaging.[1][2]

Antibody detection can be useful in a few specific circumstances, but its application is limited.[1][2][19] A positive serological test may be diagnostic in patients who are not excreting eggs, such as those with Katayama syndrome. Serological testing can be useful in field studies for defining regions of low level endemicity, where individual patients have low egg burdens, and may also be beneficial for determining whether infection has re-emerged in a region after an apparently successful control programme. It is important for diagnosis in travellers. Commercially available immunodiagnostic kits are less sensitive than multiple faecal examinations and less specific, owing to antibody cross-reactivity with antigens from other helminths.[1][19][W55-W57] Most techniques detect IgG, IgM, or IgE against soluble worm antigen or soluble egg antigen by enzyme-linked immunosorbent assay (ELISA), indirect haemagglutination, or immunofluorescence.[1][2] A cercarial antigen ELISA equivalent to the soluble egg antigen assay has been developed for serodiagnosis of schistosomiasis.[20]

Detection of circulating adult worm or egg antigens with labelled monoclonal or polyclonal antibodies in serum, urine, or sputum in infected individuals is another promising technique that may eventually supersede traditional diagnostic methods.[1][2] A commercially produced diagnostic test—the urine circulating cathodic antigen strip—is available for detection of schistosomiasis.[21] Surveillance studies and cross sectional surveys have shown that circulating cathodic antigen may be useful for screening for both *S haematobium* and *S mansoni* infections in the field but, to date, seems not to have sufficient sensitivity and/or specificity for definitive diagnosis.[W58][W59]

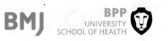

Treatment and prophylaxis for schistosomiasis. Adapted from Ross et al[8] with permission from Elsevier

Drug	Dosage regimen	Use in special groups			Main contraindication	Comments
		Pregnancy	Breast feeding	Children		
Praziquantel	S haematobium, S mansoni, S intercalatum, 40 mg/kg per day, two doses a day by mouth; S japonicum, S mekongi 60 mg/kg per day, three doses a day by mouth	Category B: usually safe, but benefits must outweigh risk	Discontinue breast feeding on day of treatment for up to 72 hours	Safe for age >4; not established for age <4	Hypersensitivity, ocular cysticercosis	Used to treat all schistosomes. Usually well tolerated. Caution while driving or performing other tasks requiring alertness on the day of treatment or the day after
Artesunate	S haematobium, S mansoni, S intercalatum, S japonicum, S mekongi, prophylaxis: 6 mg/kg every 2-4 weeks by mouth	No data, not recommended	No data, not recommended	Safe	Hypersensitivity	Prophylactic against S haematobium, S mansoni, S japonicum. Antischistosomula properties
Corticosteroids (prednisone)	Adult: 1.5-2.0 mg/kg per day by mouth for 3 weeks. Paediatric: 0.05-2.0 mg/kg per day, three doses a day by mouth	Category C: unknown effect, not recommended	Unknown effect, not recommended	Safe	Immunosuppressant	Used for treatment of Katayama syndrome (within 2 months of water contact) and treatment for sequelae of neuroschistosomiasis
Anticonvulsants	Consult neurologist	Category D: not recommended	Benefits must outweigh risk	Safe	Hypersensitivity	Treatment of seizures associated with neuroschistosomiasis

How is schistosomiasis treated?

Praziquantel

Randomised controlled trials have shown that praziquantel, a pyrazinoisoquinoline derivative, is a safe and effective oral drug that is active against all schistosome species.[22] [23] The drug is absorbed well but undergoes extensive first pass hepatic clearance. It is secreted in breast milk and is metabolised by the liver, and its metabolites (which are inactive) are excreted in the urine. The drug acts within one hour of ingestion although its precise action on adult worms is unknown. Laboratory studies have shown that it causes tetanic contractions and tegumental vacuoles, which cause worms to detach from the walls of veins and die. Schistosome calcium ion channels have been indirectly identified as the molecular target of praziquantel. In animal models, the presence of host antibodies is critical for efficacy.[1] [2] [22] [23]

Randomised controlled trials have also shown that the effective praziquantel dosage regimen is 60 mg/kg orally in divided doses over one day (3 x 20 mg/kg doses 4-hourly or 2 x 30 mg/kg either 4-hourly or 6-hourly) for S japonicum and S mekongi, and 40 mg/kg orally in divided doses over one day (2 x 20 mg/kg doses 4-hourly) for S mansoni, S haematobium, and S intercalatum.[1] [7] [19] [22] [23] [24] (table). However, a single 40 mg/kg dose is administered with 66-95% efficacy for epidemiological studies and population-based preventive chemotherapy control programmes.[2] [w60] Efficacy of 95-100% can be achieved with re-treatment four to six weeks later[25] and this second dose is advisable, especially if eosinophilia and a high antibody titre persist after primary treatment. Praziquantel has few side effects other than transient nausea, dizziness, rash, and pruritus, which are thought to be associated with the consequences of worm death rather than the drug itself.[1] [2] [22] [23] It can be used to treat young children (>4 years old) and pregnant women if breastfeeding is discontinued on the day of treatment and for the next 72 hours.[8] In patients with concurrent schistosomiasis and Taenia solium cysticercosis, praziquantel can cause irreparable eye lesions owing to the death of Taenia parasites in the ocular region, and it may also induce seizures and/or cerebral infarction owing to the intense inflammatory reactions that can be initiated by the dying Taenia cysts.[w61]

Experimental laboratory studies in mice have indicated, somewhat controversially, that resistance to praziquantel may be emerging in Africa, where there has been heavy exposure to the drug, and where, worryingly, there are reports of S mansoni and S haematobium infections that are not responsive.[1] [w62] [w63] Laboratory evidence suggests that drug tolerant schistosome worms may have an altered tegumental architecture, which could limit the effectiveness of the drug. So far, however, patients in many communities have undergone multiple courses of treatment over a period of 10 or more years without demonstrable loss of efficacy. Because worm reproduction in the mammalian host is sexual and the generation time is relatively long, resistance is likely to take many years to become an important clinical and public health issue. Nevertheless, resistance against praziquantel in the future cannot be ruled out and research should continue on developing alternative drugs—such as 4-phenyl-1,2,5-oxadiazole-3-carbonitrile-2-oxide, a new compound that has been shown to inhibit a crucial parasite enzyme, thioredoxin glutathione reductase).[26]

Adjuvant treatment

Corticosteroids (for example, prednisone 1.5-2.0 mg/kg per day for three weeks) are used to treat Katayama syndrome within two months of freshwater contact[8] [w55] [w64] (table) and for the treatment of schistosomal encephalopathy during the oviposition (egg laying) stage.[11] [12] Corticosteroids and anticonvulsants may be needed as adjuvants to praziquantel in neuroschistosomiasis, which needs specialised care.[1] Corticosteroids help to alleviate acute allergic reactions and prevent mass effects caused by excessive granulomatous inflammation in the central nervous system. Anticonvulsants are used to treat seizures associated with cerebral schistosomiasis but lifelong use is rarely indicated (table). Surgery should be preserved for particular patients, such as those with evidence of medullary compression and for those who deteriorate, despite clinical treatment.[11] [12] A ventriculoperitoneal shunt and corticosteroids are required to treat hydrocephalus and intracranial hypertension in cerebral schistosomiasis.[11] [12]

Other antiparasitic agents

Other drugs used to treat schistosomiasis are oxamniquine for S mansoni and metrifonate for S haematobium, but neither is effective against S japonicum.[1] [2] A recent randomised, exploratory open label trial of mefloquine-artesunate showed promising efficacy against S haematobium and further investigation of this approach is warranted.[27]

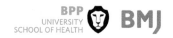

SOURCES AND SELECTION CRITERIA

Information for this clinical review was obtained from personal reference archives, personal experience, and extensive literature searches of the PubMed and Cochrane databases. We sourced English language papers that were fully published mainly between 2000 and September 2010 using appropriate index terms. Keywords included: "schistosomiasis"; "human schistosomiasis"; "schistosoma"; "schistosomiasis" with "diagnosis", "treatment", "acute", "clinical", "review", and "meta analysis"; and "schistosoma" with "diagnosis", "treatment", "acute", "clinical", "review", "meta analysis"; and "schistosome-induced pathophysiology clinical disease".

ADDITIONAL EDUCATIONAL RESOURCES

- Introduction to schistosomiasis (www.path.cam. ac.uk/~schisto/schistosoma/index.html)—Outline from the Schistosomiasis Research Group, University of Cambridge
- Health topics: schistosomiasis (www.who.int/topics/ schistosomiasis/en)—Information from the World Health Organization
- Parasites–schistosomiasis (www.cdc.gov/ncidod/dpd/ parasites/schistosomiasis/factsht_schistosomiasis.htm)— Fact sheet from the US Centers for Disease Control and Prevention
- Schistosomiasis (www.medicinenet.com/schistosomiasis/ article.htm)—Information for patients from MedicineNet

A PATIENT'S PERSPECTIVE

I am a 26 year old driver from Yueyang, China. One Sunday last summer, I drove to the Dongting Lake and fished and swam for 30 minutes. Twenty five days later, I developed a fever and cough and had a distended abdomen and diarrhoea. I was tired and had little appetite. On the third day of fever I attended a private hospital in Yueyang city. A chest x ray suggested a lung infection. I was treated for four days with antibiotics and intravenous drips, but my condition did not improve. At another local hospital, I was diagnosed with acute schistosomiasis. I returned to Yueyang to attend a special schistosomiasis hospital. Schistosome eggs were found in my stool and my blood reacted to substances in schistosome eggs. X rays showed fluid in my left lung, and my liver and spleen were enlarged. Acute schistosomiasis was confirmed. I was told all my problems were caused by *Schistosoma japonicum* and its eggs. I was prescribed a drug called praziquantel and took the tablets three times a day after meals, three pills each time, for six days. My fever was highest (41.5¢C) on the second day of my course of praziquantel. A special injection to lower my temperature was given to me and it worked well. I was discharged from hospital two days after I finished taking the drug. My stool, re-checked 10 and 20 days later, showed no more eggs. After three months, I feel well now.

Mr Yang, Yueyang, Hunan Province, People's Republic of China

Praziquantel cannot be used for chemoprophylaxis because of its short half-life (1-1.5 hours) and because it cannot kill schistosomula (migrating larvae) that are three to 21 days old. Artemether is effective against juvenile schistosomes during the first 21 days of infection in animals and humans[28] and, if given every two weeks, should kill all immature schistosomula. It has been used as a chemoprophylactic in schistosomiasis endemic areas for those at high risk of infection, such as flood relief workers and fishermen in China (table).[29] The doses required are lower than those for the treatment of malaria, but it is unlikely that artemether will be used routinely in regions where malaria is endemic because of the risk of selecting artemether resistant *Plasmodium falciparum*. Randomised controlled trials have shown that combination therapy with praziquantel plus artemether is safe and results in higher rates of worm reduction than praziquantel alone.[28] [29] However, a randomised, double blind, placebo controlled trial that evaluated combined chemotherapy for acute schistosomiasis japonica in China failed to show improved treatment efficacy compared with praziquantel alone.[24] Standard treatment with praziquantel was also more effective than artesunate with sulfalene plus pyrimethamine in the treatment of children with *S mansoni* infection in western Kenya.[30] It is unclear, therefore, whether artemether based combination therapy has a role in the treatment of schistosomiasis.[31 w65]

What are the future challenges?

The challenge for researchers who aim to improve the diagnosis and management of schistosomiasis will be to find a way to respond to environmental changes[w2] and to the threat of praziquantel resistance. New diagnostic procedures that are simple, rapid, and able to diagnose light infections (such as simple dipstick tests and PCR-based assays) need further development, as do new drugs that act effectively on both adult and larval schistosomes, and vaccines that target either the human host or, in the case of *S japonicum* or *S mekongi*, the animal reservoir hosts.

An integrated approach to the management of schistosomiasis[32 w66] that offers treatment alongside measures to reduce transmission by snail control (focal mollusciciding and environmental modification), health education and promotion, improved sanitation, and vaccination is the key to sustainable long term control of schistosomiasis.[32]

We thank Mimi Kersting and Simon Forsyth for their graphical support.

Contributors: D Gray, A Ross, Y Li and D McManus conceived and prepared the manuscript. D Gray and D McManus finalised the article.

Funding: The authors' studies on schistosomiasis have received financial support from various sources including: the UNICEF/UNDP/ World Bank/WHO Special Program for Research and Training in Tropical Diseases; the National Health and Medical Research Council of Australia; the Wellcome Trust (UK); the Sandler Foundation (USA); the Dana Foundation (USA); and the National Institute of Allergy and Infectious Diseases.

Competing interests: All authors have completed the Unified Competing Interest form at www.icmje.org/coi_disclosure.pdf (available on request from the corresponding author) and declare: all authors had financial support from the National Health and Medical Research Council of Australia for the submitted work, no financial relationships with any organisations that might have an interest in the submitted work in the previous three years, and no other relationships or activities that could appear to have influenced the submitted work.

Provenance and peer review: Not commissioned, externally peer reviewed.

1   Ross AGP, Bartley PB, Sleigh AC, Olds GR, Li Y, Williams GM, McManus DP. Schistosomiasis. *N Eng J Med* 2002;346:1212-9.
2   Gryseels B, Polman K, Clerinx J, Kestens L. Human schistosomiasis. *Lancet* 2006;368:1106-18.
3   Steinmann P, Keiser J, Bos R, Tanner M, Utzinger J. Schistosomiasis and water resources development: systematic review, meta-analysis, and estimates of people at risk. *Lancet Infect Dis* 2006;6:411-25.
4   King CH, Dickman K, Tisch DJ. Reassessment of the cost of chronic helminthic infection: a meta-analysis of disability-related outcomes in endemic schistosomiasis. *Lancet* 2005;365:561-9.
5   King CH, Dangerfield-Cha M. The unacknowledged impact of chronic schistosomiasis. *Chronic Illness* 2008;4:65-79.
6   Mas-Coma S, Valero MA, Bargues MD. Climate change effects on trematodiases, with emphasis on zoonotic fascioliasis and schistosomiasis. *Vet Parasitol* 2009;163:264-80
7   Leshem E, Meltzer E, Marva E, Schwartz E. Travel-related schistosomiasis acquired in Laos. *Emerg Infect Dis* 2009;15:1823-6.
8   Ross AG, Vickers D, Olds GR, Shah SM, McManus DP. Katayama syndrome. *Lancet Infect Dis* 2007;7:218-24.
9   Wynn TA, Thompson RW, Cheever AW, Mentink-Kane MM. Immunopathogenesis of schistosomiasis. *Immunol Rev* 2004;201:156-67.

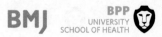

10 Burke ML, Jones MK, Gobert GN, Li YS, Ellis MK, McManus DP. Immunopathogenesis of human schistosomiasis. *Parasite Immunol* 2009;31:163-76.

11 Carod-Artal FJ. Neurological complications of *Schistosoma* infection. *Trans R Soc Trop Med Hyg* 2008;102:107-16.

12 Ferrari TC. Involvement of the central nervous system in the schistosomiasis. *Mem Inst Oswaldo Cruz* 2004;99:59-62.

13 McManus DP, Gray DJ, Li YS, Feng Z, Williams GM, Stewart D, et al. Schistosomiasis in the Peoples' Republic of China: the era of the Three Gorges Dam. *Clinic Microbiol Rev* 2010;23:442-66.

14 Katz N, Chaves A, Pellegrino J. A simple device for quantitative stool thick-smear technique for schistosomiasis mansoni. *Rev Inst Med Trop Sao Paulo* 1972;14:397-400.

15 Oliveira LM, Santos HL, Gonçalves MM, Barreto MG, Peralta JM. Evaluation of polymerase chain reaction as an additional tool for the diagnosis of low-intensity *Schistosoma mansoni* infection. *Diagn Microbiol Infect Dis* 2010;68:416-21.

16 Wichmann D, Panning M, Quack T, Kramme S, Burchard GD, Grevelding C, Drosten C. Diagnosing schistosomiasis by detection of cell-free parasite DNA in human plasma. *PLoS Negl Trop Dis* 2009;3:e422.

17 Gomes LI, Dos Santos Marques LH, Enk MJ, de Oliveira MC, Coelho PM, Rabello A. Development and evaluation of a sensitive PCR-ELISA system for detection of *Schistosoma* infection in feces. *PLoS Negl Trop Dis* 2010;4:e664.

18 Ellis MK, Li Y, Hou X, Chen H, McManus DP. sTNFR-II and sICAM-1 are associated with acute disease and hepatic inflammation in schistosomiasis japonica. *Int J Parasitol* 2008;38:717-23.

19 Bergquist R, Johansen MV, Utzinger J. Diagnostic dilemmas in helminthology: what tools to use and when? *Trends Parasitol* 2009;25:151-6.

20 Chand MA, Chiodini PL, Doenhoff MJ. Development of a new assay for the diagnosis of schistosomiasis, using cercarial antigens. *Trans R Soc Trop Med Hyg* 2010;104:255-8.

21 Stothard JR, Sousa-Figueiredo JC, Standley C, Van Dam GJ, Knopp S, Utzinger J, et al. An evaluation of urine-CCA strip test and fingerprick blood SEA-ELISA for detection of urinary schistosomiasis in schoolchildren in Zanzibar. *Acta Trop* 2009;111:64-70.

22 Doenhoff MJ, Cioli D, Utzinger J. Praziquantel: mechanisms of action, resistance and new derivatives for schistosomiasis. *Curr Opin Infect Dis* 2008;21:659-67.

23 Cioli D, Pica-Mattoccia L. Praziquantel. *Parasitol Res* 2003;90:S3-S9.

24 Hou XY, McManus DP, Gray DJ, Balen J, Luo XS, He YK, et al. A randomized, double-blind, placebo-controlled trial of safety and efficacy of combined praziquantel and artemether treatment for acute schistosomiasis japonica in China. *Bull World Health Organ* 2008;86:788-95.

25 Li Y, Sleigh AC, Williams GM, Ross AG, Forsyth SJ, Tanner M, McManus DP. Measuring exposure to *Schistosoma japonicum* in China. III. Activity diaries, snail and human infection, transmission ecology and options for control. *Acta Trop* 2000;75:279-89.

26 Sayed AA, Simeonov A, Thomas CJ, Inglese J, Austin CP, Williams DL. Identification of oxadiazoles as new drug leads for the control of schistosomiasis *Nat Med* 2008;14:407-12.

27 Keiser J, N'Guessan NA, Adoubryn KD, Silué KD, Vounatsou P, Hatz C, et al. Efficacy and safety of mefloquine, artesunate, mefloquine-artesunate, and praziquantel against *Schistosoma haematobium*: randomized, exploratory open-label trial. *Clin Infect Dis* 2010;50:1205-13.

28 Utzinger J, Xiao SH, Tanner M, Keiser J. Artemisinins for schistosomiasis and beyond. *Curr Opin Investig Drugs* 2007;8:105-16.

29 Xiao SH. Development of antischistosomal drugs in China, with particular consideration to praziquantel and the artemesinins. *Acta Trop* 2005;96:153-67.

30 Obonyo CO, Muok EM, Mwinzi PN. Efficacy of artesunate with sulfalene plus pyrimethamine versus praziquantel for treatment of *Schistosoma mansoni* in Kenyan children: an open-label randomised controlled trial. *Lancet Infect Dis* 2010;10:603-11.

31 Utzinger J, Tanner M, Keiser J. ACTs for schistosomiasis: do they act? *Lancet Infect Dis* 2010;10:579-81.

32 Gray DJ, McManus DP, Li YS, Williams GM, Bergquist R, Ross AG. Schistosomiasis elimination: lessons from the past guide the future. *Lancet Infect Dis* 2010;10:733-6.

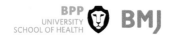

Diagnosis, treatment, and management of echinococcosis

Donald P McManus, National Health and Medical Research Council (Australia) senior principal research fellow; laboratory head[1], Darren J Gray, Australian Research Council fellow (DECRA); visiting scientist[1 2], Wenbao Zhang, senior research officer[1], Yurong Yang, Griffith University research fellow; professor; visiting scientist[1 3 4]

[1]Queensland Institute of Medical Research, Herston, Brisbane, Queensland, Australia

[2]School of Population Health, University of Queensland, Brisbane, Australia

[3]Griffith Health Institute, Griffith University, Brisbane, Australia

[4]Ningxia Medical University, Yinchuan, Ningxia Hui Autonomous Region, People's Republic of China

Correspondence to: D P McManus
don.mcmanus@qimr.edu.au

Cite this as: BMJ 2012;344:e3866

DOI: 10.1136/bmj.e3866

http://www.bmj.com/content/344/bmj.e3866

Echinococcosis (hydatid disease) is caused by the larvae of dog and fox tapeworms (cestodes) of the genus *Echinococcus* (family Taeniidae).[1 2 3] This zoonosis is characterised by long term growth of metacestode (hydatid) cysts in humans and mammalian intermediate hosts. The two major species that infect humans are *E granulosus* and *E multilocularis*, which cause cystic echinococcosis (CE) and alveolar echinococcosis (AE). A few reported cases of polycystic echinococcosis in Central and South America are caused by *E vogeli* and *E oligarthrus*.[2 W1 W2] The clinical potential of two other *Echinococcus* species (*E shiquicus* and *E felidis*) is unknown.[1 2]

Cystic echinococcosis (CE) and alveolar echinococcosis (AE) are serious chronic diseases with poor prognosis and high mortality if managed inadequately.[1 2 3] Of the estimated two to three million cases of echinococcosis globally, most are cystic.[2 4] Published reports and the Office International des Epizooties databases suggest that the global burden for human CE exceeds one million disability adjusted life years (DALYs), resulting in a loss of $760m (£490m; €612m) a year,[4] although these figures are probably underestimates.[2] Case series and small clinical trials show a mortality rate of 2-4% for CE, but this increases markedly with poor treatment and care.[5 6] There are 0.4 million cases of human AE, and survival analysis has shown that, if untreated or if treatment is limited, mortality exceeds 90% 10-15 years after diagnosis.[5 7] About 18 000 new cases of AE occur annually, with a total annual burden of 666 434 DALYs.[8]

Here, we introduce the *Echinococcus* parasites and the diseases they cause, and we discuss current methods for the diagnosis, treatment, and management of both types of echinococcosis. The life cycle characteristics of *Echinococcus* spp and the causes and immunology of echinococcosis have been described extensively.[1 2 3 9 10 11 12 13 14 W3-W16]

SUMMARY POINTS

- Echinococcosis is a parasitic zoonosis caused by *Echinococcus* cestode worms
- The two major species of medical importance are *Echinococcus granulosus* and *E multilocularis*, which cause cystic echinococcosis (CE) and alveolar echinococcosis (AE), respectively
- CE and especially AE are life threatening chronic diseases with a high fatality rate and poor prognosis if careful clinical management is not carried out
- Human CE is cosmopolitan and the more common presentation, accounting for most of the estimated two to three million global echinococcosis cases. AE has an extensive geographical range in the northern hemisphere
- Diagnosis is based on clinical findings, imaging (radiology, ultrasonography, computed axial tomography, magnetic resonance imaging), and serology
- Treatment options for CE are: surgery, percutaneous sterilisation, drugs, and observation (watch and wait). Surgery is the basis of treatment for early AE, but patients not suitable for surgery and those who have had surgical resection of parasite lesions must be treated with benzimidazoles (albendazole, mebendazole) for several years

Where and how is echinococcosis acquired?

Figure 1 shows the distribution of echinococcosis, according to statistics from the World Health Organization. *E granulosus* occurs worldwide, with high endemic areas concentrated in north east Africa, South America, and Eurasia.[10 12] *E multilocularis* is restricted to the northern hemisphere.[10 12] Figure 2 illustrates the *E granulosus* and *E multilocularis* life cycles and shows how humans become infected. Human co-infection with *E granulosus* and *E multilocularis* is not common, although these two species are co-endemic in some specific foci, notably the northwest of the People's Republic of China.[10] Figure 3 is an ultrasound image of a patient with both types of echinococcosis.

What are the clinical features of echinococcosis?

Most (>90%) CE cysts occur in liver, lung, or both organs.[12 W17] In general, the initial stages of CE do not cause symptoms—small cysts can remain asymptomatic for many years.[1] Because of the parasite's slow growth most cases are diagnosed in adults.[3] The onset of symptoms depends on the infected organ, the size and position of the cyst(s), their effect on the organ and adjacent tissues, and complications arising from the rupture of a cyst or a secondary infection.[1 12] Recurrent (secondary) CE can arise after primary cyst surgery, owing to spillage of the cyst contents, or if there is spontaneous or trauma induced cyst rupture and release of larvae, which can grow into secondary cysts.[10] Leakage or rupture of CE cysts can induce systemic immunological reactions and other complications, including cholangitis.[1 12]

AE generally has a longer latent phase (up to 15 years) before the onset of chronic disease.[1 12 W18] *E multilocularis* usually develops in the right liver lobe and AE lesions range from a few millimetres to 15-20 cm in diameter in areas of infiltration.[1 12] Extrahepatic primary disease is uncommon.[1 12 W18 W19] Metastasis formation leads to secondary AE with infiltration of the lung, spleen, or brain. Symptoms of AE usually include epigastric pain or cholestatic jaundice.[12]

How is echinococcosis diagnosed?

The box shows the best indicators of disease. The diagnosis of CE is based on clinical findings, imaging results, and serology.[1 2 3 6 7 11 12 15 16 17] Clinical manifestations may indicate cyst rupture, secondary bacterial infection, allergic reactions, or anaphylaxis.[1 17] Patients with symptoms should immediately be advised to undergo imaging and serology.

Ultrasound is a crucially important tool for the diagnosis, staging, and follow-up of abdominal CE cysts, although it has low sensitivity for detecting small cysts. The first generally accepted ultrasound classification for CE was developed in 1981.[W21] A series of meetings by a WHO informal working group on echinococcosis (WHO-IWGE) resulted in an international standardised ultrasound classification of CE

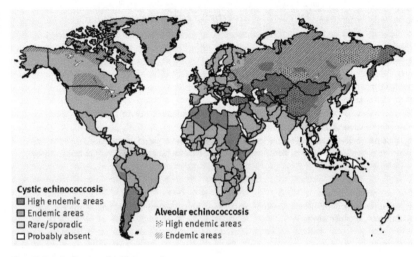

Fig 1 Global distribution of echinococcosis

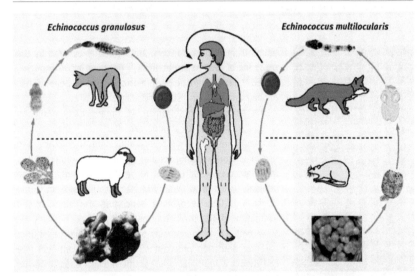

Fig 2 Life cycles of *E granulosus* and *E multilocularis*. Swallowed *Echinococcus* eggs hatch in the intestine to release oncospheres which pass through the gut wall and are carried in the blood system to various internal organs where they develop into hydatid cysts. *E granulosus* cysts are found mainly in the liver or lungs of humans and intermediate hosts. Dogs and other canines, which act as definitive hosts for *E granulosus*, become infected by eating offal with fertile hydatid cysts containing larval protoscoleces. These larvae evaginate, attach to the canine gut, and develop into sexually mature adult parasites. Eggs and gravid proglottids are released in faeces. Humans are typically "dead end" hosts, but not always.[w20] *E multilocularis* develops mainly in the liver of humans. Wild carnivores, such as the red fox (*Vulpes vulpes*) and the arctic fox (*Alopex lagopis*) are the major definitive hosts for *E multilocularis*, with small mammals acting as intermediate hosts. As with *E granulosus*, humans are exposed to *E multilocularis* eggs by handling infected definitive hosts or by eating contaminated food

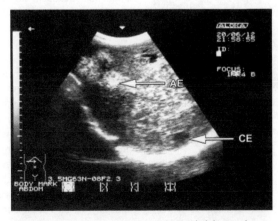

Fig 3 Ultrasound image of simultaneous alveolar (AE) (stage P3) and cystic (CE) (stage CE4) echinococcosis in the right liver of a patient from the People's Republic of China

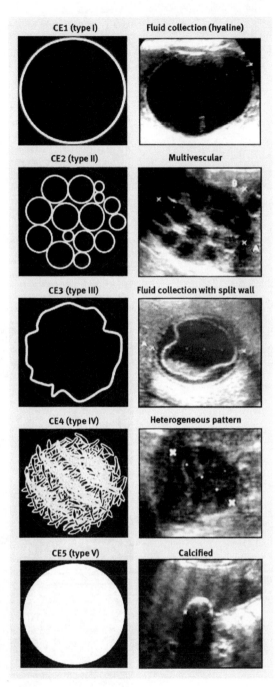

Fig 4 Ultrasound classification of CE cysts. The WHO informal working group on echinococcosis classification differs from that of Gharbi and colleagues[w21] by the addition of a "cystic lesion" (CL) stage (undifferentiated) (not shown), and by reversing the order of CE types 2 and 3. CE3 transitional cysts may be differentiated into CE3a (with detached endocyst) and CE3b (predominantly solid with daughter vesicles).[15] CE1 and CE3a are early stage cysts and CE4 and CE5 late stage cysts

cysts into three groups (fig 4).[6][12][16] Microscopy of cystic fluid for brood capsules or protoscoleces provides proof of infection and cyst viability.[6] Polymerase chain reaction (PCR) analysis of biopsy material can also provide a definitive diagnosis.[6] High field magnetic resonance spectroscopy is also useful for determining cyst viability and for staging.[1][w22]

CE serology is a helpful diagnostic adjunct and can be used to monitor patients after surgery or drug treatment. However, although used widely, particularly in developing countries where imaging techniques may not be readily available, questions remain with regard to its effectiveness

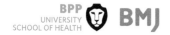

Table 1 WHO informal working group on echinococcosis PNM classification of alveolar echinococcosis

PMN	Characteristics
P	Hepatic localisation of the parasite
PX	Primary tumour cannot be assessed
Po	No detectable tumour in the liver
P1	Peripheral lesions without proximal vascular or biliary involvement
P2	Central lesions with proximal vascular or biliary involvement of one lobe*
P3	Central lesions with hilar vascular or biliary involvement of both lobes or with involvement of two hepatic veins
P4	Any liver lesion with extension along the vessels† and the biliary tree
N	Extrahepatic involvement of neighbouring organs (diaphragm, lung, pleura, pericardium, heart, gastric and duodenal wall, adrenal glands, peritoneum, retroperitoneum, parietal wall (muscles, skin, bone), pancreas, regional lymph nodes, liver ligaments, kidney)
NX	Not evaluable
No	No regional involvement
N1	Regional involvement of contiguous organs or tissues
M	The absence or presence of distant metastases (lung, distant lymph nodes, spleen, central nervous system, orbit of the eye, bone, skin, muscle, kidney, distant peritoneum, retroperitoneum)
MX	Not completely evaluated
Mo	No metastasis‡
M1	Metastasis

*For classification, the plane projecting between the bed of the gall bladder and the inferior vena cava divides the liver into two lobes.
†Inferior vena cava, portal vein, and arteries.
‡Negative on chest radiography and cerebral computed tomography.

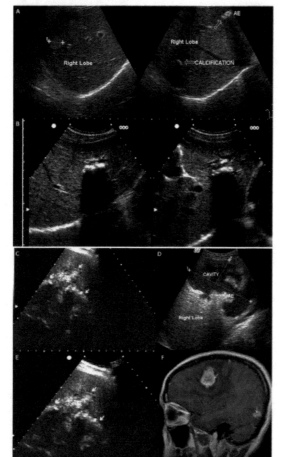

Fig 5 Staging of AE lesions according to the WHO informal working group on echinococcosis PNM classification system, based on ultrasound observations. (A) P1; (B) P2; (C) P3; (D) P4; (E) and (F) P4 NO M1—panel E shows primary lesion in the right liver lobe; panel F shows secondary metastatic lesions in the brain

for clinical detection and screening.[17] [w23] [w24] Serum antibody measurement is more sensitive than detection of circulating E granulosus antigens,[1] [11] [w8] but available tests lack standardisation.[11] [17] Current serology for human CE mainly tests for IgG antibodies against native or recombinant antigen B by enzyme linked immunosorbent assay or western blotting.[2] [11] [w25] Test specificity is affected by immunological crossreactivity with antigens found in other helminth infections, cancers, and liver cirrhosis and by the presence of anti-P1 antibodies.[2] [11] Although not thoroughly tested,[17] serodiagnostic performance seems to depend also on cyst location, cyst size, and stage.

The seriousness of human AE means early detection is crucial so that treatment can start.[1] [5] [12] Diagnosis is analogous to that for CE including clinical findings and use of imaging techniques and serology.[1] [5] [12] Ultrasound is the main diagnostic test for AE in the abdomen,[5] and the imaging based WHO-IWGE PNM classification system (table 1; fig 5) is the recognised benchmark for standardised evaluation of diagnosis and treatment.[5] [12] [18]

As with CE, serodiagnosis of AE is used as an adjunct to other detection procedures.[11] [w8] [w26] [w27] Conventional PCR can detect E multilocularis specific nucleic acids in tissue biopsies and real time PCR can be used to assess viability.[5] [w28] [w29] Notably, however, for both diseases a negative real time PCR result does not reflect complete parasite inactivity and a negative PCR cannot rule out disease.[5] [w29]

How is CE treated and managed?
The WHO-IWGE classification provides the basis for choosing basically four treatment and management options for CE: surgery, percutaneous sterilisation, drug treatment, and observation (watch and wait).[5] [6] [17] However, there is no optimum treatment for CE and no clinical trials have compared the different modalities.[5] Table 2 shows the current expert consensus on the management of liver CE.[5]

Surgery
Surgery is the classic treatment but, despite being curative, it does not totally prevent recurrence.[5] Furthermore, in the absence of specific clinical trials, the evidence for the surgical treatment of complicated liver and disseminated CE is limited.[5] [w30] Surgery is, however, the choice for large or infected cysts, cysts likely to rupture, and cysts in important organ locations.[1] [5] Surgery may not be practical for patients with multiple cysts in several organs.[1] [5] Open cystectomy, pericystectomy, partial hepatectomy or lobectomy, cyst extrusion (Barrett's technique), and drainage of infected cysts are some of the surgical options available.[1] In cases where cyst resection is incomplete, or if small lesions remain undetected, disease can recur.[1] Postoperative fatality is about 2% but can be higher if additional surgery is needed or if medical facilities are inadequate.[12] [15]

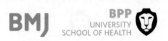

Table 2 Suggested stage specific approach to treatment of uncomplicated cystic echinococcosis of the liver. Adapted from Brunetti and colleagues,[5] with permission from Elsevier

WHO classification	Surgery	Percutaneous treatment	Drug treatment	Suggested treatment	Resource setting
CE1	No	Yes	Yes	<5 cm: albendazole	Optimal
				<5 cm: PAIR	Minimal
				>5 cm: PAIR + albendazole	Optimal
				>5 cm: PAIR	Minimal
CE2	Yes	Yes	Yes	Other PT + albendazole	Optimal
				Other PT	Minimal
CE3a	No	Yes	Yes	<5 cm: albendazole	Optimal
				<5 cm: PAIR	Minimal
				>5cm: PAIR + albendazole	Optimal
				>5cm: PAIR	Minimal
CE3b	Yes	Yes	Yes	Non-PAIR PT + albendazole	Optimal
				Non-PAIR PT	Minimal
CE4				Watch and wait	Optimal*
CE5				Watch and wait	Optimal*

*Minimal may not be applicable here because in low resourced remote endemic areas it may be impossible or too expensive to travel to the nearest hospital just to obtain a diagnosis.
PAIR= puncture, aspiration, injection, reaspiration; PT=percutaneous treatment.

Percutaneous sterilisation techniques

These include PAIR (puncture, aspiration, injection, reaspiration), which destroys the cyst's germinal layer,[w31-w33] and modified catheterisation approaches, which evacuate the complete cyst.[1 5 12] PAIR, developed in the 1980s, involves ultrasound assisted percutaneous needle puncture aspiration of the cyst, followed by injection of a suitable protoscolicide (such as 20% sodium chloride or 95% ethanol) and cyst reaspiration after 15-20 minutes.[1] Anaphylaxis is a risk. Assess cyst fluid for protoscoleces and bilirubin, and, to minimise the risk of secondary CE, co-administer benzimidazole. CE2 and CE3b stages (fig 4) are problematic because they have many compartments that require individual puncture, and these commonly relapse after PAIR.[17] Large bore catheters, combined with suitable aspiration equipment, may in future replace PAIR for these stages,[17] but their true effectiveness needs to be established.[5] The choice of between surgery or percutaneous sterilisation can be difficult. Comparison of the two procedures requires large carefully designed clinical studies, which have yet to be done.[17]

Antiparasite drug treatment

The benzimidazoles—albendazole and mebendazole— are generally regarded as the most effective drugs for treating uncomplicated CE cysts and as an alternative to invasive surgery. Mebendazole was used in the 1970 and 1980s, but albendazole is now the drug of choice. It is administered in 10 mg/kg doses (usually 400 mg) twice daily; mebendazole (40-50 mg/kg a day in three doses) is less effective than albendazole.[19] However, studies carried out with both drugs have been small, and heterogeneity in methodology has prevented meta-analysis.[17] Furthermore, a recent pooled study of individual data from patients with CE (six treatment centres; five countries) suggested that the overall efficacy of these drugs may have been overstated.[20] Systematic randomised controlled trials that compare standardised treatment with benzimidazoles at different cyst stages with other options are needed,[20] especially as these drugs seem to work better against some cyst stages (such as small CE1 cysts). Indeed, benzimidazoles are not effective against large cysts (>10 cm), being diluted by the volume of fluid present.[5] The degree and type of side effects of sustained use of benzimidazoles also warrant rigorous study.[5] Benzimidazoles should not be used in early pregnancy or against cysts at risk of rupture.[1 5] Thorough

assessment of other anthelmintics (such as praziquantel and nitazoxanide) and combinations of anthelmintics (such as albendazole plus praziquantel) that have been used to treat CE is also needed.[w34-w37]

Watch and wait

Leaving uncomplicated cyst types (CE4 and CE5) untreated and just monitoring them by imaging (particularly ultrasound) is a logical management option given that a proportion of cysts calcify over time and become completely inactive; such cysts do not compromise organ function or cause discomfort.[15 w38] Such an approach is attractive but requires systematic study to define fully its indications and limitations.

How is AE treated and managed?

Table 3 details a stage specific approach to treating AE. Historically, surgery has been the recommended treatment for early disease.[1 5] Early diagnosis reduces the need for radical surgery and results in fewer unresectable lesions.[1 5] Long term treatment with benzimidazoles is essential for patients with inoperable AE or after resection of *E multilocularis* lesions.[1 5 12] Benzimidazoles are parasitostatic—they inhibit larval proliferation but do not kill metacestodes.[w39] They should be given for a minimum of two years and patients monitored for at least 10 years for relapse.[w40] Benzimidazoles are not recommended before surgery.[5] As for CE, the drugs are given orally with fat-rich meals (10-15 mg/kg/day, in two doses), although they have been given at a higher dose of 20 mg per kg per day for 4.5 years.[5] Continuous treatment with albendazole is tolerated well, having been used for more than 20 years in some patients; intermittent use is not recommended.[5] Mebendazole, given at a dose of 40-50 mg per kg per day over three days with a fatty meal, is an alternative to albendazole.[5] Figure 6 shows the effect of albendazole treatment on a P4 AE lesion. Neither praziquantel nor nitazoxanide is clinically effective against AE.[5 w41-w43]

Allotransplantation of the liver has been carried out in patients with end stage AE.[w44-w46] However, the essential use of immunosuppressive treatment can stimulate the proliferation of parasitic remnants in the lung or brain.[w45] A long term prospective follow-up of patients with AE treated by palliative liver transplantation in the 1980s found that some patients survived for 20 years.[21] Ex vivo liver resection, followed by autotransplantation of AE-free lateral

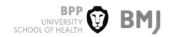

Table 3 Suggested stage specific approach to treatment of alveolar echinococcosis. Adapted from Brunetti and colleagues,[5] with permission from Elsevier

WHO classification	Surgery	Interventional treatment	Drug treatment	Suggested treatment	Resource setting
P1N0M0	Yes	No	Yes	Radical resection (R0); benzimidazoles for 2 years; PET/CT controls	Optimal
				Radical resection (R0); benzimidazoles for 3 months	Minimal
P2N0M0	Yes	No	Yes	Radical resection (R0); benzimidazoles for 2 years	Optimal
				Radical resection (R0); benzimidazoles for 3 months	Minimal
P3N0M0	No	No	Yes	Benzimidazoles continuously; PET/CT /MRI scan initially and at 2 year intervals	Optimal
				Benzimidazoles continuously	Minimal
P3N1M0	No	Yes	Yes	Benzimidazoles continuously; PET/CT/MRI scan initially and at 2 year intervals	Optimal
				Surgery if indicated	Minimal
P4N0M0	No	Yes	Yes	Benzimidazoles continuously; PET/CT/MRI scan initially and at 2 year intervals	Optimal
				Surgery, if indicated	Minimal
P4N1M1	No	Yes	Yes	Benzimidazoles continuously; PET/CT/MRI scan initially and at 2 year intervals	Optimal
				Surgery if indicated	Minimal

CT=computed tomography; MRI=magnetic resonance imaging; PET=positron emission tomography; R0=complete removal of alveolar echinococcosis lesion.

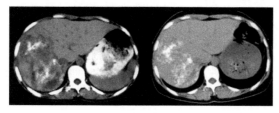

Fig 6 Computed tomography scan of the liver showing a large irregular AE lesion in the right lobe containing scattered calcifications and liquefactions (left panel). After five years of treatment with albendazole, the lesion had not changed in size but the areas of calcification had increased and those of liquefaction had decreased (right panel)

segments,[22] may offer a radical approach to improving prognosis, but this procedure needs to be fully evaluated.

What are the future challenges?

Considerable recent progress has been made in the diagnosis, treatment, and management of echinococcosis, but challenges remain. Clinical trial data systematically evaluating existing treatments are not available and ideal treatment options are lacking. Treatment indicators are often complicated, being based on cyst characteristics, availability of medical and surgical expertise and equipment, and patient compliance in long term monitoring programmes.[5]

Comparable and standardised procedures and terminology need to be established by the medical fraternity.[5] PAIR should be undertaken only by experienced doctors and trained teams capable of managing anaphylactic shock.[1] PAIR needs to be studied systematically, via randomised controlled trials, to assess its efficacy compared with surgery and other available options for treatment of uncomplicated hepatic cysts.[23]

Given recent concerns about the cost and treatment efficacy of the benzimidazoles,[17] new drugs are needed to combat both AE and CE. Strategies aimed at defining new compounds need to be pursued.[24]

The WHO-IWGE consensus recommendations for the ultrasound imaging based classification of CE cysts need to be more wider disseminated to clinicians because they are useful when choosing treatment options.[5] Similarly, the WHO-IWGE classification for AE should be advocated as the international classification because it can help determine

whether an *E multilocularis* lesion should be excised or otherwise treated, give some indications for improved prognosis, and help determine the best treatment option for the individual patient.[5]

The current clinical diagnosis of AE and CE relies mainly on the detection of parasite lesions by imaging methods, but the procedures are expensive and are generally not available in resource poor settings. Furthermore, they are not useful for detecting the early stages of infection, which is a major disadvantage because earlier diagnosis results in more effective and successful treatment. Serodiagnosis can play a role in early detection because specific anti-*Echinococcus* antibodies appear in the blood system four to eight weeks after infection. Most available immunodiagnostic techniques have been used in the diagnosis of echinococcosis.[11] However, most of these tests have not been systematically compared by independent laboratories, they are mainly used for research purposes, and few have found general acceptance by clinicians.

We thank Mimi Kersting and Simon Forsyth for graphical support and Hawys McManus for help in editing drafts of the manuscript.

Contributors: DPMcM conceived the manuscript and is guarantor. DPMcM, DJG, WZ, and YY prepared individual sections of the article and jointly prepared drafts of the paper. DPMcM and DJG finalised the article. All authors approved the final version of the manuscript.

Funding: The authors' studies on echinococcosis have received financial support from the National Health and Medical Research Council of Australia and the Queensland Institute of Medical Research.

Competing interests: All authors have completed the ICMJE uniform disclosure form at www.icmje.org/coi_disclosure.pdf (available on request from the corresponding author) and declare: all authors had financial support from the National Health and Medical Research Council of Australia for the submitted work; no financial relationships with any organisations that might have an interest in the submitted work in the previous three years; no other relationships or activities that could appear to have influenced the submitted work.

Provenance and peer review: Commissioned; externally peer reviewed.

Patient consent obtained.

1 McManus DP, Zhang W, Li J, Bartley PB. Echinococcosis. *Lancet* 2003;362:1295-304.
2 Craig PS, McManus DP, Lightowlers MW, Chabalgoity JA, Garcia HH, Gavidia CM, et al. Prevention and control of cystic echinococcosis. *Lancet Infect Dis* 2007;7:385-94.
3 Moro P, Schantz PM. Echinococcosis: a review. *Int J Infect Dis* 2009;13:125-33.
4 Budke CM, Deplazes P, Torgerson PR. Global socioeconomic impact of cystic echinococcosis. *Emerg Infect Dis* 2006;12:296-303.

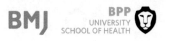

SOURCES AND SELECTION CRITERIA

We obtained information from personal reference archives, personal experience, and extensive literature searches of the PubMed and Cochrane databases. We sourced English language papers that were fully published mainly between 2000 and March 2012 using appropriate index terms. Keywords included: "*Echinococcus*", "*Echinococcus granulosus*", "*Echinococcus multilocularis*", "echinococcal cysts", "hydatid cysts", "hydatid disease", "cystic echinococcosis", "alveolar echinococcosis", "hydatidosis", "hydatid", "surgery", "liver transplant", "mebendazole", "albendazole", "benzimidazole", "chemotherapy", "PAIR", "percutaneous treatment", "percutaneous drainage", "ultrasound"; and "*Echinococcus*" with "diagnosis", "serology", "treatment", "clinical", "review", "meta analysis"; and "echinococcosis" with diagnosis", "serology", "treatment", "clinical", "review", and "meta analysis".

KEY INDICATORS FOR A POSITIVE DIAGNOSIS OF ECHINOCOCCOSIS

Medical history

- Have you travelled to or emigrated from an endemic country (about five to 10 years ago)? If so, from where? (fig 1)
- Have you had contact with dogs, foxes, or livestock during the past five to 10 years?
- Have you worked in a pastoral area where you may have had contact with wildlife during the past five to 10 years?
- Have you worked in an abattoir during the past five to 10 years?

Cystic echinococcosis

- Upper abdominal discomfort
- Poor appetite

Alveolar echinococcosis

- Vague abdominal pain (right upper quadrant; 30% cases) (most cases originate in the liver)
- Jaundice (25% cases)
- Fatigue, weight loss, fever, chills

Physical examination

Cystic echinococcosis

- On palpation of the abdomen a mass may be found on the surface of organs (the liver is affected in two thirds of patients); hepatomegaly or abdominal distension may also be seen
- Chest pain, cough, and haemoptysis can be indicative of cysts in the lung; cyst rupture into the bronchi may result in the expulsion of hydatid material and cystic membranes
- Cyst rupture can induce fever, urticaria, eosinophilia, and anaphylactic shock

Alveolar echinococcosis

- On palpation of the abdomen, hepatomegaly may be detected
- Splenomegaly may be present in cases complicated by portal hypertension
- Collateral circulation between the inferior and superior vena cava may be present on the skin in the thoracic and abdominal regions in advanced cases
- Other physical symptoms are dictated by the location of metastatic legions (see lung involvement for cystic echinococcosis)

Laboratory investigations

- General laboratory investigations show non-specific results
- Serology can help form a definitive diagnosis
- Ultrasound guided fine needle biopsy can also be used to examine hydatid cyst fluid for the presence of protoscoleces or DNA using molecular techniques (polymerase chain reaction)

Radiology

- Ultrasound (figs 4 and 5), computed tomography, and magnetic resonance imaging are the procedures of choice for the definitive diagnosis of echinococcosis
- Imaging should be used to examine not only the liver but also the entire abdomen and thorax, and they are able to determine metastatic locations in alveolar echinococcosis

A PATIENT'S PERSPECTIVE

I am a 31 year old farmer of the Hui minority from Ningxia, China. I was first admitted to hospital in May 2003 with extreme fatigue, cough, and difficulty breathing. A chest radiograph showed that my lungs were scattered with dark shadows and the doctors diagnosed me with a form of cancer and sent me home. In September 2003 a specialist doctor reviewed my case and asked me to come back to the hospital for further tests. The specialist doctor asked me many questions, performed a physical examination, and ran some tests including an ultrasound. The ultrasound and blood test showed that I did not have cancer but had alveolar echinococcosis. The parasite started in my liver and had spread to my lungs. I was given daily treatment with a drug called albendazole and after six months another chest radiograph showed that my lungs were clear and I felt much better. I was told to continue taking the drug to stop the parasite spreading from my liver to other organs. Today I am still taking albendazole and am feeling well.

Zhang Yin Gui, Xiji County, Ningxia Hui Autonomous Region, Peoples' Republic of China

TIPS FOR NON-SPECIALISTS

- Refer symptomatic patients who travelled to, or emigrated from, an echinococcosis endemic area about five to 10 years ago, and had contact with dogs or wildlife, to an infectious disease physician
- Serology provides supportive information for diagnosis but imaging studies provide the definitive diagnosis
- Differential diagnosis is important because alveolar echinococcosis often presents with cancer-like symptoms
- Imaging studies should examine the entire thorax and abdomen, not just the liver
- Treatment may involve the use of drugs (albendazole, mebendazole) or surgery (or both)

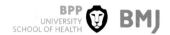

ADDITIONAL EDUCATIONAL RESOURCES

- Wikipedia (http://en.wikipedia.org/wiki/Echinococcosis)—Information on the *Echinococcus* parasites and echinococcosis for patients and the public
- Wikipedia (http://en.wikipedia.org/wiki/Alveolar_hydatid_disease)—Brief fact sheet on alveolar echinococcosis for patients and the public
- US Centers for Disease Control and Prevention (http://www.cdc.gov/parasites/echinococcosis/)—Fact sheet on the *Echinococcus* parasites and echinococcosis for professionals, patients, and the public
- US Centers for Disease Control and Prevention (www.dpd.cdc.gov/dpdx/HTML/Echinococcosis.htm)—Description of the *Echinococcus* parasites and echinococcosis for professionals, patients, and the public
- Patient.co.uk (www.patient.co.uk/doctor/Hydatid-Disease.htm)—Fact sheet of the *Echinococcus* parasites and echinococcosis for professionals, patients and the public
- Nunnari G, Pinzone MR, Gruttadauria S, Celesia BM, Madeddu G, Malaguarnera G, et al. Hepatic echinococcosis: clinical and therapeutic aspects. *World J Gastroenterol* 2012;18:1448-58. Review of the clinical and therapeutic aspects of hepatic echinococcosis for professionals

5   Brunetti E, Kern P, Vuitton DA; Writing Panel for the WHO-IWGE. Expert consensus for the diagnosis and treatment of cystic and alveolar echinococcosis in humans. *Acta Trop* 2010;114:1-16.
6   Brunetti E, Junghanss T. Update on cystic hydatid disease. *Curr Opin Inf Dis* 2009;22:497-502.
7   Torgerson PR, Schweiger A, Deplazes P, Pohar M, Reichen J, Ammann RW, et al. Alveolar echinococcosis: from a deadly disease to a well-controlled infection. Relative survival and economic analysis in Switzerland over the last 35 years. *J Hepatol* 2008;49:72-7.
8   Torgerson PR, Keller K, Magnotta M, Ragland N. The global burden of alveolar echinococcosis. *PLoS Negl Trop Dis* 2010;4:e722.
9   Thompson R, McManus DP. Towards a taxonomic revision of the genus Echinococcus. *Trends Parasitol* 2002;18:452-7.
10 Eckert J, Deplazes P. Biological, epidemiological, and clinical aspects of echinococcosis, a zoonosis of increasing concern. *Clin Microbiol Rev* 2004;17:107-35.
11 Zhang W, McManus DP. Recent advances in the immunology and diagnosis of echinococcosis. *FEMS Immunol Med Microbiol* 2006;47:24-41.

12 Pawlowski ZS, Eckert DA, Vuitton DA, Ammann RW, Kern P, Craig PS, et al. Echinococcosis in humans: clinical aspects, diagnosis and treatment. In: Eckert J, Gemmell MA, Meslin F-X, Pawlowski ZS, eds. WHO/OIE manual on echinococcosis in humans and animals: a public health problem of global concern. World Organisation for Animal Health, 2001:20-72.
13 McManus DP. Echinococcosis with particular reference to Southeast Asia. *Adv Parasitol* 2010;72C: 267-303.
14 Zhang W, Ross AG, McManus DP. Mechanisms of immunity in hydatid disease: implications for vaccine development. *J Immunol* 2008;181:6679-85.
15 Junghanss T, da Silva AM, Horton J, Chiodini PL, Brunetti E. Clinical management of cystic echinococcosis: state of the art, problems, and perspectives. *Am J Trop Med Hyg* 2008;79:301-11.
16 WHO Informal Working Group on Echinococcosis. International classification of ultrasound images in cystic echinococcosis for application in clinical and field epidemiological settings. *Acta Trop* 2003;85:253-61.
17 Brunetti E, Garcia HH, Junghanss T; International CE Workshop in Lima, Peru, 2009. Cystic echinococcosis: chronic, complex, and still neglected. *PLoS Negl Trop Dis* 2011;5:e1146.
18 Kern P, Wen H, Sato N, Vuitton DA, Gruener B, Shao Y, et al. WHO classification of alveolar echinococcosis: principles and application. *Parasitol Int* 2006;55(suppl):S283-7.
19 Horton R. Albendazole for the treatment of echinococcosis. *Fundam Clin Pharmacol* 2003;17:205-12.
20 Stojkovic M, Zwahlen M, Teggi A, Vutova K, Cretu CM, Virdone R, et al. Treatment response of cystic echinococcosis to benzimidazoles: a systematic review. *PLoS Negl Trop Dis* 2009;3:e524.
21 Bresson-Hadni S, Blagosklonov O, Knapp J, Grenouillet F, Sako Y, Delabrousse E, et al. Should possible recurrence of disease contraindicate liver transplantation in patients with end-stage alveolar echinococcosis? A 20-year follow-up study. *Liver Transpl* 2011;17:855-65.
22 Wen H, Dong J-H, Zhang J-H, Zhao J-M, Shao Y-M, Duan W-D, et al. Ex vivo liver resection followed by autotransplantation for end-stage hepatic alveolar echinococcosis. *Chin Med J* 2011;124: 2813-7.
23 Nasseri-Moghaddam S, Abrishami A, Taefi A, Malekzadeh R. Percutaneous needle aspiration, injection, and re-aspiration with or without benzimidazole coverage for uncomplicated hepatic hydatid cysts. *Cochrane Database Syst Rev* 2011;1:CD003623.
24 Hemphill A, Müller J. Alveolar and cystic echinococcosis: towards novel chemotherapeutical treatment options. *J Helminthol* 2009;83:99-111.

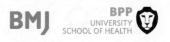

Management of chronic hepatitis B infection

Vinay Sundaram, assistant medical director of liver transplantation[1], Kris Kowdley, director of the Swedish Liver Care Network, research director of the organ care program[2]

[1]Department of Medicine and Comprehensive Transplant Center, Cedars-Sinai Medical Center, Los Angeles, CA, USA

[2]Liver Care Network, Swedish Medical Center, Seattle, WA 98104, USA

Correspondence to: K Kowdley Kris. Kowdley@swedish.org

Cite this as: *BMJ* 2015;351:h4263

DOI: 10.1136/bmj.h4263

http://www.bmj.com/content/351/bmj.h4263

ABSTRACT

Hepatitis B virus (HBV) is a global health problem that can lead to cirrhosis and hepatocellular carcinoma (HCC). Although HBV vaccination has reduced the prevalence Of HBV infection, the burden of disease remains high. Treatment with antiviral drugs reduces the risk of liver disease and the development of HCC, and it can even reverse liver fibrosis. However, challenges remain regarding optimal timing, as well as the modality and duration of treatment. Currently approved drugs include pegylated interferon and nucleos(t)ide analogs. Nucleos(t)ide analogs are better tolerated and provide excellent viral suppression with a low risk of antiviral resistance, but pegylated interferon offers the benefit of a finite duration of treatment. Monitoring of hepatitis B surface antigen (HBsAg) levels may help to predict the likelihood of response to treatment, particularly for pegylated interferon. Prolonged treatment is usually needed with oral antiviral agents, and relapse is common if treatment is discontinued. New treatments that result in sustained clearance of HBV DNA and the clearance of HBsAg are needed.

Introduction

Hepatitis B virus (HBV) is a major global health burden—240 million patients are estimated to be chronically infected.[1] [2] About 30% of patients with chronic HBV develop liver cirrhosis, and nearly 23% of these decompensate within five years.[3] [4] (fig 1) Research on the long term efficacy of HBV treatment, the impact of treatment on the progression of liver disease and regression of cirrhosis, the utility of combination therapy, and strategies to manage patients coinfected with HIV and hepatitis delta virus (HDV) is ongoing. This research will inform decisions about the optimal timing of treatment initiation, the appropriateness of treatment withdrawal, and the role of serologic markers in predicting the response to treatment.

This review will focus on the clinical management of chronic HBV infection. It will discuss the epidemiology and life cycle of the disease, the accuracy of non-invasive testing for fibrosis in HBV, when to start treatment, which treatment modalities to use, the effect of treatment on the development of HBV related complications, and when to consider stopping treatment. Management in special populations infected with HBV, future treatments, and the potential for viral eradication will also be reviewed.

Incidence and prevalence

About 240 million people are infected with HBV worldwide and nearly 780000 people die from HBV related complications each year.[5] Furthermore, nearly 50% of the mortality secondary to hepatocellular carcinoma (HCC) in 2010 was associated with HBV.[6] In the United States alone nearly 704000 people have HBV infection.[7]

A systematic review from 2012 estimated that nearly 1.32 million people with HBV infection in the US were foreign born, with 58% having emigrated from Asia.[8] Regions of the world considered to have high prevalence (>7%) include China, South East Asia, Africa, the Pacific Islands, parts of the Middle East, and the Amazon basin.[9] Areas of intermediate prevalence (2-7%) include south central and southwest Asia, eastern and southern Europe, Russia, Central America, and South America. Countries of low prevalence (<2%) are primarily the US, western Europe, Australia, and Japan.[2]

Because of the low likelihood of symptoms related to chronic HBV infection, the true incidence is difficult to determine.

In areas of the world with a high prevalence of HBV, perinatal transmission is the main mode of spread, whereas in countries with lower prevalence sexual exposure is principally responsible for transmission.[2] The risk of infection is greater in those with a high number of sexual partners, homosexual males, and those with other sexually transmitted diseases.[10] Blood borne transmission of HBV may still occur in developing countries.[2]

The availability of the HBV vaccine since 1981 has led to a substantial decrease in the incidence of HBV infection and its sequelae such as HCC.[11] Population studies have shown that the proportion of children in Taiwan who are hepatitis B surface antigen (HBsAg) positive decreased from 10% in 1984 to 0.9% in 2009,[12] while in the US, the prevalence of HBV infection decreased in people aged 6-19 years (from 1.9% to 0.6%; P<0.01) and 20-49 years of age (5.9% to 4.6%; P<0.01).[13]

Sources and selection criteria

We used the terms "hepatitis B", "hepatitis B treatment", "antiviral resistance", "transient elastography", "surface antigen", "hepatocellular carcinoma", "nucleos(t)ide analog", "pregnancy", "hepatitis delta", "human immunodeficiency virus", "chemotherapy", and "future therapies" alone and in combination to search PubMed and Google Scholar from the year 2000 to 1 April 2015. Landmark studies before that date were also included. In addition, we searched bibliographies of articles for relevant studies. Where relevant, we incorporated practice guidelines from the American Association for Study of Liver Diseases (AASLD, 2009), European Association for the Study of the Liver (EASL, 2012), and the Asian Pacific Association for Study of the Liver (APASL, 2012).[10] [14] [15] We also reviewed abstracts from the 65th annual meeting of the American Association for the Study of Liver Diseases (Boston, November 2014), and the 49th annual meeting of the European Association for the Study of the Liver (London, April 2014). Evidence was obtained primarily from randomized controlled trials.

Diagnosis and initial evaluation

The serologic indicators for HBV infection include HBsAg, hepatitis B surface antibody (anti-HBs), hepatitis B e antigen (HBeAg), hepatitis B e antibody (anti-HBe), and hepatitis B

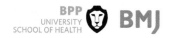

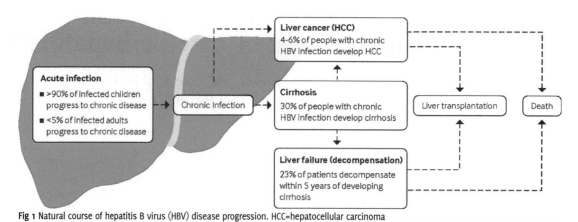

Fig 1 Natural course of hepatitis B virus (HBV) disease progression. HCC=hepatocellular carcinoma

---

SEROLOGIC INDICATORS OF HEPATITIS B VIRUS (HBV) INFECTION

- Hepatitis B surface antigen (HBsAg): viral envelope surface protein, primary marker of HBV infection
- Hepatitis B surface antibody (anti-HBs): antibody that recognizes HBsAg; indicator of immunity to HBV
- Hepatitis B core antibody (anti-HBc): antibody that recognizes the intracellular core antigen
- Anti-HBc IgM: marker of acute infection (may also be raised in acute exacerbation of chronic HBV)
- Anti-HBc IgG: marker of chronic infection
- Hepatitis B e antigen (HBeAg): secretory protein produced by translation of the precore region of the HBV genome
- Hepatitis B e antibody (anti-HBe): antibody that recognizes HBeAg

core antibody (IgM and IgG; (anti-HBc)) (box). Serum HBsAg is the primary marker of infection. Once the diagnosis of HBV has been made on the basis of positive HBsAg, further evaluation should be performed by measuring alanine aminotransferase (ALT), HBV DNA, and anti-HBc IgG, as well as assessing HBeAg status and liver fibrosis.[10] [14] [15] Screening for coinfection with HIV and hepatitis C virus is also recommended.[14]

Phases of HBV infection

The natural course of chronic HBV infection can be broadly classified into four stages: immune tolerance, immune clearance, inactive carrier state, and reactivation or HBeAg negative chronic hepatitis B. Figure 2 depicts the immune tolerance, immune clearance, and inactive carrier phases.

HBeAg negative chronic HBV

After HBeAg seroconversion, a subset of patients may enter a disease state of viral reactivation, known as HBeAg negative chronic HBV. Similar to the inactive carrier phase, this condition is also denoted by the absence of HBeAg. The main reason for HBeAg negativity is the presence of the precore stop codon mutation (G1896A), which is selected during the immune clearance phase and becomes dominant, while the wild-type e antigen producing virus is eliminated.[17] Patients with HBeAg negative disease have double the risk of progressing to cirrhosis than those with HBeAg positive infection.[18] It is therefore crucial that the inactive carrier state is accurately differentiated from HBeAg negative HBV, because those with HBeAg negative HBV will benefit from treatment.

In addition, the double A1762T/G1764A mutation, also known as the basal core promoter mutation, is associated with HBeAg negativity owing to decreased production of the precore mRNA, which leads to reduced levels of HBeAg.[19] [20]

People with HBeAg negative disease associated with the basal core promoter mutation are at increased risk of progression to cirrhosis[21] and HCC,[22] [23] independent of HBV DNA level.

Occult HBV infection

Occult HBV infection is defined as the presence of HBV DNA in the liver and the absence of detectable HBsAg using currently available assays, with or without the presence of HBV DNA in the serum.[24] HBV DNA levels are often less than 200 IU/mL. Occult HBV infection is more common in patients with hepatitis C virus (HCV) infection. In these patients it is associated with a greater risk of progression to cirrhosis and development of HCC, as well as a shorter survival time.[25] [26] Patients with negative HBsAg but with serum HBV DNA levels comparable to those found in overt HBV are classified as having false occult HBV infection as a result of infection with HBV escape mutants that are not recognized by commercial HBsAg assays.[27] [28] Such patients should be treated in the same manner as those with overt HBV infection.[28]

Assessment of liver fibrosis

Because treatment is indicated for those with stage 2 fibrosis or greater, it is often necessary to stage the degree of hepatic fibrosis. Furthermore, patients aged 30 years or more can have stages 2-4 liver fibrosis even with persistently normal ALT concentrations.[10] [14] [29] The measurement of serum ALT may therefore not be a reliable way to determine the extent of liver injury, and a recent meta-analysis of nine studies showed that 27.8% of patients had stages 2-4 fibrosis even with normal ALT concentrations.[30]

Although liver biopsy is considered the gold standard for this indication there are concerns regarding sampling error—discordance in fibrosis stage occurs in up to 33% of biopsies. In addition, complications such as hemorrhage occur in up to 1/2500 biopsies, and pain occurs in up to 84% of patients.[31] Non-invasive evaluation of liver fibrosis can be considered as an alternative to biopsy.

Serologic biomarkers

Among serologic biomarkers of liver fibrosis, the aspartate aminotransferase-to-platelet ratio index (APRI) and fibrosis index based on the four factors (FIB-4) have been most widely studied in patients with HBV.

APRI is based on the ratio of aspartate aminotransferase (AST) concentration to platelet count.[32] FIB-4 was initially derived as a measure of fibrosis in a cohort of patients infected with both HCV and HIV using the formula: (age (years)×AST (U/L))/((platelets (10^9/L))×(ALT (U/L)$^{1/2}$).[33]

A meta-analysis of 39 studies published in 2015 evaluated the efficacy of APRI and FIB-4 in accurately assessing liver

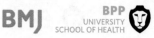

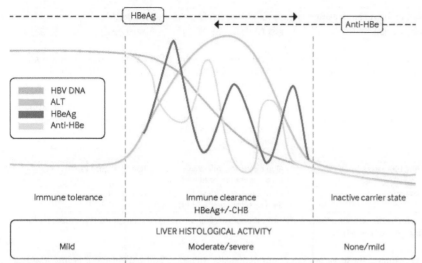

Fig 2 Phases of HBV infection. The immune tolerance phase occurs in patients who acquire HBV infection perinatally or in childhood and may last for 20-30 years. It is characterized by HBeAg positivity, high HBV DNA levels (>20000 IU/mL), normal ALT values, and high HBsAg levels >100000 IU/mL). During this phase, the virus is not cytopathic and minimal hepatic inflammation occurs. In the immune clearance phase, the host immune system attempts to eliminate infected hepatocytes through a T cell mediated immune response to viral antigens, leading to hepatocyte apoptosis. Subsequently ALT levels rise above normal, HBV DNA levels fluctuate, and hepatic inflammation occurs. The immune response may ultimately lead to HBeAg seroconversion, defined as loss of HBeAg and development of anti-HBe. The inactive carrier state occurs after the immune clearance phase and is characterized by the presence of HBsAg in serum, HBeAg seroconversion, low levels of serum HBV DNA (<2000 IU/mL), and normal ALT concentrations. The inactive carrier state may last indefinitely and potentially lead to loss of HBsAg. Abbreviations: ALT=alanine aminotransferase; anti-HBe=hepatitis B e antigen antibody; CHB=chronic hepatitis B infection; HBeAg=hepatitis B e antigen; HBsAg=hepatitis B surface antigen; HBV=hepatitis B virus Reproduced, with permission, from Yim and Lok[16]

fibrosis in HBV. When the APRI threshold was set at 0.5, sensitivity to predict advanced fibrosis was 73.0% and specificity was 54.5%; at a threshold of 1.0, sensitivity was 50.0% and specificity was 83.0%; and at a threshold of 1.5, sensitivity was 33.0% and specificity was 91.0%. With regard to FIB-4 for detecting advanced fibrosis, a threshold of below 1.45 and above 3.25 yielded a sensitivity of 78.6% and a specificity of 98.0%.[34] The meta-analysis concluded that these tests have moderate diagnostic accuracy for predicting fibrosis in chronic HBV infection.

Transient elastography
Transient elastography uses ultrasound elastography to assess the amount of liver stiffness as a surrogate of hepatic fibrosis.[35] The outcome is measured in kPa and ranges from 2.5 kPa to 75 kPa, with 5 kPa often designated as normal and 13.4 kPa or more as cirrhosis.[36] [37] [38]

Several studies have investigated the utility of this test in determining the degree of liver fibrosis in patients with HBV. A study of 202 patients with HBV found that this measure correlated well with stage of fibrosis on liver biopsy (r=0.65).[39] In a meta-analysis of 50 studies assessing the reliability of transient elastography for all causes of liver cirrhosis, the mean area under the receiver operating characteristic (AUROC) curve for the diagnosis of cirrhosis was 0.94, with an optimal cut-off value of 13.01 kPa. This indicates that transient elastography is a reliable technique for detecting cirrhosis regardless of the cause.[40] Another meta-analysis published in 2012 of 18 studies of patients with HBV, found that the mean AUROC curve was 0.93 for liver cirrhosis. A cut-off value of 11.7 yielded a sensitivity and specificity for liver cirrhosis of 84.6% and 81.5%, respectively.[41]

Treatment initiation

The decision to begin treatment is based on the goals of treatment, including suppression of HBV DNA levels, normalization of ALT, and HBeAg seroconversion in HBeAg positive patients as well as patient characteristics, including presence or absence of cirrhosis and hepatitis B inactive carrier state.

People with cirrhosis

In patients with cirrhosis, guidelines agree that those with decompensated cirrhosis should be treated with a nucleos(t)ide analogs, regardless of HBV DNA or ALT level.[10] [14] [15] However, the approach to the treatment of patients with compensated cirrhosis differs.

EASL recommendations state that treatment should be considered in all patients with compensated cirrhosis irrespective of ALT concentration or HBV viral load.[14] However, both AASLD and APASL recommendations suggest that patients with compensated cirrhosis and a viral load 2000 IU/mL or more should be treated, whereas monitoring of ALT and HBV DNA values can be considered for those with a viral load less than 2000 IU/mL.[10] [15]

People without cirrhosis

In people without cirrhosis, recommendations from guidelines and from a panel of experts suggest that for those in the immune tolerant phase, observation and monitoring of ALT and HBV DNA values every three to six months is appropriate, given the lack of data showing a benefit of treatment and the potential for antiviral resistance.[10] [14] [15] [42] In addition, a recent double blind randomized controlled trial of 126 immune tolerant patients, as determined by HBeAg and normal ALT concentration, showed an HBeAg seroconversion rate of less than 5% after four years of nucleos(t)ide analog treatment.[43]

People in the inactive carrier state

The same guidelines also recommend that close monitoring rather than treatment is appropriate for people in the inactive carrier state.[10] [14] [15] Although patients in this phase usually have a low risk of disease progression, a cohort study of 146 inactive carriers over a 23 years of follow-up found that 43 patients had increases in ALT levels to above normal, one had spontaneous reactivation to the HBeAg negative state, and two developed HCC.[44] In a larger cohort of 20069 patients in the inactive carrier phase, the annual incidence rates of HCC and liver related death were 0.06% and 0.04%, respectively, compared with 0.02%, and 0.02% for controls. Furthermore, the hazard ratios were 4.6 (95% confidence interval 2.5 to 8.3) for the development of HCC and 2.1 (1.1 to 4.1) for liver related mortality compared with controls.[45] These findings emphasize the importance of continued surveillance of carriers with inactive disease for HCC. Furthermore, given the potential for liver related complications during the inactive carrier state even in people without cirrhosis, treatment should be considered in all patients with cirrhosis, regardless of HBV DNA level.

Other patients

In the remainder of patients the decision to start therapy should be based on a variety of factors including HBeAg status, ALT concentration, HBV viral load, age (<40 v >40

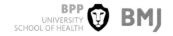

Table 1 Guideline recommendations on treatment initiation in patients with hepatitis B virus (HBV) infection

Patient characteristics	AASLD (2009)	EASL (2012)	APASL (2012)
HBeAg status			
Positive	HBV DNA >20 000 IU/mL and ALT >2× upper limit of normal	HBV DNA > 2000 IU/mL with ALT > upper limit of normal or biopsy with moderate fibrosis or inflammation	HBV DNA >20 000 IU/mL and ALT >2× upper limit of normal
Negative	HBV DNA >2000 IU/mL and ALT > upper limit of normal or stage 2 fibrosis	HBV DNA >2000 IU/mL with ALT > upper limit of normal or biopsy with moderate fibrosis or inflammation	HBV DNA >2000 IU/mL and ALT > upper limit of normal or stage 2 fibrosis
Cirrhosis			
Compensated	HBV DNA >2000 IU/mL	All patients regardless of decompensation or HBV DNA level	HBV DNA >2000 IU/mL
Decompensated	All patients	All patients regardless of decompensation or HBV DNA level	All patients

AASLD=American Association for Study of Liver Diseases; ALT=alanine aminotransferase; APASL=Asian Pacific Association for Study of the Liver; EASL=European Association for the Study of the Liver; HBeAg=hepatitis B e antigen.

years), and stage of liver fibrosis. Among these variables, ALT concentration, HBV viral load, and HBeAg status are the most important. An ALT concentration of 30 U/L in men and 19 U/L in women with HBV should be considered the upper limit of normal.[46] Table 1 shows recommendations from the AASLD, EASL, and APASL guidelines on when to start HBV therapy.

Predictors of treatment outcome

Evidence has consistently shown that the most important outcome of treatment is suppression of HBV viral load because this parameter strongly correlates with the risk of progression to cirrhosis and development of HCC.[47]

In the Risk Evaluation of Viral Load Elevation and Associated Liver Disease/Cancer-HBV (REVEAL-HBV) cohort study, Cox regression adjusting for ALT concentration and HBeAg status showed that increasing HBV DNA level was the strongest independent predictor of progression to cirrhosis.[48] Additional data from this cohort showed that greater than 2000 IU/mL HBV DNA was the strongest risk factor for HCC, when controlling for HBeAg status, ALT concentration, and cirrhosis.[49] Furthermore, patients whose HBV DNA dropped to less than 2000 IU/mL from baseline had a significantly lower risk of developing HCC (hazard ratio 2.25, 0.68 to 7.37 compared with controls) than those whose HBV DNA level persisted at 2000-20000 IU/mL (3.12, 1.09 to 8.89), 20000-200000 IU/mL (8.85, 3.85 to 20.35), or greater than 200000 IU/mL (16.78, 7.33 to 38.29).[50]

Currently available treatments

Two therapeutic approaches are available for both HBeAg positive and HBeAg negative patients: finite therapy and long term suppressive therapy. The goal of the first strategy is sustained suppression of viral replication after the completion of treatment through the induction of the inactive carrier state of HBV. This is designated by normal ALT concentrations, HBV DNA less than 2000 IU/mL, and, specifically for HBeAg positive patients, seroconversion of HBeAg to anti-HBeAg. This strategy uses treatment with pegylated interferon for 48 weeks. The second approach aims to obtain rapid and long term viral suppression with the use of oral nucleos(t)ide analogs, although the duration of treatment may be indefinite.

Pegylated interferon

The purpose of using pegylated interferon is to provide the patient with a finite duration of treatment. Because pegylated interferon is associated with multiple toxicities, including fatigue, a flu-like reaction, anemia, pancytopenia,

and depression (in 20-30% of patients),[51] it is important to determine which patients will respond to this drug before starting treatment. Characteristics indicating a favorable response include low HBV DNA levels, high levels of ALT and HBV, presence of the HBV genotype A or B, and lack of advanced liver disease.[52] [53] The *IL28B* polymorphism may also predict response to interferon based therapy because studies have indicated greater decreases in HBV DNA and higher rates of HBeAg to anti-HBe seroconversion or HBsAg loss in those who have the CC genotype rather than the CT or TT polymorphism.[54]

In one of the largest trials to evaluate the efficacy of pegylated interferon in HBV, 814 HBeAg positive patients were given pegylated interferon, lamivudine, or a combination of both for 48 weeks and followed up for 24 weeks after treatment was discontinued. Compared with patients assigned to lamivudine alone, the HBeAg to anti-HBeAg seroconversion rate was significantly greater in those taking pegylated interferon monotherapy (32% v 19%; P<0.001) or combination therapy (27% v 19%; P=0.02).[55] In addition, 16 patients given interferon seroconverted from HBsAg to anti-HBsAg, compared with none who received lamivudine (P=0.001). In a retrospective analysis of 808 patients, HBeAg positive patients with HBV genotype A, high ALT concentration, and low HBV DNA level had a 54% predicted probability of a sustained response to pegylated interferon, defined as HBeAg seroconversion and HBV DNA level less than 2000 IU/mL[52]

Because interferon seems to be successful in only a third of patients, studies have assessed how to improve the efficacy of interferon based therapy, including combination therapy with nucleos(t)ide analogs. However, regimens involving interferon combined with nucleos(t)ide analogs or ribavirin did not improve the response in HBeAg positive and HBeAg negative patients with HBV.[55] [56] [57]

Regarding the duration of treatment, the NEPTUNE randomized trial showed that among 544 patients with HBeAg positive HBV, the highest response was associated with pegylated interferon at a dosage of 180 μg once weekly for 48 weeks (36.2% HBeAg seroconversion rate) rather than 180 μg or 90 μg for 24 weeks (25.8% and 14.1%, respectively; P values not provided).[58] Another randomized controlled trial of 128 HBeAg negative patients, 94% of whom had HBV genotype D, compared 48 weeks of pegylated interferon (180 μg/week; n=51); 96 weeks of pegylated interferon (48 weeks at 180 μg/week then 48 weeks at 135 μg/week; n=52); and 48 weeks of pegylated interferon (180 μg/week) plus lamivudine (100 mg/day) then 48 weeks of pegylated interferon alone (135 μg/week) (n=25). It found that 48

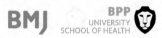

Table 2 Guideline recommendations for management of antiviral resistance in patients with hepatitis B virus infection

Drug	AASLD (2009)	EASL (2012)
Lamivudine	Add adefovir or tenofovir	Switch to tenofovir or add adefovir if tenofovir not available
Telbivudine	Add adefovir or tenofovir; switch to emtricitabine	Switch to or add tenofovir
Adefovir	Add lamivudine; switch to or add entecavir; switch to or add tenofovir	Switch to entecavir or tenofovir if naive to lamivudine; switch to tenofovir and add nucleoside analogue if has been exposed to lamivudine
Entecavir	Switch to tenofovir or tenofovir + emtricitabine	Switch to or add tenofovir

AASLD=American Association for Study of Liver Diseases; EASL=European Association for the Study of the Liver.

weeks after finishing treatment, HBV DNA was less than 2000 IU/mL in significantly more patients who were treated for 96 weeks with pegylated interferon alone than in those treated for 48 weeks with pegylated interferon monotherapy (28.8% v 11.8%; P=0.03). The rate of normalization of ALT was also higher in the group receiving 96 weeks of pegylated interferon monotherapy, but this was not significant (25% v 11.8%; P=0.08).[59] Furthermore, the addition of lamivudine during the first 48 weeks of treatment did not lead to significantly higher rates of sustained HBV DNA suppression to less than 2000 IU/mL at 48 weeks after stopping treatment (28.8% for monotherapy v 20% for combination treatment). Adverse effects associated with pegylated interferon were seen in 20-30% of patients, but data on the rate of individual side effects were seldom reported in the above trials.

Nucleos(t)ide analogs

Several nucleos(t)ide analogs are available for the treatment of HBV including lamivudine, adefovir, telbivudine, entecavir, and tenofovir disoproxil fumarate. However, international guidelines recommend only entecavir and tenofovir as first line therapy for nucleos(t)ide analog naive patients with HBV.[10 14 15] Both of these drugs are well tolerated overall with minimal adverse effects.

Entecavir

Registration trials that compared lamivudine with entecavir in HBeAg positive and HBeAg negative treatment naive patients showed that entecavir had significantly greater efficacy in reducing HBV DNA to undetectable levels and normalizing ALT over 48 weeks.[60 61] A randomized controlled trial of 715 HBeAg positive patients showed that entecavir significantly increased the proportion of patients with undetectable HBV DNA (67% v 36%; P<0.001) and normalization of ALT (68% v 60%; P=0.02).[60] Reported rates of adverse events were 86% in the entecavir arm and 84% in the lamivudine arm (not significant). Common adverse events included diarrhea, fatigue, abdominal pain, and cough.

A separate randomized controlled trial of 648 HBeAg negative patients randomized to entecavir or lamivudine found that entecavir significantly increased the proportion of patients with undetectable HBV DNA levels (90% v 72%; P<0.001) and ALT normalization (78% v 71%; P=0.045).[61] Rates of adverse events, including fatigue, headache, diarrhea, and nausea, were similar between the two study groups—76% in people taking entecavir and 79% in those taking lamivudine. However, 6% of those taking entecavir and 9% of those taking lamivudine discontinued treatment.

These findings were confirmed in a randomized controlled trial that compared lamivudine with entecavir in 709 HBeAg positive patients over 96 weeks. This trial demonstrated superiority of entecavir in the reduction of HBV DNA (80% v 39%; P<0.001) and normalization of ALT (87% v 79%; P=0.005), although cumulative HBeAg seroconversion was similar between the two groups.[62] No patients taking entecavir developed resistance during the study period.

Regarding HBeAg negative patients, a randomized controlled trial of 648 patients showed that entecavir significantly increased the proportion of patients with undetectable HBV DNA compared with lamivudine (90% v 72%; P<0.001) and with normalization of ALT (78% v 71%; P=0.045).[61] Follow-up of this cohort for five years detected entecavir resistance in one patient, HBeAg seroconversion in 23% of patients, and loss of HBsAg in 1.4%.[63]

An observational study reported a 1.2% cumulative probability of entecavir resistance in treatment naive patients, whereas patients refractory to lamivudine had a lower barrier to developing resistance mutations, leading to a 51% cumulative probability of developing resistance mutations over five years.[64] These findings were similar to a more recent prospective study that reported a cumulative 1.2% incidence of entecavir resistance in HBeAg positive, treatment naive patients over three years' duration.[65]

Regarding the safety profile of entecavir, one retrospective study identified five cases of lactic acidosis among 16 entecavir treated patients with decompensated liver disease, all of whom had MELD (model for end stage liver disease) scores of 22 or greater.[66] In two subsequent studies of patients with decompensated cirrhosis, no cases of lactic acidosis were reported.[67 68]

Tenofovir disoproxil fumarate

Initial randomized controlled trial data comparing tenofovir with adefovir in 846 HBeAg positive and 603 HBeAg negative patients showed that tenofovir significantly increased normalization of ALT (68% v 54%; P=0.03) and loss of HBsAg (3% v 0%; P=0.02) without evidence of resistance to tenofovir.[69] After eight years of follow-up of this patient cohort, no resistance mutations have been detected in HBeAg positive or HBeAg negative patients receiving long term tenofovir, with most cases of virologic breakthrough being caused by non-adherence.[70]

Studies of combination therapy with two nucleos(t)ide analogs have found marginal benefit over monotherapy overall. One randomized trial of 379 treatment naive patients compared entecavir monotherapy with combined entecavir and tenofovir in naive HBeAg positive and negative patients. It found that entecavir was as effective as combination therapy, although patients with HBV DNA levels greater than 10^8 IU/mL had a significantly greater likelihood of having undetectable DNA levels at 100 weeks.[71] Additional studies have shown that tenofovir monotherapy has comparable efficacy to tenofovir combined with emtricitabine (Truvada) in both naive and lamivudine experienced patients.[43 72]

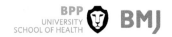

Antiviral resistance

Treatment of antiviral resistance involves selection of an agent without cross resistance to the mutation, thereby reducing the risk of selecting viral strains with mutations that lead to multidrug resistance. This is best accomplished by switching to a drug with a high barrier to resistance instead of adding extra drug (table 2).[14] [15]

Switching to tenofovir is appropriate in patients with lamivudine resistance. In a study of 131 patients in whom treatment with lamivudine or adefovir alone, sequentially, or in combination was ineffective, tenofovir was an effective rescue therapy and nearly 80% of patients given tenofovir monotherapy achieved an undetectable HBV DNA level.[73] Resistance was shown in 62% of patients taking lamivudine and 19% taking adefovir.[73] Entecavir has also been shown to be effective in people who are resistant to adefovir. One cohort study of 161 patients, of whom 34% had been previously treated with nucleos(t)ide analogs, found that treatment with adefovir did not reduce the efficacy of entecavir even in those who had developed adefovir resistance mutations.[74] Although resistance to entecavir is rare, treatment of this condition with tenofovir monotherapy is comparable to tenofovir and entecavir combination therapy, with 71% and 73% of patients obtaining an undetectable HBV DNA level at 48 weeks.[75]

Monitoring surface antigen level

HBsAg has traditionally been used to diagnose HBV infection and two commercially available assays for measuring HBsAg—the Architect HBsAg assay (Abbott Diagnostics)[76] and the Elecsys HBsAg II quant assay (Roche Diagnostics)[77]—have recently been developed. Recent studies suggest that the measurement of HBsAg titers may also be useful for predicting the course of HBV infection and assessing treatment response.[78]

Several studies have demonstrated the utility of measuring HBsAg to establish the patient's clinical course. In HBeAg positive patients in the immune tolerant phase, a HBsAg value of greater than 25000 IU/mL yielded a 90% positive predictive value for mild liver fibrosis.[79] Another study showed that in HBeAg positive patients, HBsAg levels of 38500 IU/mL or less were associated with moderate to severe fibrosis.[80]

HBsAg levels may also help distinguish between inactive carriers and chronic active HBeAg negative infection. Several studies showed that inactive carriers have lower HBsAg levels, with HBsAg less than 1000 U/mL having a 87.9% positive predictive value and 96.7% negative predictive value for the patient having HBV DNA less than 2000 IU/mL.[81] The REVEAL-HBV study group showed that HBsAg less than 1000 IU/mL is associated with a lower risk of developing HCC.[47]

With regard to HBsAg and treatment response, data suggest that lower pretreatment HBsAg values are associated with a greater response to pegylated interferon, and that HBsAg titers may be used as an on-treatment marker for sustained treatment response to this drug.[82] A reduction in HBsAg to 300 IU/mL or less after six months of treatment correlates with a sustained response at 12 months after completion of therapy, defined as anti-HBe seroconversion and HBV DNA less than 2000 IU/mL.[83] Furthermore, patients who do not have a reduction in HBsAg levels at week 12 of pegylated interferon treatment have a low likelihood of sustained response or HBsAg loss.[84]

One study of 48 HBeAg negative patients treated with pegylated interferon for 48 weeks found that people whose HBsAg dropped by greater than 0.5 log IU/mL at week 12 and greater than 1 log IU/mL at week 24 had an 89% and 92% positive predictive value, respectively, of having a sustained response after completing treatment. By contrast, patients in whom HBsAg did not drop had only a 10% chance of response, defined as undetectable HBV DNA at 24 weeks after treatment stopped.[85]

Treatment withdrawal

Evidence from a randomized controlled trial of 548 patients supports the notion that pegylated interferon should be stopped in any of the following scenarios: absence of a decline in HBV DNA level to 20000 IU/mL or less, lack of a reduction of HBsAg to less than 1500 U/mL at week 12 or 24,[58] and completion of 48 weeks of treatment.[10]

Withdrawal of nucleos(t)ide analogs can be considered six to 12 months after anti-HBe seroconversion in patients who are HBeAg positive before they start treatment, and after HBsAg loss in those who are HBeAg negative at the start of treatment.[10] [14] [15] However, published findings suggest that relapse rates may be high after withdrawal of treatment.

HBeAg positive patients

A single center prospective cohort study of 132 HBeAg positive patients showed that HBeAg seroconversion occurred in 46 patients (35%) receiving nucleos(t)ide analogs after a median duration of 26 months of treatment. Of nine patients who discontinued treatment after seroconversion and six months of consolidation therapy, only two had a sustained treatment response.[86]

In another retrospective study of 178 Korean patients with HBeAg positive HBV treated with lamivudine monotherapy who had attained a complete response (undetectable HBV DNA level, normalization of ALT, and loss of HBeAg), the cumulative rate of relapse within five years of stopping treatment was 30.2%. Relapse occurred in 33 of the 40 patients within the first two years.[87]

HBeAg negative patients

Studies on treatment withdrawal in HBeAg negative patients have typically been conducted in small samples. In an observational cohort study of 33 Greek patients treated for four or five years with adefovir, six years after stopping treatment, 18 patients had an HBV DNA value less than 2000 IU/mL and 13 of them achieved HBsAg loss.[88]

A larger study evaluated relapse rates after withdrawal of entecavir in 184 HBeAg negative patients with an undetectable HBV DNA level for more than two years. It reported high relapse rates of 74.1% and 91.4% at 24 and 48 weeks, respectively, after stopping treatment.[89] In a randomized controlled study of vaccine therapy in patients with HBV and undetectable HBV DNA after a median of three years of treatment with nucleos(t)ide analogs, discontinuation of treatment was associated with HBV reactivation in 97%, indicating that vaccination does not reduce the risk of relapse after discontinuation of nucleos(t)ide analogs.[90] Given the relatively high rate of relapse after withdrawal of nucleos(t)ide analogs, treatment discontinuation should be undertaken cautiously, particularly in HBeAg negative patients.

Outcomes of HBV treatment

Long term treatment with third generation nucleos(t)ide analogs may lead to improvement in liver fibrosis and potentially reversal of cirrhosis. A five year study of entecavir treated patients documented the histological

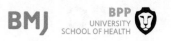

reversal of cirrhosis in four of 10 cases.[63] Another study found that, among 96 patients with cirrhosis, 71 patients had regression of cirrhosis after five years of treatment with tenofovir and successful viral suppression.[91]

With regard to the effect of HBV treatment on the progression of liver disease and development of HCC, a landmark study in patients with advanced fibrosis from East Asia and the Pacific showed that a response to lamivudine delays progression of HBV related liver disease in terms of hepatic decompensation, liver related mortality, and development of HCC.[92] The study randomized 651 patients to receive lamivudine or placebo; 7.8% of patients receiving lamivudine versus 17.7% of those receiving placebo reached an end point of disease progression (hazard ratio 0.45; P=0.001), and 3.9% of patients receiving lamivudine versus 7.4% of those receiving placebo developed HCC (P=0.047).[92]

Evidence on the effectiveness of entecavir and tenofovir in preventing complications of HBV has come primarily from observational studies. In a Japanese observational study, the cumulative five year incidence of HCC was significantly lower in 472 patients treated with entecavir than in 1143 treatment naive patients (adjusted hazard ratio 0.37; P=0.03).[93]

Another retrospective-prospective cohort study that compared 1446 entecavir treated patients with 424 untreated historical controls found no difference in hepatic events in patients without cirrhosis. However, entecavir reduced liver related mortality (hazard ratio 0.51, 0.34 to 0.78; P=0.002), occurrence of HCC (0.55, 0.31 to 0.99; P=0.049), and liver related mortality (0.26, 0.13 to 0.55; P<0.001) in patients with cirrhosis as determined by Cox proportional hazard regression.[94]

In a Taiwanese national cohort study of more than 21000 patients, treatment with nucleos(t)ide analogs was associated with a significantly lower seven year incidence of HCC.[95] Notably, however, most studies showing that nucleos(t)ide analogs reduce the risk of HCC have been performed in Asian people, and studies that look at the effects of nucleos(t)ide analog treatment on risk of HCC are also needed in white people.[96]

HIV coinfection

Among the estimated 40 million people infected with HIV worldwide, two to four million are chronically infected with HBV. HIV infection worsens the natural course of HBV infection by impairing the innate and adaptive immune responses to the virus.[97] [98] This may lead to increased rates of chronic HBV after acute infection and lower rates of HBeAg seroconversion or HBsAg loss with treatment.[99] [100]

In the Multicenter Cohort Study of 5293 homosexual men, liver related mortality was higher in coinfected patients than in those with HIV or HBV monoinfection, especially when CD4 cell nadir counts were low.[101] The Euro-SIDA cohort also showed greater liver related mortality in coinfected patients, with mortality increasing from 8% in HBV negative to 18% in HBV positive people.[102]

When both HIV and HBV infections need to be treated, antiretroviral therapy using the combination of tenofovir and emtricitabine or lamivudine is preferred.[14] [15] A retrospective study of 65 HBV and HIV coinfected patients showed that tenofovir was effective in patients with wild-type and lamivudine resistant HBV infection, indicating that tenofovir can be used as a component of HIV therapy even in those exposed to lamivudine.[103] A meta-analysis of 23 studies also demonstrated the efficacy of tenofovir in the suppression

of HBV viremia, with no impact of previous lamivudine exposure or combination with emtricitabine.[104] Although evidence from this study suggests that tenofovir may have similar efficacy to combined tenofovir and emtricitabine, combination therapy is still the preferred treatment for coinfected patients.[14]

Hepatitis delta

HDV is a human RNA virus that encodes the delta antigen, which is subsequently encased in an envelope within HBsAg.[105] Although HDV infection suppresses HBV replication, it can lead to severe liver disease including fulminant liver failure, end stage liver disease, and HCC. HDV infection occurs as a coinfection, when both HBV and HDV are acquired simultaneously, or as a superinfection, whereby HDV infection occurs in a patient with HBV infection.

Interferon based therapy is the primary treatment for HDV. The Hep-Net International Delta Hepatitis Intervention Study (HIDIT) group published a randomized trial that compared pegylated interferon alone (n=29), adefovir alone (n=30), or combination therapy (n=31) for treating HDV. It found that pegylated interferon, with or without adefovir, led to sustained HDV clearance in 28% of patients 24 weeks after treatment.[106] However, long term follow-up of this patient cohort found that more than half of those with a sustained response 24 weeks after the end of treatment relapsed, as defined by HDV ribonucleic acid positive testing.[107] The randomized double blind trial HIDIT-2 study evaluated prolonged treatment with pegylated interferon, with (n=59) or without tenofovir (n=61), for 96 weeks. Both treatments had similar efficacy with regard to sustained response 24 weeks after treatment (23-30%), and the presence of cirrhosis was associated with a higher response rate on multivariate analysis.[108]

Pregnancy

In women of childbearing age, treatment aims to reduce HBV transmission to the infant because the risk of developing chronic HBV infection is high in those exposed during birth.[109] Active-passive immunoprophylaxis reduces mother to child transmission rates by 95%.[110] The standard regimen involves administration of hepatitis B immune globulin and hepatitis B vaccination to the infant. However, transmission may still occur even with immunoprophylaxis in mothers who have an HBV DNA level greater than 10[7] IU/mL.[111]

In women who are pregnant or planning pregnancy in the near future, nucleos(t)ide analogs should be used with caution because of the risk of mitochondrial toxicity.[10] However, in women with advanced fibrosis or cirrhosis it has been suggested that treatment should be initiated and continued throughout pregnancy.[109]

A population based study that compared 339 women with cirrhosis with 6625 age matched controls found that those with underlying cirrhosis have the highest risk of HBV associated decompensation in pregnancy, with an associated mortality risk of 1.8% for mothers and 5.2% for the fetus.[112]

Women without advanced fibrosis and with HBV DNA levels greater than 10[7] IU/mL can be considered for treatment in the third trimester to prevent fetal transmission. Interferon should be avoided because animal studies suggest that it may lead to fetal abortion and data from humans are not available.[113] If nucleos(t)ide analogs are used, telbivudine and tenofovir are pregnancy category B drugs. It has been shown that administration of either of these drugs to highly

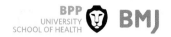

Table 3 Emerging treatments for hepatitis B virus (HBV) infection

Treatment	Mechanism of action	Phase	Comments
Myrcludex-B[131] [132]	Viral entry inhibitor	Ia	Targets sodium taurocholate cotransporting polypeptide, a receptor for HBV entry
Bay 41-4109[133]	Viral nucleocapsid inhibitor	I	Part of the heteroaryldihydropyrimidine family, which decreases stability of the viral capsid by misdirecting its assembly
GLS 4[134]	Viral nucleocapsid inhibitor	I	Heteroaryldihydropyrimidine family
REP 9 AC[135]	HBsAg release inhibitor	Ib	Blocks secretion of non-infectious subviral particles that may act as decoys to immune system; in combination with immune therapy may lead to HBsAg clearance
GS-9620[136]	Toll-like receptor 7 agonist	I	Activation of toll-like receptor-7 induces innate immunity to inhibit HBV replication
DV-601[137]	Therapeutic vaccine	Ib	Stimulates T cell and B cell antibody response against HBsAg; comprises HBsAg and HBcAg
Zinc finger proteins[138]	Block transcription of cccDNA	Preclinical	
Disubstituted sulfonamides (CCC-0975 and CCC-0346)[139]	Reduce cccDNA levels	Preclinical	Inhibit cccDNA production

cccDNA=covalently closed circular DNA; HBcAg=hepatitis B core antigen; HBsAg=hepatitis B surface antigen.

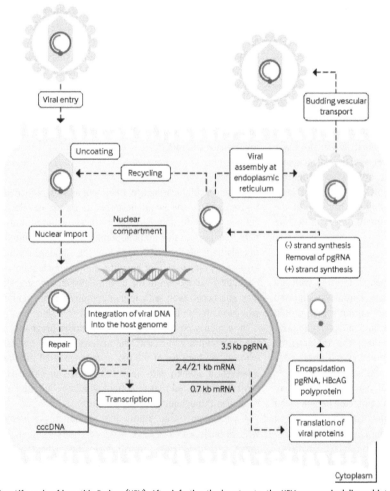

Fig 3 Life cycle of hepatitis B virus (HBV). After infecting the hepatocyte, the HBV genome is delivered into the nucleus where cellular enzymes repair the viral genome into covalently closed circular DNA (cccDNA). cccDNA acts as a template for transcription of pregenomic and pre-core mRNA. The pregenomic RNA (pgRNA) is encapsulated by the core particle and reverse transcribed by viral polymerase to form a single strand DNA molecule. Subsequently, the pre-genome is degraded and the negative strand DNA acts as a template for synthesis of a positive strand DNA molecule. The HBV genome is then either encapsulated by the envelope to produce virions that are secreted out of the hepatocyte or recycled back to the nucleus as cccDNA, resulting in the formation of a steady state of 5-50 copies of cccDNA molecules per infected hepatocyte. Abbreviations: HBcAg=hepatitis B core antigen. Reproduced, with permission, from Jayalakshmi and colleagues[128]

viremic mothers leads to 0% HBV transmission to the fetus, compared with about 8% transmission in controls.[114] [115] [116]

If antiviral therapy is started during pregnancy it should be discontinued postpartum in mothers who intend to breast feed. Even though these drugs are secreted at low levels in breast milk, studies on the long term safety in infants who were breast fed by mothers taking HBV antiviral drugs are lacking.[117]

HBV reactivation after immunosuppression

Patients infected with HBV who receive immunosuppressive therapy are at risk of viral reactivation. Such patients include those who undergo bone marrow, stem cell, or solid organ transplantation and those receiving chemotherapy, anti-CD20 antibodies, or biologic agents (tumor necrosis factor α inhibitors).[118] [119] [120] Rates of HBV reactivation range from 38% in those receiving tumor necrosis factor α inhibitors to as high as 80% in those undergoing stem cell or solid organ transplantation and those receiving anti-CD20 antibodies.[121] Presentation varies from a mild increase in aminotransferase to fulminant liver failure.[118] Because HBV reactivation is preventable with appropriate screening and treatment, testing all patients for HBsAg and anti-HBc, followed by an HBV DNA level if positive, is recommended before immunosuppressive therapy is started.[122]

HBsAg positive patients

Two randomized controlled trials have compared the efficacy of prophylactic versus pre-emptive antiviral therapy in preventing HBV reactivation. In the first study, 30 HBsAg positive patients undergoing chemotherapy received lamivudine prophylactically or pre-emptively—that is, when a 10-fold increase in HBV DNA occurred or HBV DNA was present in those who had undetectable HBV DNA at baseline. HBV reactivation occurred in 53% of the patients receiving pre-emptive lamivudine but none of those receiving prophylactic lamivudine (P=0.002).[123]

The second study of 51 HBsAg positive patients also showed that fewer patients receiving prophylactic lamivudine had HBV reactivation (12% v 56%; P=0.001).[124] Because more than 50% of HBsAg positive patients have viral reactivation in this setting, we suggest that all HBsAg positive patients should receive nucleos(t)ide analogs before immunosuppression and then for 12 weeks after discontinuation of immunosuppressive therapy, regardless of DNA level.[14]

Lamivudine is an appropriate and cost effective drug in this setting, particularly if treatment is expected to be of finite duration.[125] However, entecavir or tenofovir is recommended in those in whom treatment might be for an indefinite period, and entecavir may be preferable because of reduced renal toxicity.[119]

HBsAg negative, anti-HBc positive patients

Patients who are HBsAg negative but anti-HBc positive can also be considered for prophylactic nucleos(t)ide analog therapy, even though reactivation (reverse seroconversion) rates are lower than in HBsAg positive patients, ranging from 5% in patients receiving biologic agents to 20% in those receiving immunosuppression for stem cell transplantation. In a randomized trial of 80 HBsAg negative and anti-HBc positive patients receiving chemotherapy, the rate of HBV reactivation was significantly lower in those receiving entecavir prophylactically (n=41) than in those on pre-emptive treatment (n=39) (2% v 18%; P<0.05).[126] However, a

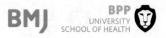

ABBREVIATIONS

- AASLD: American Association for Study of Liver Diseases
- ALT: Alanine aminotransferase
- Anti-HBc: Hepatitis B core antibody
- Anti-HBe: Hepatitis B e antibody
- Anti-HBs: Hepatitis B surface antibody
- APASL: Asian Pacific Association for Study of the Liver
- AST: Aspartate aminotransferase
- APRI: Aspartate aminotransferase to platelet ratio index
- AUROC: Area under receiver operating characteristic
- EASL: European Association for the Study of the Liver
- FIB-4: Fibrosis index based on the four factors
- HBeAg: Hepatitis B e antigen
- HBsAg: Hepatitis B surface antigen
- HBV: Hepatitis B virus
- HCC: Hepatocellular carcinoma
- HCV: Hepatitis C virus
- HDV: Hepatitis delta virus
- REVEAL-HBV: Risk Evaluation of Viral Load Elevation and Associated Liver Disease/Cancer-HBV

prospective cohort study evaluating pre-emptive entecavir for HBV flares in 150 anti-HBc positive patients found that after rituximab based chemotherapy, the incidence of HBV reactivation and HBV related hepatitis flares was 10.4 and 6.4 per 100 person year and that only four patients had a severe HBV flare without prophylactic entecavir treatment.[127] Currently, studies evaluating the cost effectiveness of prophylactic versus pre-emptive nucleos(t)ide analog therapy in anti-HBc positive patients are lacking.

Emerging treatments

Despite improvements in the treatment of chronic HBV infection, treatment is currently directed towards inhibition of viral replication rather than complete elimination of HBV. Future treatments that aim to inhibit various aspects of the HBV life cycle are in development (fig 3). There are several potential therapeutic targets in the HBV life cycle, including inhibition of viral entry into the hepatocyte, disruption of the viral nucleocapsid, degeneration of covalently closed circular DNA, prevention of HBsAg release, and immune based therapies including toll-like receptor agonists and therapeutic vaccines (table 3).[129 130]

Conclusion

HBV infection represents a global health burden that is associated with serious morbidity and mortality if untreated. Treatment strategies include pegylated interferon for a finite duration or long term suppressive therapy with nucleos(t)ide analogs. Pegylated interferon therapy has lower rates of sustained response after treatment is stopped, and combination therapy with nucleos(t)ide analogs does not improve efficacy. Nucleos(t)ide analogs provide excellent suppression of HBV DNA and potential for regression of fibrosis but low rates of HBeAg seroconversion and a high

risk of relapse after treatment is withdrawn. Monitoring of HBsAg values can be used as a guide to response to therapy. Treatment aimed at alternative targets that may ultimately lead to a cure for HBV infection is currently under development.

Guidelines

HBV diagnosis and treatment guidelines are available from the American Association for the Study of Liver Disease (2009; www.aasld.org), European Association for the Study of Liver Diseases (2012; www.easl.eu), and the Asian Pacific Association for Study of the Liver (2012; www.apasl.info). All guidelines are of high quality, and we have cited recommendations from these guidelines on evaluation, treatment initiation, and management of antiviral resistance.

Contributors: VS and KK contributed equally to conceptualization and study design, including literature search, and drafting and critical revision of the manuscript. Both authors are guarantors.

Competing interests: We have read and understood BMJ policy on declaration of interests and declare the following interests: VS: speakers bureau: Salix (makes no products related to this review and has no relationship to the subject matter); advisory board: Gilead, Abbvie, Janssen. KK: grants/research: Evidera, Gilead, Immuron, Intercept, Tobira; advisory board: Abbvie, Achillion, BMS, Evidera, Gilead, Merck, Novartis, Trio Health; consultant: Abbvie, Gilead.

Provenance and peer review: Commissioned; externally peer reviewed.

1   Goldstein ST, Zhou F, Hadler SC, et al. A mathematical model to estimate global hepatitis B disease burden and vaccination impact. Int J Epidemiol2005;34:1329-39.
2   Trepo C, Chan HL, Lok A. Hepatitis B virus infection. Lancet2014;384:2053-63.
3   Fattovich G, Giustina G, Schalm SW, et al. Occurrence of hepatocellular carcinoma and decompensation in western European patients with cirrhosis type B. The EUROHEP Study Group on Hepatitis B Virus and Cirrhosis. Hepatology1995;21:77-82.
4   Moyer LA, Mast EE. Hepatitis B: virology, epidemiology, disease, and prevention, and an overview of viral hepatitis. Am J Prevent Med1994;10(suppl):45-55.
5   WHO. Hepatitis B. Fact sheet 204. 2015. www.who.int/mediacentre/factsheets/fs204/en.
6   Lozano R, Naghavi M, Foreman K, et al. Global and regional mortality from 235 causes of death for 20 age groups in 1990 and 2010: a systematic analysis for the Global Burden of Disease Study 2010. Lancet2012;380:2095-128.
7   Ioannou GN. Hepatitis B virus in the United States: infection, exposure, and immunity rates in a nationally representative survey. Ann Intern Med2011;154:319-28.
8   Kowdley KV, Wang CC, Welch S, et al. Prevalence of chronic hepatitis B among foreign-born persons living in the United States by country of origin. Hepatology2012;56:422-33.
9   Te HS, Jensen DM. Epidemiology of hepatitis B and C viruses: a global overview. Clin Liver Dis2010;14:1-21, vii.
10   Lok AS, McMahon BJ. Chronic hepatitis B: update 2009. Hepatology2009;50:661-2.
11   Chang MH, You SL, Chen CJ, et al. Decreased incidence of hepatocellular carcinoma in hepatitis B vaccinees: a 20-year follow-up study. J Natl Cancer Inst2009;101:1348-55.
12   Ni YH, Chang MH, Wu JF, et al. Minimization of hepatitis B infection by a 25-year universal vaccination program. J Hepatol2012;57:730-5.
13   Wasley A, Kruszon-Moran D, Kuhnert W, et al. The prevalence of hepatitis B virus infection in the United States in the era of vaccination. J Infect Dis2010;202:192-201.
14   European Association for the Study of the Liver. EASL clinical practice guidelines: management of chronic hepatitis B virus infection. J Hepatol2012;57:167-85.
15   Liaw YF, Leung N, Kao JH, et al. Asian-Pacific consensus statement on the management of chronic hepatitis B: a 2012 update. Hepatol Int2012;6:531-61.
16   Yim HY, Lok AS-F. Natural history of chronic hepatitis B virus infection: what we knew in 1981 and what we know in 2005. Hepatology2006;43(suppl 1):S173-81.
17   Hadziyannis SJ, Vassilopoulos D. Hepatitis B e antigen-negative chronic hepatitis B. Hepatology2001;34:617-24.
18   Fattovich G, Bortolotti F, Donato F. Natural history of chronic hepatitis B: special emphasis on disease progression and prognostic factors. J Hepatol2008;48:335-52.
19   Kurosaki M, Enomoto N, Asahina Y, et al. Mutations in the core promoter region of hepatitis B virus in patients with chronic hepatitis B. J Med Virol1996;49:115-23.

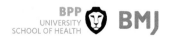

20 Sato S, Suzuki K, Akahane Y, et al. Hepatitis B virus strains with mutations in the core promoter in patients with fulminant hepatitis. Ann Intern Med1995;122:241-8.

21 Chu CM, Lin CC, Chen YC, et al. Basal core promoter mutation is associated with progression to cirrhosis rather than hepatocellular carcinoma in chronic hepatitis B virus infection. Br J Cancer2012;107:2010-5.

22 Liu CJ, Chen BF, Chen PJ, et al. Role of hepatitis B virus precore/core promoter mutations and serum viral load on noncirrhotic hepatocellular carcinoma: a case-control study. J Infect Dis2006;194:594-9.

23 Liu CJ, Chen BF, Chen PJ, et al. Role of hepatitis B viral load and basal core promoter mutation in hepatocellular carcinoma in hepatitis B carriers. J Infect Dis2006;193:1258-65.

24 Raimondo G, Allain JP, Brunetto MR, et al. Statements from the Taormina expert meeting on occult hepatitis B virus infection. J Hepatol2008;49:652-7.

25 Cacciola I, Pollicino T, Squadrito G, et al. Occult hepatitis B virus infection in patients with chronic hepatitis C liver disease. N Engl J Med1999;341:22-6.

26 Squadrito G, Cacciola I, Alibrandi A, et al. Impact of occult hepatitis B virus infection on the outcome of chronic hepatitis C. J Hepatol2013;59:696-700.

27 Gerlich WH, Glebe D, Schuttler CG. Deficiencies in the standardization and sensitivity of diagnostic tests for hepatitis B virus. J Viral Hepatitis2007;14(suppl 1):16-21.

28 Raimondo G, Pollicino T, Cacciola I, Squadrito G. Occult hepatitis B virus infection. J Hepatol2007;46:160-70.

29 Lai M, Hyatt BJ, Nasser I, et al. The clinical significance of persistently normal ALT in chronic hepatitis B infection. J Hepatol2007;47:760-7.

30 Chao DT, Lim JK, Ayoub WS, et al. Systematic review with meta-analysis: the proportion of chronic hepatitis B patients with normal alanine transaminase ≤40 IU/L and significant hepatic fibrosis. Aliment Pharmacol Ther2014;39:349-58.

31 Rockey DC, Caldwell SH, Goodman ZD, et al; American Association for the Study of Liver Diseases. Liver biopsy. Hepatology2009;49:1017-44.

32 Wai CT, Greenson JK, Fontana RJ, et al. A simple noninvasive index can predict both significant fibrosis and cirrhosis in patients with chronic hepatitis C. Hepatology2003;38:518-26.

33 Sterling RK, Lissen E, Clumeck N, et al. Development of a simple noninvasive index to predict significant fibrosis in patients with HIV/HCV coinfection. Hepatology2006;43:1317-25.

34 Xiao G, Yang J, Yan L. Comparison of diagnostic accuracy of aspartate aminotransferase to platelet ratio index and fibrosis-4 index for detecting liver fibrosis in adult patients with chronic hepatitis B virus infection: a systemic review and meta-analysis. Hepatology2015;61:292-302.

35 Yeh WC, Li PC, Jeng YM, et al. Elastic modulus measurements of human liver and correlation with pathology. Ultrasound Med Biol2002;28:467-74.

36 Colombo S, Belloli L, Zaccanelli M, et al. Normal liver stiffness and its determinants in healthy blood donors. Dig Liver Dis 2011;43:231-6.

37 Kim SU, Choi GH, Han WK, et al. What are "true normal" liver stiffness values using FibroScan? A prospective study in healthy living liver and kidney donors in South Korea. Liver Int 2010;30:268-74.

38 Roulot D, Czernichow S, Le Clesiau H et al. Liver stiffness values in apparently healthy subjects: influence of gender and metabolic syndrome. J Hepatol2008;48:606-13.

39 Marcellin P, Ziol M, Bedossa P, et al. Non-invasive assessment of liver fibrosis by stiffness measurement in patients with chronic hepatitis B. Liver Int 2009;29:242-7.

40 Friedrich-Rust M, Ong MF, Martens S, et al. Performance of transient elastography for the staging of liver fibrosis: a meta-analysis. Gastroenterology2008;134:960-74.

41 Chon YE, Choi EH, Song KJ, et al. Performance of transient elastography for the staging of liver fibrosis in patients with chronic hepatitis B: a meta-analysis. PloS One2012;7:e44930.

42 Jonas MM, Block JM, Haber BA, et al. Treatment of children with chronic hepatitis B virus infection in the United States: patient selection and therapeutic options. Hepatology2010;52:2192-205.

43 Chan HL, Chan CK, Hui AJ, et al. Effects of tenofovir disoproxil fumarate in hepatitis B e antigen-positive patients with normal levels of alanine aminotransferase and high levels of hepatitis B virus DNA. Gastroenterology2014;146:1240-8.

44 Tong MJ, Trieu J. Hepatitis B inactive carriers: clinical course and outcomes. J Digest Dis2013;14:311-7.

45 Chen JD, Yang HI, Iloeje UH, et al. Carriers of inactive hepatitis B virus are still at risk for hepatocellular carcinoma and liver-related death. Gastroenterology2010;138:1747-54.

46 Prati D, Taioli E, Zanella A, et al. Updated definitions of healthy ranges for serum alanine aminotransferase levels. Ann Intern Med2002;137:1-10.

47 Chen CJ, Yang HI, Iloeje UH, et al. Hepatitis B virus DNA levels and outcomes in chronic hepatitis B. Hepatology2009;49:S72-84.

48 Iloeje UH, Yang HI, Su J, et al. Predicting cirrhosis risk based on the level of circulating hepatitis B viral load. Gastroenterology2006;130:678-86.

49 Chen CJ, Yang HI, Su J, et al. Risk of hepatocellular carcinoma across a biological gradient of serum hepatitis B virus DNA level. JAMA2006;295:65-73.

50 Chen CF, Lee WC, Yang HI, et al. Changes in serum levels of HBV DNA and alanine aminotransferase determine risk for hepatocellular carcinoma. Gastroenterology2011;141:1240-8, 8 e1-2.

51 Feeney ER, Chung RT. Antiviral treatment of hepatitis C. BMJ2014;348:g3308.

52 Buster EH, Hansen BE, Lau GK, et al. Factors that predict response of patients with hepatitis B e antigen-positive chronic hepatitis B to peginterferon-alfa. Gastroenterology2009;137:2002-9.

53 Santantonio TA, Fasano M. Chronic hepatitis B: Advances in treatment. World J Hepatol2014;6:284-92.

54 Sonneveld MJ, Wong VW, Woltman AM, et al. Polymorphisms near IL28B and serologic response to peginterferon in HBeAg-positive patients with chronic hepatitis B. Gastroenterology2012;142:513-20 e1.

55 Lau GK, Piratvisuth T, Luo KX, et al. Peginterferon alfa-2a, lamivudine, and the combination for HBeAg-positive chronic hepatitis B. N Engl J Med2005;352:2682-95.

56 Marcellin P, Lau GK, Bonino F, et al. Peginterferon alfa-2a alone, lamivudine alone, and the two in combination in patients with HBeAg-negative chronic hepatitis B. N Engl J Med2004;351:1206-17.

57 Rijckborst V, ter Borg MJ, Cakaloglu Y, et al. A randomized trial of peginterferon alfa-2a with or without ribavirin for HBeAg-negative chronic hepatitis B. Am J Gastroenterol2010;105:1762-9.

58 Liaw YF, Jia JD, Chan HL, et al. Shorter durations and lower doses of peginterferon alfa-2a are associated with inferior hepatitis B e antigen seroconversion rates in hepatitis B virus genotypes B or C. Hepatology2011;54:1591-9.

59 Lampertico P, Vigano M, Di Costanzo GG, et al. Randomised study comparing 48 and 96 weeks peginterferon alpha-2a therapy in genotype D HBeAg-negative chronic hepatitis B. Gut2013;62:290-8.

60 Chang TT, Gish RG, de Man R, et al. A comparison of entecavir and lamivudine for HBeAg-positive chronic hepatitis B. N Engl J Med2006;354:1001-10.

61 Lai CL, Shouval D, Lok AS, et al. Entecavir versus lamivudine for patients with HBeAg-negative chronic hepatitis B. N Engl J Med2006;354:1011-20.

62 Gish RG, Lok AS, Chang TT, et al. Entecavir therapy for up to 96 weeks in patients with HBeAg-positive chronic hepatitis B. Gastroenterology2007;133:1437-44.

63 Chang TT, Lai CL, Kew Yoon S, et al. Entecavir treatment for up to 5 years in patients with hepatitis B e antigen-positive chronic hepatitis B. Hepatology2010;51:422-30.

64 Tenney DJ, Rose RE, Baldick CJ, et al. Long-term monitoring shows hepatitis B virus resistance to entecavir in nucleoside-naive patients is rare through 5 years of therapy. Hepatology2009;49:1503-14.

65 Yuen MF, Seto WK, Fung J, Wong DK, Yuen JC, Lai CL. Three years of continuous entecavir therapy in treatment-naive chronic hepatitis B patients: VIRAL suppression, viral resistance, and clinical safety. Am J Gastroenterol2011;106:1264-71.

66 Lange CM, Bojunga J, Hofmann WP, et al. Severe lactic acidosis during treatment of chronic hepatitis B with entecavir in patients with impaired liver function. Hepatology2009;50:2001-6.

67 Liaw YF, Sheen IS, Lee CM, et al. Tenofovir disoproxil fumarate (TDF), emtricitabine/TDF, and entecavir in patients with decompensated chronic hepatitis B liver disease. Hepatology2011;53:62-72.

68 Shim JH, Lee HC, Kim KM, et al. Efficacy of entecavir in treatment-naive patients with hepatitis B virus-related decompensated cirrhosis. J Hepatol2010;52:176-82.

69 Marcellin P, Heathcote EJ, Buti M, et al. Tenofovir disoproxil fumarate versus adefovir dipivoxil for chronic hepatitis B. N Engl J Med2008;359:2442-55.

70 Corsa AC, Liu Y, Flaherty JF, et al. No detectable resistance to tenofovir disoproxil fumarate (TDF) in HBeAg+ and HBeAg patients with chronic hepatitis B (CHB) after eight years of treatment. Hepatology2015;1707.

71 Lok AS, Trinh H, Carosi G, et al. Efficacy of entecavir with or without tenofovir disoproxil fumarate for nucleos(t)ide-naive patients with chronic hepatitis B. Gastroenterology2012;143:619-28 e1.

72 Fung S, Kwan P, Fabri M, et al. Randomized comparison of tenofovir disoproxil fumarate vs emtricitabine and tenofovir disoproxil fumarate in patients with lamivudine-resistant chronic hepatitis B. Gastroenterology2014;146:980-8.

73 Van Bommel F, de Man RA, Wedemeyer H, et al. Long-term efficacy of tenofovir monotherapy for hepatitis B virus-monoinfected patients after failure of nucleoside/nucleotide analogues. Hepatology2010;51:73-80.

74 Reijnders JG, Deterding K, Petersen J, et al. Antiviral effect of entecavir in chronic hepatitis B: influence of prior exposure to nucleos(t)ide analogues. J Hepatol2010;52:493-500.

75 Lim YS, Byun KS, Yoo BC, et al. Tenofovir monotherapy versus tenofovir and entecavir combination therapy in patients with entecavir-resistant chronic hepatitis B with multiple drug failure: results of a randomised trial. Gut2015.

76 Deguchi M, Yamashita N, Kagita M, et al. Quantitation of hepatitis B surface antigen by an automated chemiluminescent microparticle immunoassay. J Virologic Methods2004;115:217-22.

77 Zacher BJ, Moriconi F, Bowden S, et al. Multicenter evaluation of the Elecsys hepatitis B surface antigen quantitative assay. Clin Vaccine Immunol2011;18:1943-50.

78 Honer Zu Siederdissen C, Cornberg M. The role of HBsAg levels in the current management of chronic HBV infection. Ann Gastroenterol 2014;27:105-12.

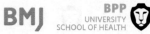

79 Seto WK, Wong DK, Fung J, et al. High hepatitis B surface antigen levels predict insignificant fibrosis in hepatitis B e antigen positive chronic hepatitis B. PloS One2012;7:e43087.

80 Martinot-Peignoux M, Carvalho-Filho R, Lapalus M, et al. Hepatitis B surface antigen serum level is associated with fibrosis severity in treatment-naive, e antigen-positive patients. J Hepatol2013;58:1089-95.

81 Brunetto MR, Oliveri F, Colombatto P, et al. Hepatitis B surface antigen serum levels help to distinguish active from inactive hepatitis B virus genotype D carriers. Gastroenterology2010;139:483-90.

82 Takkenberg RB, Jansen L, de Niet A, et al. Baseline hepatitis B surface antigen (HBsAg) as predictor of sustained HBsAg loss in chronic hepatitis B patients treated with pegylated interferon-alpha2a and adefovir. Antiviral Ther2013;18:895-904.

83 Chan HL, Wong VW, Chim AM, et al. Serum HBsAg quantification to predict response to peginterferon therapy of e antigen positive chronic hepatitis B. Aliment Pharmacol Ther2010;32:1323-31.

84 Sonneveld MJ, Rijckborst V, Boucher CA, et al. Prediction of sustained response to peginterferon alfa-2b for hepatitis B e antigen-positive chronic hepatitis B using on-treatment hepatitis B surface antigen decline. Hepatology2010;52:1251-7.

85 Moucari R, Mackiewicz V, Lada O, et al. Early serum HBsAg drop: a strong predictor of sustained virological response to pegylated interferon alfa-2a in HBeAg-negative patients. Hepatology2009;49:1151-7.

86 Reijnders JG, Perquin MJ, Zhang N, et al. Nucleos(t)ide analogues only induce temporary hepatitis B e antigen seroconversion in most patients with chronic hepatitis B. Gastroenterology2010;139:491-8.

87 Lee HW, Lee HJ, Hwang JS, et al. Lamivudine maintenance beyond one year after HBeAg seroconversion is a major factor for sustained virologic response in HBeAg-positive chronic hepatitis B. Hepatology2010;51:415-21.

88 Hadziyannis SJ, Sevastianos V, Rapti I, et al. Sustained responses and loss of HBsAg in HBeAg-negative patients with chronic hepatitis B who stop long-term treatment with adefovir. Gastroenterology2012;143:629-36 e1.

89 Seto WK, Hui AJ, Wong VW, et al. Treatment cessation of entecavir in Asian patients with hepatitis B e antigen negative chronic hepatitis B: a multicentre prospective study. Gut2015;64:667-72.

90 Fontaine H, Kahi S, Chazallon C, et al. Anti-HBV DNA vaccination does not prevent relapse after discontinuation of analogues in the treatment of chronic hepatitis B: a randomised trial-ANRS HB02 VAC-ADN. Gut2015;64:139-47.

91 Marcellin P, Gane E, Buti M, et al. Regression of cirrhosis during treatment with tenofovir disoproxil fumarate for chronic hepatitis B: a 5-year open-label follow-up study. Lancet2013;381:468-75.

92 Liaw YF, Sung JJ, Chow WC, et al. Lamivudine for patients with chronic hepatitis B and advanced liver disease. N Engl J Med2004;351:1521-31.

93 Hosaka T, Suzuki F, Kobayashi M, et al. Long-term entecavir treatment reduces hepatocellular carcinoma incidence in patients with hepatitis B virus infection. Hepatology2013;58:98-107.

94 Wong GL, Chan HL, Mak CW, et al. Entecavir treatment reduces hepatic events and deaths in chronic hepatitis B patients with liver cirrhosis. Hepatology2013;58:1537-47.

95 Wu CY, Lin JT, Ho HJ, et al. Association of nucleos(t)ide analogue therapy with reduced risk of hepatocellular carcinoma in patients with chronic hepatitis B: a nationwide cohort study. Gastroenterology2014;147:143-51 e5.

96 Papatheodoridis GV, Chan HL, Hansen BE, et al. Risk of hepatocellular carcinoma in chronic hepatitis B: assessment and modification with current antiviral therapy. J Hepatol2015;62:956-67.

97 Phung BC, Sogni P, Launay O. Hepatitis B and human immunodeficiency virus co-infection. World J Gastroenterol2014;20:17360-7.

98 McGovern BH. The epidemiology, natural history and prevention of hepatitis B: implications of HIV coinfection. Antiviral Ther2007;12(suppl 3):H3-13.

99 Thio CL. Hepatitis B and human immunodeficiency virus coinfection. Hepatology2009;49:S138-45.

100 Puoti M, Torti C, Bruno R, et al. Natural history of chronic hepatitis B in co-infected patients. J Hepatol2006;44:S65-70.

101 Thio CL, Seaberg EC, Skolasky R, Jr., et al. HIV-1, hepatitis B virus, and risk of liver-related mortality in the Multicenter Cohort Study (MACS). Lancet2002;360:1921-6.

102 Konopnicki D, Mocroft A, de Wit S, et al. Hepatitis B and HIV: prevalence, AIDS progression, response to highly active antiretroviral therapy and increased mortality in the EuroSIDA cohort. AIDS2005;19:593-601.

103 Benhamou Y, Fleury H, Trimoulet P, et al. Anti-hepatitis B virus efficacy of tenofovir disoproxil fumarate in HIV-infected patients. Hepatology2006;43:548-55.

104 Price H, Dunn D, Pillay D, et al. Suppression of HBV by tenofovir in HBV/HIV coinfected patients: a systematic review and meta-analysis. PloS One2013;8:e68152.

105 Noureddin M, Gish R. Hepatitis delta: epidemiology, diagnosis and management 36 years after discovery. Curr Gastroenterol Rep2014;16:365.

106 Wedemeyer H, Yurdaydin C, Dalekos GN, et al. Peginterferon plus adefovir versus either drug alone for hepatitis delta. N Engl J Medic2011;364:322-31.

107 Heidrich B, Yurdaydin C, Kabacam G, et al. Late HDV RNA relapse after peginterferon alpha-based therapy of chronic hepatitis delta. Hepatology2014;60:87-97.

108 Wedemeyer H, Yurdaydin C, Ernst S, et al. Prolonged therapy of hepatitis delta for 96 weeks with pegylated-interferon-a-2a plus tenofovir or placebo does not prevent HDV RNA relapse after treatment: the HIDIT-2 study. 49th European Association for the Study of the Liver International Liver Congress (EASL 2014). London, April 9-13, 2014. Abstract 04. http://hepatitis-delta.org/assets/DownloadPage/000000/2014-04-HIDIT-II-EASL-Homepage.pdf.

109 Patton H, Tran TT. Management of hepatitis B during pregnancy. Nat Rev Gastroenterol Hepatol2014;11:402-9.

110 US Department of Health and Human Services. MMWR: a comprehensive immunization strategy to eliminate transmission of hepatitis B virus infection in the United States. 2005. www.cdc.gov/mmwr/preview/mmwrhtml/rr5416a1.htm.

111 Zou H, Chen Y, Duan Z, et al. Virologic factors associated with failure to passive-active immunoprophylaxis in infants born to HBsAg-positive mothers. J Viral Hepatitis2012;19:e18-25.

112 Shaheen AA, Myers RP. The outcomes of pregnancy in patients with cirrhosis: a population-based study. Liver Int 2010;30:275-83.

113 Peginterferon alfa-2b pregnancy and breastfeeding warnings. www.drugs.com/pregnancy/peginterferon-alfa-2b.html.

114 Pan CQ, Mi LJ, Bunchorntavakul C, et al. Tenofovir disoproxil fumarate for prevention of vertical transmission of hepatitis B virus infection by highly viremic pregnant women: a case series. Dig Dis Sci2012;57:2423-9.

115 Pan CQ, Han GR, Jiang HX, et al. Telbivudine prevents vertical transmission from HBeAg-positive women with chronic hepatitis B. Clin Gastroenterol Hepatol 2012;10:520-6.

116 Han GR, Cao MK, Zhao W, et al. A prospective and open-label study for the efficacy and safety of telbivudine in pregnancy for the prevention of perinatal transmission of hepatitis B virus infection. J Hepatol2011;55:1215-21.

117 Ehrhardt S, Xie C, Guo N, Nelson K, Thio CL. Breastfeeding while taking lamivudine or tenofovir disoproxil fumarate: a review of the evidence. Clin Infect Dis 2015;60:275-8.

118 Hoofnagle JH. Reactivation of hepatitis B. Hepatology2009;49:S156-65.

119 Hwang JP, Lok AS. Management of patients with hepatitis B who require immunosuppressive therapy. Nat Rev Gastroenterol Hepatol2014;11:209-19.

120 Vassilopoulos D, Calabrese LH. Management of rheumatic disease with comorbid HBV or HCV infection. Nat Rev Rheumatol2012;8:348-57.

121 Di Bisceglie AM, Lok AS, Martin P, et al. Recent US Food and Drug Administration warnings on hepatitis B reactivation with immune-suppressing and anticancer drugs: just the tip of the iceberg? Hepatology2015;61:703-11.

122 Reddy KR, Beavers KL, Hammond SP, et al. American gastroenterological association institute guideline on the prevention and treatment of hepatitis B virus reactivation during immunosuppressive drug therapy. Gastroenterology2015;148:215-9.

123 Lau GK, Yiu HH, Fong DY, et al. Early is superior to deferred preemptive lamivudine therapy for hepatitis B patients undergoing chemotherapy. Gastroenterology2003;125:1742-9.

124 Hsu C, Hsiung CA, Su IJ, et al. A revisit of prophylactic lamivudine for chemotherapy-associated hepatitis B reactivation in non-Hodgkin's lymphoma: a randomized trial. Hepatology2008;47:844-53.

125 Saab S, Dong MH, Joseph TA, et al. Hepatitis B prophylaxis in patients undergoing chemotherapy for lymphoma: a decision analysis model. Hepatology2007;46:1049-56.

126 Huang YH, Hsiao LT, Hong YC, et al. Randomized controlled trial of entecavir prophylaxis for rituximab-associated hepatitis B virus reactivation in patients with lymphoma and resolved hepatitis B. J Clin Oncol 2013;31:2765-72.

127 Hsu C, Tsou HH, Lin SJ, et al. Chemotherapy-induced hepatitis B reactivation in lymphoma patients with resolved HBV infection: a prospective study. Hepatology2014;59:2092-100.

128 Jayalakshmi MMK, Kalyanaraman N, Pitchappan R. Hepatitis B virus genetic diversity: disease pathogenesis, viral replication. In: Rosas-Acosta G, ed. Immunology and microbiology "viral replication." InTech, 2013. www.intechopen.com/books/viral-replication/hepatitis-b-virus-genetic-diversity-disease-pathogenesis.

129 Kapoor R, Kottilil S. Strategies to eliminate HBV infection. Future Virol2014;9:565-85.

130 Wang XY, Chen HS. Emerging antivirals for the treatment of hepatitis B. World J Gastroenterol2014;20:7707-17.

131 Petersen J, Dandri M, Mier W, et al. Prevention of hepatitis B virus infection in vivo by entry inhibitors derived from the large envelope protein. Nat Biotechnol2008;26:335-41.

132 Volz T, Allweiss L, Ben MM, et al. The entry inhibitor myrcludex-B efficiently blocks intrahepatic virus spreading in humanized mice previously infected with hepatitis B virus. J Hepatol2013;58:861-7.

133 Stray SJ, Zlotnick A. BAY 41-4109 has multiple effects on Hepatitis B virus capsid assembly. J Mol Recogn2006;19:542-8.

134 Wang XY, Wei ZM, Wu GY, et al. In vitro inhibition of HBV replication by a novel compound, GLS4, and its efficacy against adefovir-dipivoxil-resistant HBV mutations. Antiviral Ther2012;17:793-803.

135 Mahtab MA, Bazinet M, Patient R, et al. REP 9 AC: a potent HBsAg release inhibitor that elicits durable immunological control of chronic HBV infection. Hepatology2011;54(suppl S1): 478A.

136 Lanford RE, Guerra B, Chavez D, et al. GS-9620, an oral agonist of Toll-like receptor-7, induces prolonged suppression of hepatitis B virus in chronically infected chimpanzees. Gastroenterology2013;144:1508-17, 17 e1-10.

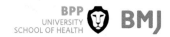

137 Spellman M, Martin JT. Treatment of chronic hepatitis B infection with DV-601, a therapeutic vaccine. J Hepatol2011;54(suppl 1):s302.

138 Zimmerman KA, Fischer KP, Joyce MA, et al. Zinc finger proteins designed to specifically target duck hepatitis B virus covalently closed circular DNA inhibit viral transcription in tissue culture. J Virol2008;82:8013-21.

139 Cai D, Mills C, Yu W, et al. Identification of disubstituted sulfonamide compounds as specific inhibitors of hepatitis B virus covalently closed circular DNA formation. Antimicrob Agents Chemother2012;56:4277-88.

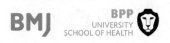

The role of pathogen genomics in assessing disease transmission

Vitali Sintchenko, associate professor, director[1][2], Edward C Holmes, professor[1][3]

[1]Marie Bashir Institute for Infectious Diseases and Biosecurity and Sydney Medical School, University of Sydney, Sydney, Australia

[2]Centre for Infectious Diseases and Microbiology-Public Health, Institute of Clinical Pathology and Medical Research-Pathology West, Westmead Hospital, Sydney, NSW 2145, Australia

[3]School of Biological Sciences, Charles Perkins Centre, University of Sydney, Sydney, Australia

Correspondence to: V Sintchenko vitali.sintchenko@sydney.edu.au

Cite this as: BMJ 2015;350:h1314

DOI: 10.1136/bmj.h1314

http://www.bmj.com/content/350/bmj.h1314

ABSTRACT

Whole genome sequencing (WGS) of pathogens enables the sources and patterns of transmission to be identified during specific disease outbreaks and promises to transform epidemiological research on communicable diseases. This review discusses new insights into disease spread and transmission that have come from the use of WGS, particularly when combined with genomic scale phylogenetic analyses. These include elucidation of the mechanisms of cross species transmission, the potential modes of pathogen transmission, and which people in the population contribute most to transmission. Particular attention is paid to the ability of WGS to resolve individual patient to patient transmission events. Importantly, WGS data seem to be sufficiently discriminatory to target cases linked to community or hospital contacts and hence prevent further spread, and to investigate genetically related cases without a clear epidemiological link. Approaches to combine evidence from epidemiological with genomic sequencing observations are summarised. Ongoing genomic surveillance can identify determinants of transmission, monitor pathogen evolution and adaptation, ensure the accurate and timely diagnosis of infections with epidemic potential, and refine strategies for their control.

Introduction

Recent advances in nucleic acid sequencing technology have made rapid whole genome sequencing (WGS) of pathogens technically and economically feasible.[1][2][3][4] DNA sequencing has advantages over other methods of pathogen identification and characterisation used in microbiology laboratories. Firstly, it provides a universal solution with high throughput, speed, and quality and can be applied to any micro-organism.[3][4] Secondly, it produces data that can be compared at national and international levels. Finally, its usefulness has been augmented by the rapid growth of public databases containing reference genomes,[2][3][5][6] which can be linked to equivalent databases that contain additional clinical and epidemiological metadata (for example, the influenza research database www.fludb.org/).

The ability to focus on pathogen genomes at the scale of individual outbreaks is a major leap forward in biomedical science.[3][7] It follows two previous breakthroughs in the investigation and understanding of communicable diseases. The first was the foundation of spatial epidemiology by John Snow, whose quasi case-control study identified the Broad Street water pump as the source of a cholera outbreak in London in 1854 (fig 1). An array of methods for the spatial and temporal analyses of infectious diseases is now available.

The second breakthrough was the invention of solid culture media by Robert Koch three decades later, which enabled the identification of numerous bacterial pathogens as agents of human and animal disease. This revolutionised our understanding of the causes and pathogenesis of infectious diseases and facilitated the development of laboratory diagnostics, antimicrobials, and vaccines.

The ability to analyse the genomes of pathogens enables more rapid and precise identification than ever before as well as assessment of their virulence and drug resistance potential. In addition, phylogenetic and related methods of evolutionary analysis can be used to infer the origin and emergence of pathogen. Advances in pathogen genomics open a new frontier in biomedical science by moving the study of disease spread and transmission from the population level to the (individual) patient level, and from the estimation of potential sources of disease to the accurate identification of transmission chains.

Next generation sequencing refers to high throughput sequencing methods that allow the process to be performed in parallel, producing thousands or millions of sequences at once. This encompasses several different technologies that include but are not limited to sequence by synthesis, terminator based sequencing, and ligation based sequencing. The sequence by synthesis approach, notably pyrosequencing, means that nucleotide sequence data are generated during DNA synthesis rather than from the analysis of amplicons after synthesis, as is the case with traditional Sanger sequencing. Another technology based on the sequence by synthesis approach is semiconductor sequencing, which is used by the Ion Torrent system, where parallel sequencing reactions are carried out in 1.2 million microwells on the surface of a semiconductor chip. By contrast, sequencing by Illumina (Solexa) systems relies on reversible dye terminators. DNA molecules are first attached to primers on a slide and amplified so that local clonal colonies are formed. Four types of reversible terminator bases are added and non-incorporated nucleotides are washed away, allowing the fluorescently labelled nucleotides to be captured by a camera.[8] More technical details can be found in recent reviews and will not be discussed here.[2][4][5][8]

This review summarises recent advances in WGS in relation to communicable disease transmission. These developments have the potential to substantially improve the detection and control of disease. Emerging areas of research and clinical research translation are also briefly discussed. The review also evaluates the added value of next generation sequencing in the control of communicable diseases and associated translational research. New insights into mechanisms of spread and transmission of bacterial and viral diseases are also discussed.

Sources and selection criteria

We searched PubMed and Google Scholar from January 2005 to August 2014 using the terms "whole genome sequencing" and "next generation sequencing", with the filters "infection", "infectious disease", "communicable disease", "transmission", "spread", "molecular epidemiology", and "disease emergence". The evidence was appraised for validity and relevance to public health practice. Priority was given to human and clinical studies over experimental,

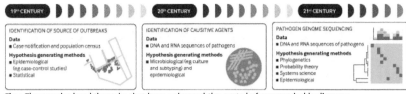

Fig 1 Three major breakthroughs that have enhanced the control of communicable diseases

---

ONGOING RESEARCH QUESTIONS

- How does identification of the factors that drive cross species transmission and establishment in new hosts influence the emergence of new pathogens and the design of effective control strategies?
- Does phylogenetics have sufficient resolution to accurately reconstruct transmission pathways and to date transmission events within community outbreaks and the transmission of newly emerged pathogens?
- Can phylogenetic and molecular clock dating studies discover unsuspected epidemiological links and identify the time scales of disease outbreaks?
- Is the extent of intra-host diversity in microbial populations affected by modes of transmission?
- How can next generation sequencing data further enhance models that can infer the environmental source of food borne bacteria (that is, source attribution models for foodborne diseases)?
- What are the most appropriate models and techniques to infer patient to patient transmission networks from whole genome sequencing data?
- What are the ethical and medico-legal implications of identifying sources of disease outbreaks among asymptomatic carriers and healthcare workers?

---

infection transmission modelling or animal studies, and to original research about pathogens with epidemic potential over review type publications. We also searched bibliographies of articles for relevant studies and selected translational medicine studies where possible. We also examined abstracts from the Wellcome Trust conference "Applied Bioinformatics and Public Health" (Cambridge, May 2013).

How has clinical medicine benefited from pathogen genomics?

Old and new definitions of pathogen diversity
Genomic studies have shown that microbial populations carry more genetic diversity, often in more complex forms, than previously thought. So how should the diversity of pathogens be defined?

A commonly used term in this context is "strain," which has been defined as a group of isolates that share a particular set of phenotypic traits, although usually it simply refers to any phylogenetically distinct entity. However, with the increase in resolution provided by WGS, strains can now be further subdivided into genotypes, clones, lineages, and variants.

Classic microbiology has often viewed pathogen diversity in the guise of fixed or static "types," whereas evolutionary and epidemiological studies depict pathogen genomic variation as a dynamic process,[9][10] in which genetic diversity changes in time and space. Given our ability to sequence pathogen genomes in "real time" during disease outbreaks, the dynamic view of pathogen diversity is likely to be more appropriate.

The dynamic view of pathogen genomes is also supported by the growing body of literature showing that pathogen populations can experience rapid and profound changes in genetic structure that reflect and may affect their epidemiology.[11][12] For example, selective sweeps (see Glossary) of advantageous mutations, such as those mediating escape from population immunity or those that confer antimicrobial resistance lead to wide

ranging (and sometimes genomic scale) reductions in genetic diversity.[13] A good example of this process would be the gradual development of drug resistance in *Mycobacterium tuberculosis* during treatment. In the case of bacteria, population diversity can be represented by the "pathogenome" concept. This concept combines a "core genome," which depicts a set of genes conserved among all strains, with a "dispensable genome," which consists of partially shared or unique, strain specific genes (see Glossary).[14] The larger the dispensable genome the greater the pathogen's capacity to survive in hostile ecological niches and to be effectively transmitted to susceptible hosts.[15]

Genomic differences in pathogen virulence and transmissibility
Evidence suggests that pathogen lineages (see Glossary) may differ in virulence or transmission potential, or both.[15] For example, the Beijing lineage of *Mycobacterium tuberculosis* seems to be more transmissible than other lineages and to be associated with pulmonary tuberculosis in younger patients.[16] Although such differences have generally been harder to pin point in viruses,[17] partly because of the speed with which genetic diversity is generated in these organisms, some examples have been identified,[18][19][20] and more are likely to be found in the future with improved links between genotypic and phenotypic data.

The chikungunya virus is interesting because a single mutation enables human transmission through the highly successful anthropophilic vector *Aedes aegypti*, thereby increasing epidemic potential.[21] Ultimately, analyses of this type may enable a form of "genomic risk assessment" involving the surveillance of mutations that affect virulence, transmission, or both, which in turn may guide intervention strategies. A high profile example is the identification of those mutations that facilitate the human to human transmission of highly pathogenic influenza A H5N1 virus,[22][23] and similar risk assessment tools can probably be applied to other emerging pathogens.

Investigating the origin and spread of high impact pathogens
Pathogen genomics has provided new and more detailed explanations for the origin, patterns, and dynamics of spread of several important human pathogens.[24] For example, the virtual absence of the meticillin resistant *Staphylococcus aureus* (MRSA) II sequence type 5 bacteria (which carry staphylococcal toxic shock toxin) from Germany indicated that most of these clinically important micro-organisms originated recently (within the past 15 years) from a very small imported population.[25]

The origin of and factors responsible for the emergence of the devastating influenza pandemic of 1918-19, as well as its relatively high mortality in young adults are still unclear,[26] whereas the origins of the pandemic A/H1N1 2009 influenza outbreak were rapidly reconstructed through genomics.[27] Furthermore, the genome-wide analysis of *Streptococcus pneumoniae* identified 147 genes needed for survival in human saliva and transmission by droplet spread, including those involved in cell envelope synthesis and cell transport.[28]

On an entirely different time scale, the sequencing of *Yersinia pestis* bacteria isolated from teeth disinterred from the east Smithfield Black Death burial ground in London dating to 1348 showed that the plague strains associated

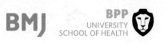

Applications of pathogen genome sequencing to communicable disease control

Application	Actionable information about infectiousness or transmissibility generated by pathogen genome sequencing	Pathogens†
Direct culture independent microbiological diagnosis	Identification of fastidious pathogens at the species and lineage levels	*Leptospira* spp[11], *Mycobacterium tuberculosis*[31 32]
Detection of cross species transmission and host adaptation in emerging pathogens	Genomic risk assessment of host adaptive mutations; discovery and impact of recombination events	Human influenza virus A H7/N9,[33-35] MERS-coronavirus,[36] *Staphylococcus aureus*,[37 38] *Salmonella typhimurium*,[39] *Streptococcus pneumoniae*,[28 40] *Enterococcus* spp[41]
Pathogen risk assessment	Identification of targets for assays differentiating highly virulent pathogen strains	Influenza virus H5/N1,[22 23] *Chlamydia trachomatis*[42 43]
	Distinguishing recent from pre-existing (chronic) infection	*Mycobacterium tuberculosis*[44 45]
	Redefining periods of transmissibility	MRSA,[46] group A streptococcus[47]
Detection, monitoring, and control of hospital acquired outbreaks	Identification of new clones associated with hospital acquired pathogens	*Acinetobacter baumannii*,[48 49] *S aureus*,[50] *Escherichia coli*,[51 52] *Pseudomonas aeruginosa*[53]
	Near real time identification of transmission events (patient to patient, healthcare staff to patient, environment to patient)*	*S aureus*,[53-59] *Clostridium difficile*,[53-55 60] *Klebsiella pneumoniae*[61]
	Monitoring transmission and (antimicrobial resistance) gene flow between healthcare institutions	*C difficile*,[56] *S aureus*,[62] HIV,[63] norovirus,[64] human influenza virus[65]
Improved resolution of regional, national, and global public health laboratory surveillance	Detection of outbreaks, covert clusters, and associated risk factors	*Neisseria meningitidis*,[66] *Salmonella enterica*,[67] enterohaemorrhagic *E coli*,[51 68] *M tuberculosis*[4 69 70]
	Reconstruction of outbreak origins, transmission pathways and dating of transmission events within community outbreaks (person to person contact, water and food borne modes of direct transmission)*	Ebola virus,[71] enterovirus,[72] *Vibrio cholerae*,[73 74] *Mycobacterium tuberculosis*,[4 46 75-78] group A streptococcus,[48 79 80] *Shigella* spp,[81-83] *Legionella* spp[84]
	Source attribution and detecting the spatial spread (phylogeography) of disease outbreaks	MERS-coronavirus,[85] *C difficile*,[86] *Vibrio cholerae*[74]
	Epidemiological scale evolution and dispersal, contribution of intra-host and inter-host dynamics to pathogen evolution (person to person; environment to person modes of direct transmission; exposure to blood and vectors)*	Hepatitis C virus,[87 88] *E coli*,[89] *Helicobacter pylori*,[90] *S aureus*,[91] *Salmonella typhimurium*,[40 92] human influenza virus,[93] *Cryptococcus gattii*,[94] norovirus,[64] *Campylobacter* spp,[95] *S pneumoniae*,[96] *Neisseria meningitidis*,[66 97] arboviruses[98 99]

*Modes of transmission of pathogens under study are indicated in parenthesis.
†MERS=Middle East respiratory syndrome; MRSA=meticillin resistant *Staphylococcus aureus*.

with this pandemic were similar to those currently circulating, although associated mortality was far greater.[29] This is compatible with the idea that the high mortality seen in the medieval plagues (and the sixth century Plague of Justinian[30]) was more likely to be associated with epidemiological circumstances (overcrowding, poor general health and living conditions) than with bacterial encoded virulence.

New insights into disease spread and transmission provided by genome sequencing

The table lists the main applications of genome sequencing, with specific examples of the added value that it brings to communicable disease control. It shows that studies undertaken so far have focused on infections that are directly transmitted through contact, food, or water. More complex microbial transmission pathways involving zoonotic and environmental reservoirs and intermediate hosts still await systematic examination at the genomic scale.

Cross species transmission and host adaptation

Advances in genomics have been instrumental in identifying the factors that facilitate the successful cross species transmission of emerging pathogens. One of the main observations is that more host adaptive mutations are needed, often in multiple genes, as the phylogenetic distance (see Glossary) between the donor and recipient species increases.[100] Hence, despite the rapidity of microbial evolution, it may be a major adaptive challenge to acquire the multiple changes needed to increase host range (see Glossary), and recombination (see Glossary) (or reassortment (see Glossary) in the case of influenza virus) might be a more efficient way to place host adaptive mutations in the same genotype.

Once cross species transmission of a pathogen has occurred various outcomes are possible. These range from infections controlled by a host's immune system to lethal disease, both of which are likely to result in

"spill over" (or dead end) infections with no subsequent transmission, as well as those in which the pathogen is able to evolve sustained (epidemic) transmission in the human population.[100] Clearly, to assess the risks of the emergence of new strains and to design effective control strategies, it is important to identify the factors that drive the efficacy of cross species transmission. However, the genomic basis of the pathogen host range has been resolved in only a small number of cases, which indicates that further research is needed.[10 17]

Work in this area has also confirmed the role of co-infection (simultaneous infection) and superinfection (second infection superimposed on an earlier one) as facilitators of lateral gene transfer (see Glossary).[101] For example, individual patients can be colonised with multiple strains of *Acinetobacter baumannii*, which are then capable of recombining. The movement of patients and staff between healthcare facilities also contributes to strain mixing and diversification,[48] and it has been an important factor in the rise of antimicrobial resistance.

Intra-host and inter-host pathogen evolution and transmission

The genetic and phenotypic variation present in bacteria and viruses is generated within individual hosts and, in the case of some bacteria, in the environment. The rate at which genetic and phenotypic diversity is generated is central to understanding the ability of pathogens to adapt to and spread within host populations.[78 87 102] This rate depends on four major factors: the population size of the pathogen; its mutation rate; the frequency of replication (assuming that mutations occur during replication); and the fitness of the mutations produced, with advantageous mutations fixed faster than neutral ones.

Replication can occur for extended periods in immunocompromised people, and such people may represent an important reservoir for the emergence of genetically and phenotypically distinct variants.[64 103] About

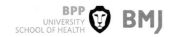

one mutation occurs in every replication cycle in RNA viruses, so these viruses are expected to be particularly rapid generators of genetic variation, even though most mutations will be deleterious.[10]

Despite this propensity to generate genetic variation, population bottlenecks are probably common during inter-host transmission and this will greatly restrict genetic diversity. In some cases, such as certain modes of HIV-1 transmission, infections can be initiated by a single viable virus particle,[104] and this will put a strong brake on adaptive evolution at the epidemiological scale, although wider bottlenecks are seen in other viruses such as influenza virus and foot and mouth disease virus.[105 106] Also, rates of pathogen evolution may vary within and among hosts, reflecting the different selection pressures in these circumstances. For example, evolutionary rates in HIV-1 are consistently lower at the epidemiological (inter-host) scale than within individual hosts.[9] Similarly, although inter-host transmission is often initiated by a randomly generated variant in the donor host, it is possible that the variant transmitted may not be representative of the donor's viral population or that specific variants may preferentially outgrow in the new host.

Non-invasive bacterial disease and colonisation as enablers of transmission

One of the most striking features of disease transmission is the varying infectiousness of individual hosts, which has a major impact at the epidemiological scale. Indeed, the roles of chance and genetics in the progression from carriage to invasive disease are yet to be fully determined in most cases.[107] Recent epidemiological studies using comparative genomics have emphasised the relative contribution of asymptomatic colonisation in disease transmission. For example, comparison of *Clostridium difficile* genomes suggested that many infections were not caused by recent transmission from a symptomatic person, highlighting the potential importance of asymptomatic carriage or multiple introductions from an environmental source.[60] The same is true of many blood borne viral infections, such as HIV, hepatitis B virus, and hepatitis C virus.

Intra-host heterogeneity and modes of transmission

It is also possible that the analysis of intra-host heterogeneity during outbreaks may provide important clues to potential modes of pathogen transmission, especially when microbial cultures of implicated micro-organisms from environmental samples are not available. For example, exposure to a large inoculum of a pathogen (such as uncooked food heavily contaminated with salmonella or hepatitis A virus in raw sewage) is expected to result in productive infection by a large and potentially heterogeneous microbial population.[108 109]

By contrast, exposure to a relatively small infectious dose of micro-organisms, such as that transmitted through an aerosol or insect vector, would probably lead to infection by a smaller and more homogeneous microbial population.[108 109] Thus, the sequencing of the genomes of pathogens obtained from patients during outbreaks may offer additional clues to the precise mode of pathogen transmission, especially when microbial cultures of implicated micro-organisms from environmental samples are not available.

As another example, in a 3.6 year study of *C difficile* isolates from 1200 patients residing in a defined geographical area, 75% of infections were not transmitted from symptomatic patients, indicating that numerous sources of infection should be targeted to prevent exposure.[55] WGS data also seemed to be sufficiently discriminatory to target cases linked to community or hospital contacts and prevent further spread, and to investigate genetically related cases without a clear epidemiological link to uncover novel routes of transmission.[55] Clearly, however, additional studies are needed to fully resolve the association between intra-host microbial diversity and mode of transmission, and how much inferential power this provides. WGS is unlikely to be informative in the case of RNA viruses in which genetic diversity accumulates so rapidly.

Case study: the evolution and transmission pathways of hospital acquired MRSA

New methods of genome sequencing have helped answer old questions in the clinical diagnosis and epidemiology of MRSA, one of the most important public health problems in developed countries.[38] For example, some studies have used the "molecular clock" analysis of genome sequence data (based on the assumption that nucleotide substitutions accumulate at a constant rate) to estimate the time to the most common recent ancestor (TMCRA) of specific MRSA lineages and hence the dates of presumed transmission events.[110 111] Accordingly, the mean substitution rate is estimated at 3.3×10^{-6} to 7.6×10^{-5} substitutions per site per year, which corresponds to about one new single nucleotide polymorphism (SNP) in the core MRSA genome every six weeks.[62]

Figure 2 shows the information that can be derived from analyses of this kind. In this example, the TMCRA for isolates 3 and 4 had to be after infection of patient 3 but before transmission to patient 4. Similarly, because nosocomial MRSA infections probably occur on a time scale of weeks rather than months, direct transmission links can be excluded if the TMCRA of a pair of isolates is estimated to occur over long time scales.[58 59]

This approach was verified in investigations of MRSA outbreaks, which confirmed an important role for asymptomatic carriers.[59] Although these types of analyses are potentially powerful they make several simplifying assumptions:

- That a single genome is the founder of each new infection (which is probably true for MRSA)[58 59 75]
- No recombination has occurred
- Neutral evolution (an absence of natural selection on fixed mutations)
- The rate of nucleotide substitution is constant, particularly in the core genome regions.

Obviously, these assumptions will not be valid in all cases, and this may lead to erroneous estimates. For example, it has been postulated that the evolutionary rate of MRSA differs between patients with systemic infection and asymptomatic carriers. In support of this notion, rapidly evolving "hyper-mutating" MRSA-15 strains have been described during an outbreak in a neonatal intensive care unit.[110]

WGS has also provided important insights into the origin and regional spread of a healthcare associated epidemic MRSA-15 clone belonging to sequence type 22 (ST22), which was highly transmissible and produced sustained infection.[38] Phylogenetic analysis of 193 sequenced isolates showed that the currently circulating MRSA-15 clone is descended from an MRSA epidemic in English hospitals, which emerged from a community associated meticillin sensitive population

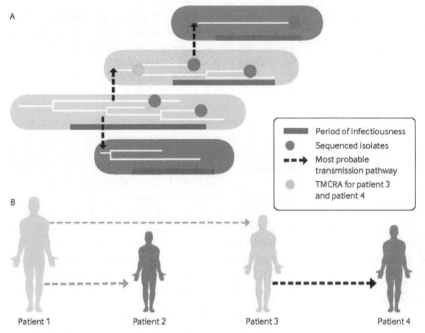

Fig 2 Putative relationships between patients and their pathogen genomes. (A) Each infection is caused by a population of genetic variants within an individual host. Transmission events between patients are indicated by dotted black arrows. A colonising population may evolve between the time of infection and the onset of symptoms (in the same patient), when a strain is usually isolated (blue dot). The time to the most common recent ancestor (TMCRA) of two isolates is shown as a green dot. (B) Most probable transmission pathways—size of the patient reflects the heterogeneity of the population (observed within host diversity based on sampled isolates) and the thickness of the arrow represents the likelihood of the link (inversely proportional to the number of single nucleotide polymorphisms in sequenced genomes)

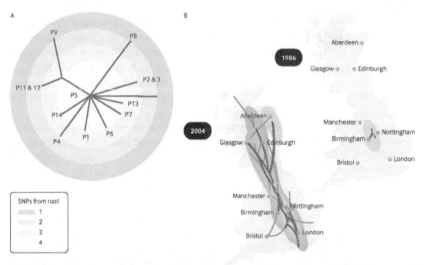

Fig 3 Visualisation of micro-evolution and regional spread of successful pathogens. (A) Phylogenetic tree based on whole genome sequencing of meticillin resistant *Staphylococcus aureus* (MRSA) isolates associated with the outbreak in an intensive care unit. Sequences of isolates obtained from 14 patients (P1-14) show low levels of genomic variation (as measured by single nucleotide polymorphisms; SNPs) of MRSA within the outbreak that lasted around 220 days (adapted, with permission, from Harris and colleagues).[56] (B) Reconstruction of the spread of sequence type 22 (ST22) in the UK. A continuous spatial diffusion model was used to reconstruct the finer scale geographical dispersal of ST22-A2 within the UK and to predict the origin of fluoroquinolone resistance. Lines indicate the inferred routes of spread with 80% Bayesian credible intervals for the latitude and longitude of spread shown as green ovals. The timing of transmission events isrepresented by red (oldest) or black (more recent) lines and light to dark green oval shading (adapted, with permission, from Holden and colleagues)[38]

of *S aureus*. Modelling of the spread of a fluoroquinolone resistant variant of MRSA ST22 suggested that it originated in the Midlands in the 1980s, and was initially restricted to this geographical region. It then spread rapidly to the north, reaching Scotland, and also to the south, arriving in London five years later.[38] The epidemic had spread across

the United Kingdom through multiple routes by 2000, and then globally (fig 3).

Importantly, the use of MRSA genome sequencing in infection control enables comprehensive and rapid identification of transmission pathways in hospital and community settings.[10 53] Its advantages include:

- Resolution is high enough to assess transmission events indicated by conventional methods of MRSA typing and to identify otherwise unsuspected transmission events[58 59]
- Hospital acquired outbreaks can be identified months earlier than when identification is based on epidemiological clustering of cases
- It can benchmark the accuracy of infection control investigations of MRSA outbreaks
- It can identify or confirm carriage of MRSA that allows the outbreak to persist.[59]

In one hospital based study, 26 MRSA isolates were successfully sequenced and analysed within five days of culture, leading to the identification of two outbreaks.[53] In both outbreaks most sequences were indistinguishable and the others had only three mutations, while epidemiologically unrelated strains were genetically distinct (>20 SNPs).[53] An evaluation of nosocomial transmission of *S aureus* in an endemic setting of a critical care unit using WGS identified 44 acquisition events, with only a minority explained by patient to patient transmission.[59] Finally, genome sequencing has helped to define the transmission of MRSA within hospitals for use in clinical trials (existing definitions relied on the recovery of MRSA from two or more patients within 10 days, two weeks, or a three week transmission period in the same ward).[47]

Analysis of the spread of pathogens at different scales

Real time outbreak analysis

Bench top sequencers allow a rapid proactive approach to pathogen surveillance that can identify recently accumulated genetic variation. Such studies look at pathogen "microevolution," which occurs over weeks or months of transmission,[112] as opposed to long term "macroevolution," which reflects the process of microbial speciation that occurs over thousands or millions of years. Because of its short time frame, the analysis of pathogen microevolution requires high resolution genomic data—for example, data that can discern differences in several nucleotides between two bacterial genomes of more than 3 Mb in length. This new capacity to provide (near) real time data on the origin and transmission dynamics of pathogens could provide a major public health benefit.[113]

The 2014-15 outbreak of Ebola virus in west Africa provides a recent and high profile example. WGS has shown that this outbreak derives from a single transmission from a natural zoonotic (bat) reservoir that probably occurred in early 2014 (fig 4A).[71] It is currently unclear whether the genotype of this particular Ebola virus facilitates more extensive human to human transmission or whether it represents an initially early seeding of the virus in urban populations in west Africa. However, the rapid production of genome sequence data will enable this question to be answered more quickly. These data may also provide important information on the major sources of transmission, which will in turn inform disease control strategies.

Similar real time analysis of the recently emerged Middle East respiratory syndrome coronavirus in Saudi Arabia identified the patterns of spread.[36] With respect to bacteria,

A

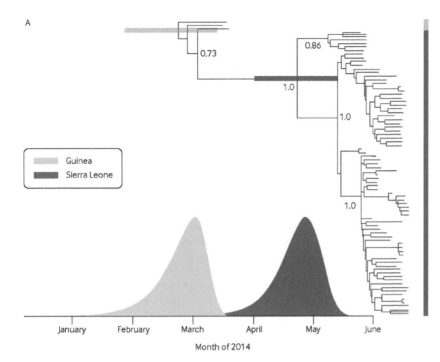

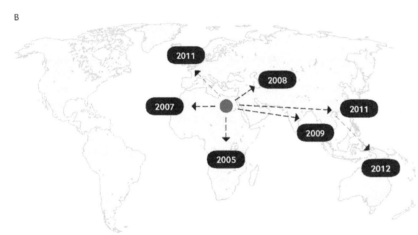

B

Fig 4 Global and regional spread of successful epidemic lineages. (A) Phylogenetic tree depicting the ongoing regional spread of Ebola virus in west Africa in 2014, and the molecular clock dating of the time to the most common recent ancestor of the 2014 outbreak (95% credible intervals of 27 January to 14 March 2014) and that of the Sierra Leone viral lineages (95% credible intervals of 2 April to 13 May 2014). Posterior probability distributions of the estimated times to the most common recent ancestor are overlaid below (adapted, with permission, from Gire and colleagues).[71] (B) Worldwide spread of *Salmonella enterica* serovar Kentucky ST198 CIP[R] clone. The clone originated in Egypt (adapted, with permission, from Le Hello and colleagues)[114]

increases).[80] This forms the basis of molecular contact tracing: for example, the recovery of identical sequences in different patients is compatible (although not confirmative) of direct transmission between them.

The reconstruction of transmission networks is plausible for Gram positive bacteria with the relative rarity of backward mutations and homoplasy (see Glossary).[70 92 96] By contrast, the extreme rapidity of RNA virus evolution potentially allows individual transmission events (who infected whom) to be determined with accuracy, particularly if the intra-host variation (a common output of next generation sequencing at high coverage) can be incorporated into an analysis to improve phylogenetic resolution (see Glossary).[117 118]

Some studies have defined thresholds for the number of SNPs shared by independent isolates needed to infer involvement in the same transmission cluster.[4 45 53 64] However, because the mutation rate of different lineages of the same species may differ,[75] and threshold values could be affected by the times of infection and sampling, these "rules" should be used with caution.

Several studies have inferred disease transmission from rich WGS datasets that identify microbial diversity not captured by traditional typing methods.[117 118 119] These studies highlight important differences in the interpretation and characteristics of phylogenetic and transmission trees. For example, the timing of nodes (see Glossary) in the transmission tree corresponds to the point of transmission, whereas the timing of nodes in phylogenetic trees of genomic data reflect branching events (see Glossary) that may have taken place before transmission. Hence, intra-host and inter-host evolution change the association between transmission and phylogenetic trees.[120] Although Bayesian methods have been developed that jointly estimate transmission and phylogenetic trees and capture within host pathogen dynamics,[117 118 119] in many cases there may be too much uncertainty to resolve person to person transmission networks, even with WGS data.

Summary

In summary, pathogen genomics provides a new line of evidence that complements existing epidemiological tools in the reconstruction of transmission networks, including the identification of previously unrecognised epidemiological links. Figure 5 shows how genomic data can be mapped to epidemiological curves to make inferences in this area. It combines two ways of organising information from outbreaks: the number of cases over time that satisfy the epidemiological case definition of the outbreak, and phylogenetic trees that show the evolutionary and putative transmission relationships between pathogen genomes obtained from outbreak cases. Through such genomic analyses it is possible to determine the origin of disease outbreaks and transmission dynamics in hospital and community settings; estimate the timing of patient to patient transmission events; and differentiate cases of recurrent or relapsing infection (failure of treatment) from reinfection (failure of public health).[44]

Clinical applications of developments in pathogen genomics

Active high resolution public health laboratory surveillance
The effectiveness of public health interventions for the control of communicable disease is limited by the low resolution of current surveillance methods and an

the study of the global spread of *Salmonella enterica* serotype Kentucky ST198 clone serves as another example of how the analysis of pathogen genomes provides data of international public health importance.[115] In particular, this clone originated in the Middle East (fig 4B) and has been associated with fluoroquinolone resistance.[114 115]

Analysis of person to person transmission networks
One of the most important benefits stemming from the use of WGS in an epidemiological context is the ability to resolve individual patient to patient transmission events. Recent pathogen transmission between patients in densely sampled outbreaks can be inferred when they cluster together on phylogenetic trees (see Glossary) (if a sufficiently large sample of background lineages has been obtained) or from the genomic distances between genomes of pathogens isolated from them.[116 117]

Genetic distance between strains increases with time (as the number of individual transmission events also

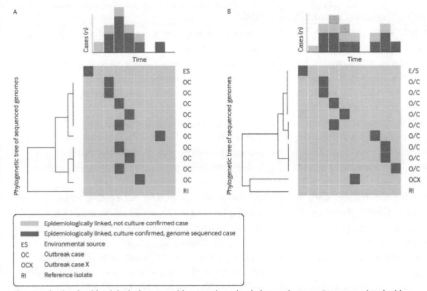

Fig 5 Synthesis of epidemiological curves with genomic scale phylogenetic trees. Cases associated with a specific outbreak are ordered in the matrix according to the phylogeny of genomes recovered from culture confirmed cases and displayed along the left. (A) The shape of the epidemic curve (histogram) suggests a point source outbreak in which all cases are exposed within one incubation period. (B) The epidemic curve shows an example of a propagated (ongoing) outbreak, in which secondary person to person spread occurs with successive peaks, distanced one incubation period apart. The phylogenetic tree suggests that case X may not be part of this outbreak because it is more closely related to the reference isolate than those from the outbreak cases

incomplete understanding of disease spread, which is largely based on retrospective outbreak investigation.

Importantly, WGS enhanced surveillance allows cases that are misclassified by other surveillance methods to be implicated or ruled out of an outbreak. For example, a comparison of WGS with conventional typing methods in the investigation of an outbreak of *Shigella sonnei* in the Orthodox Jewish community in the UK showed that the strains originally implicated in the outbreak formed three phylogenetically distinct clusters. One cluster represented cases associated with recent exposure to a single strain, whereas the other two represented distinct (although related) strains of *S sonnei* circulating in the UK. These observations informed infection control measures within local schools and allowed a stronger public health message to be passed to the local community.[82]

Genomics enhanced surveillance with radically improved resolution appeals to public health professionals dealing with increasingly complex outbreaks where trace back is complicated and labour intensive.[121] Genomics enhanced surveillance relies on the assumption that the epidemiological link between patients can be reliably inferred from the similarity between pathogen genomes. Although this is feasible, particularly when combined with phylogenetic methods that enable transmission pathways to be inferred in detail,[116 117 118 119] the identification of epidemiological links is a process of statistical inference, and hence comes with an associated sampling error.

Studies in this area depend heavily on the quality of genome sequencing, assembly, and the choice of reference genomes, but they have been instructive in the deciphering of different outbreaks.[6] In addition, frequent recombination can greatly complicate the inference of evolutionary history and estimates of times of origin, so that all such estimates should be treated with caution.[96 122] However, when the assumptions are upheld and sampling is representative, phylogenetic analyses help identify the temporal and geographical origin of epidemics and the dominant transmission routes responsible for the global

dissemination of pathogens.[7 13] This knowledge is important for risk assessment of future pandemic variants, public health interventions, and the design of effective vaccines.

Proactive disease control guided by the identification of transmission pathways

WGS guided surveillance promises the rapid and precise identification of bacterial transmission pathways in hospital[49 53 113] and community settings,[51 68 70 76] with concomitant reductions in infections, morbidity, and costs.[59 91] Because WGS offers unprecedented resolution for determining degrees of relatedness among bacterial and viral isolates, it complements existing epidemiological tools by allowing reconstruction of recent transmission chains and identification of sequential acquisitions and otherwise unrecognised epidemiological links.[45 76]

For example, investigations of hospital outbreaks of MRSA and *C difficile* by WGS have allowed discrimination between apparently similar isolates collected within a short time frame.[53 110] Recent studies have also shown that WGS can detect super spreaders (see Glossary), predict the existence of undiagnosed cases and intermediates in transmission chains,[4 46 48 58 60] suggest likely directionality of transmission, and identify unrecognised risk factors for onward transmission.[58 61] Such data can help stop or minimise outbreaks, inform the design and evaluation of intervention programs, and optimise the allocation of public health resources.[121]

A growing body of statistical methods is aimed at inferring transmission networks and contact structures from pathogen genomic data, with and without contextual epidemiological information.[116 117 118 119 120] These methodological developments provide new opportunities for proactive laboratory surveillance and a better understanding of the epidemiology of high burden infectious diseases.[3 12 65 122 123]

For example, examination of the genomic diversity of *Salmonella typhimurium* in co-located human and animal populations in the UK showed that a large proportion of transmissions occurred between humans, challenging the current belief that human to human transmission is uncommon in the developed world.[92 122] WGS enabled reconstruction of transmission networks also suggested that branched transmissions—where one case causes more than one secondary case—are more common than linear stepwise case to case transmissions.[92] It also identified more potential super spreaders than previously assumed.[77 78]

Genomics based estimation of likely transmission pathways can greatly improve the practice of tracking transmissions,[108] and it reduces dependency on epidemiological data, which are more difficult to collect and often incomplete. For example, phylogenetic analysis has been integrated into forensic-style analyses to identify transmission events and the sources of specific outbreaks. Phylogenetic analysis combined with molecular clock dating (see Glossary) of hepatitis C virus was used to reconstruct a large scale outbreak of hepatitis that stemmed from a single anaesthetist in Spain. Notably, dates of infection predicted from the molecular clock analysis correlated well with dates of infection estimated from patient medical records.[124]

Genomics enhanced clinical risk assessment

The genomes of viruses, bacteria, fungi, and parasites can be rapidly identified and characterised directly in clinical specimens or from laboratory cultures.[31 32] WGS of these pathogens can also inform management decisions in complex cases. For example, patients requiring prosthetic devices who are chronically colonised with Shiga-like toxin producing *Escherichia coli* (STEC) may be denied function saving surgery because of the potential risk for the development of STEC associated haemolytic uraemic syndrome caused by the perioperative use of broad spectrum antimicrobial prophylaxis.[125] In such circumstances, analysis of the core and especially dispensable genomes of isolates from individual patients can help ascertain the patient's risk of progression from long term colonisation to haemolytic uraemic syndrome. For example, patients with an uncommon serotype and sequence type of STEC identified by genetic diversity within the somatic antigen encoding operon, flagellin genes, and MLST genes are at lower risk. The presence or absence of marker genes at the *LEE* locus or in pathogenicity islands (see Glossary), which are associated with a high virulence of STEC in humans, can also be useful in such assessments.[125]

Research is accumulating on radically new bioengineering approaches to controlling microbial infections with virulence altering drugs that can disrupt genes and gene complexes.[126] Genes and mobile genetic elements can be readily shared among microbial clones, and the identification of genomic markers of drug resistance represents another important element of clinical risk assessment.[127]

Pathogen genome sequencing

The challenges of data analysis and integration

Although pathogen genomics offers much to medical science, it also presents serious challenges for data analysis, storage, and sharing, as well as the interpretation and management of data by clinicians and public health authorities. The full power of genomic sequence data will not be fully realised until the data are combined with clinical and epidemiological metadata, and the linking of these data types presents several important technical challenges.[128]

Particular attention has to be paid to the time of the sampling (a patient might have been infected with different strains over time) and the completeness of the sampling frame (undiagnosed cases might be responsible for transmission). In addition, several aspects of quality control are important for the harmonisation of sequencing data analysis. Firstly, the accuracy of identifying variants depends on the depth of sequence coverage. Increased coverage improves variant calling (see Glossary), whereas low coverage increases the risk of missing variants (false negatives) and assigning incorrect allelic states (false positives). Although relatively low sequencing coverage and the analyses of only the core genome might be acceptable for the identification of pathogens, higher coverage is expected for the WGS of bacterial pathogens of public health concern as part of ongoing laboratory surveillance or outbreak investigation.[121] [129] [130] Higher coverage is also needed for the reliable detection of genomic sequences from potentially mixed cultures, including those that contain drug susceptible and resistant versions of the same strain.

Secondly, an increasing number of commercial and "open source" programs with different performance characteristics are available for the mapping and assembly of short reads.[131] However, it is not certain that public health laboratories will converge towards a few "validated" pipelines. The (often complex) assembly, alignment, filtering, and SNP calling processes must be fully disclosed for a study to

---

GLOSSARY

- **Backward mutation:** Change in a mutated gene that restores the original sequence
- **Branching events:** Lineage splitting events that produce two or more separate genotypes
- **Core genome:** Genes that are conserved among all strains of a pathogen
- **Dispensable genome:** Partially shared or unique strain specific genes
- **Homoplasy:** Similarity between sequences that is not due to their shared ancestry, in contrast to homology, which is similarity derived from a common ancestor
- **Host range:** Collection of hosts that a pathogen can infect
- **Lateral gene transfer:** Exchange of genetic material between bacteria not associated with reproduction
- **Molecular clock dating:** Approximation of the dates of branching events using the "molecular clock" hypothesis that changes in the amino acid sequences, which can occur during evolution, take place at a regular rate
- **Nodes:** Connection points in a network
- **Pathogen lineage:** A subpopulation of microbial species with a defined virulence or ecological niche that differs from other subpopulations
- **Pathogen phylogeography:** Spatial distribution of different phylogenetic lineages of pathogens
- **Pathogenicity island:** Distinct genetic element on the chromosome of a pathogen that is responsible for its capacity to cause disease
- **Phylogenetic distance:** Genetic distance between genomes of related pathogens represented as the number of mutations or evolutionary events on a phylogenetic tree
- **Phylogenetic resolution:** Capacity to identify distinct lineages on a phylogenetic tree
- **Phylogenetic tree:** Branching diagram that shows the evolutionary inter-relations of a group of pathogens usually derived from a common ancestor
- **Reassortment:** Mixing of the genetic material into new combinations in different strains of the same pathogen
- **Recombination:** Process of transfer and incorporation of genetic material from a donor cell to a recipient cell to increase diversity and adaptation potential
- **Selective sweeps:** The reduction of genetic variation around the mutation site as the result of strong positive selection
- **Statistical machine learning:** A field of computer science/artificial intelligence that enables computers to discover new associations between data without being explicitly programmed
- **Super spreaders:** A highly infectious person who spreads the pathogen to many other susceptible people
- **Systems science:** An interdisciplinary field that studies the nature of systems—from simple to complex—in nature, society, and science itself
- **Variant calling:** Identification of sites of difference (such as nucleotide polymorphisms), usually using computational algorithms

---

be reproducible and investigation methods comparable between laboratories.

Thirdly, the choice of reference genomes for sequence alignment can greatly affect interpretation.[129] Indeed, phylogenetic and other analyses may need to be repeated in light of initial results to select references that provide the highest resolution for an outbreak cluster. Fortunately, several international initiatives support proficiency testing in microbial genome sequencing for public health.[122] [132]

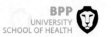

Sharing genome sequence data to "crowd source" epidemic analysis

The speed at which genomic data are being generated and increased access to public databases have aided global responses to newly emerging diseases. Equally importantly, this has shifted the bottleneck in bioscience capacity from the generation of data to its analysis. Major advances in the development and provision of online resources for storing and sharing genome sequencing data (http://epidemic.bio. ed.ac.uk/), including rapid publication avenues such as *PLoS Currents Outbreaks* (http://currents.plos.org/outbreaks/), will be of great importance in epidemic situations. Despite this, sequencing data alone may not be sufficient to identify transmission events and pathways accurately, and genomic data should routinely be analysed in conjunction with other types of epidemiological and clinical evidence.[7][11][128][133] Such data synthesis will require stronger collaboration between epidemiologists, microbiologists, and specialist bioinformaticians.

System science's (see Glossary) view of hosts and pathogens and their interactions has been replacing the reductionism that dominated biomedicine for several centuries. Instead, there is a growing awareness that diseases are often caused by multiple pathogens, rather than the paradigm that a single disease is caused by a single microbial species or strain that has dominated microbiology since the time of Robert Koch.

It is also possible that statistical machine learning (see Glossary) and network approaches to studying technological, social, and biological systems and their quantifiable organising principles may offer new opportunities to examine processes of disease transmission.[129][130][134][135] Similarly, recent advances in phylogenetic methodology allow increasingly complex characteristics to be inferred from the analysis of pathogen genomes, enable explicit links to be made between pathogen genotype and phenotype, and have greatly improved pathogen phylogeography (see Glossary).[128][136][137][138]

Conclusion

The availability of bench top WGS analysers has facilitated combined genomic and epidemiological approaches to investigating outbreaks and infection control. Ongoing genomic surveillance can identify determinants of transmission, monitor pathogen evolution and adaptation, ensure accurate diagnosis of infections with epidemic potential, and refine strategies for their control. Crucially, the evolutionary analysis of pathogen genome sequence data allows epidemiological hypotheses to be tested, potentially in real time, and this will greatly enhance the management and control of communicable diseases.

Pathogen genomics has revolutionised our understanding of the mechanisms of disease transmission. We have moved from the view that all forms of disease spread are alike in that they are chiefly mechanical extensions of human contact or of contact between a sick animal and a human body. Instead, we now understand that transmission is an evolutionary event that can have a major impact on the extent and structure of genetic diversity as it flows through the population. Overall, the insights provided by pathogen genomics have fundamentally changed our collective understanding of long term global and short term local spread of communicable diseases and have opened up potential new strategies of disease control and prevention.

Both authors were supported by the Australian National Health and Medical Research Council.

Contributors: Both authors had full access to the content of this review, wrote the manuscript, and are guarantors.

Competing interests: We have read and understood BMJ policy on declaration of interests and declare the following interests: none.

Provenance and peer review: Commissioned; externally peer reviewed.

1 Köser CU, Ellington MJ, Cartwright EJP, et al. Routine use of microbial whole genome sequencing in diagnostic and public health microbiology. PLoS Pathog2012;8:e1002824.
2 Didelot X, Bowden R, Wilson DJ, et al. Transforming clinical microbiology with bacterial genome sequencing. Nat Rev Genet2012;13:601-12.
3 Relman DA. Microbial genomics and infectious diseases. N Engl J Med2011;365:347-57.
4 Walker TM, Ip CL, Harrell RH, et al. Whole-genome sequencing to delineate Mycobacterium tuberculosis outbreaks: a retrospective observational study. Lancet Infect Dis2013;13:137-46.
5 Barzon L, Lavezzo E, Costanzi G, et al. Next-generation sequencing technologies in diagnostic virology. J Clin Virol2013;58:346-50.
6 Lipkin WI. The changing face of pathogen discovery and surveillance. Nat Rev Microbiol 2013;11:133-41.
7 Kao RR, Haydon DT, Lycett SJ, et al. Supersize me: how whole-genome sequencing and big data are transforming epidemiology. Trends Microbiol2014;22:282-91.
8 Buchan BW, Ledeboer NA. Emerging technologies for the clinical microbiology laboratory. Clin Microbiol Rev2014;27:783-22.
9 Pybus OG, Rambaut A. Evolutionary analysis of the dynamics of viral infectious disease. Nat Rev Genet2009;10:540-50.
10 Holmes EC. The evolutionary genetics of emerging viruses. Annu Rev Ecol Evol Syst 2009;40:353-72.
11 Wilson MR, Naccache SN, Samayoa E, et al. Actionable diagnosis of neuroleptospirosis by next-generation sequencing. N Engl J Med2014;370:2408-17.
12 Ypma RJF, Donker T, van Ballegooijen WM, et al. Finding evidence for local transmission of contagious disease in molecular epidemiological datasets. PLoS One2013;8:e69875.
13 Holt KE, Thieu Nga TV, Thanh DP, et al. Tracking the establishment of local endemic populations of an emergent enteric pathogen. Proc Natl Acad Sci U S A2013;110:17522-7.
14 Chen C, Zhang W, Zheng H, et al. Minimum core genome sequence typing of bacterial pathogens: a unified approach for clinical and public health microbiology. J Clin Microbiol2013;51:2582-91.
15 Palmer GH, Brayton KA. Antigenic variation and transmission fitness as drivers of bacterial strain structure. Cell Microbiol2013;15:1969-75.
16 Iwamoto T, Grandjean L, Arikawa K, et al. Genetic diversity and transmission characteristics of Beijing family strains of Mycobacterium tuberculosis in Peru. PLoS One 2012;7:e49651.
17 Holmes EC. RNA virus genomics: a world possibilities. J Clin Invest 2009;119:2488-95.
18 Leitmeyer KC, Vaughn DW, Watts DM, et al. Dengue virus structural differences that correlate with pathogenesis. J Virol 1999;73:4738-47.
19 Weaver SC, Salas R, Rico-Hesse R, et al. Re-emergence of epidemic Venezuelan equine encephalomyelitis in South America. VEE Study Group. Lancet1999;348:436-40.
20 Anishchenko M, Bowen RA, Paessler S, et al. Venezuelan encephalitis emergence mediated by a phylogenetically predicted viral mutation. Proc Natl Acad Sci USA2006;103:4994-9.
21 Tsetsarkin KA, Vanlandingham DL, McGee CE, et al. A single mutation in chikungunya virus affects vector specificity and epidemic potential. PLoS Pathog2007;3:e201.
22 Herfst S, Schrauwen EJ, Linster M, et al. Airborne transmission of influenza A/H5N1 virus between ferrets. Science 2012;336:1534-41.
23 Imai M, Watanabe T, Hatta M, et al. Experimental adaptation of an influenza H5 HA confers respiratory droplet transmission to a reassortant H5 HA/H1N1 virus in ferrets. Nature 2012;486:420-8.
24 Barry JD, Hall JP, Plenderleith L. Genome hyperevolution and the success of a parasite. Ann N Y Acad Sci2012;1267:11-7.
25 Monecke S, Enright R, Slickers P, et al. Intra-strain variability of methicillin-resistant Staphylococcus aureus strains ST228-MRSA-I and ST5-MRSA-II. Eur J Clin Microbiol Infect Dis2009;28:1381-90.
26 Morens DM, Taubenberger JK, Fauci AS. The persistent legacy of the 1918 influenza virus. N Engl J Med2009;361:225-9.
27 Smith GJ, Vijaykrishna D, Bahl J, Lycett SJ, et al. Origin and evolutionary genomics of the 2009 swine-origin H1N1 influenza A epidemic. Nature 2009;459:1122-5.
28 Verhagen LM, de Jonge MI, Burghout P, et al. Genome-wide identification of genes essential for the survival of Streptococcus pneumoniae in human saliva. PLoS One2014;9:e89541.
29 Bos KI, Schuenemann VJ, Golding GB, et al. A draft genome of Yersinia pestis from victims of the Black Death. Nature 2011;478:506-10.
30 Wagner DM, Klunk J, Harbeck M, et al. Yersinia pestis and the Plague of Justinian 541-543 AD: a genomic analysis. Lancet Infect Dis2014;14:319-26.
31 Doughty EL, Sergeant MJ, Adetifa I, et al. Culture-independent detection and characterisation of Mycobacterium tuberculosis and M africanum in sputum samples using shotgun metagenomics on a benchtop sequencer. Peer J2014;2:e585.

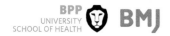

32   Hasman H, Saputra D, Sicheritz-Ponten T, et al. Rapid whole-genome sequencing for detection and characterization of microorganisms directly from clinical samples. J Clin Microbiol 2014;52:139-46

33   Chen Y, Liang W, Yang S, et al. Human infections with the emerging avian influenza A H7N9 virus from wet market poultry: clinical analysis and characterization of viral genome. Lancet2013;381:1916-25.

34   Munier S, Moisy D, Marc D, et al. Interspecies transmission, adaptation to humans and pathogenicity of animal influenza viruses. Pathol Biol (Paris)2010;58:e59-68.

35   Liu Q, Zhou B, Ma W, et al. Analysis of recombinant H7N9 wild-type and mutant viruses in pigs shows that the Q226L mutation in HA is important for transmission. J Clin Microbiol2014;88:8153-65.

36   Azhar EI, El-Kafrawy SA, Farraj SA, Hassan AM, et al. Evidence for camel-to-human transmission of MERS coronavirus. N Engl J Med2014;370(26):2499-505.

37   Lowder BV, Guinane CM, Ben Zakour NL, et al. Recent human-to-poultry host jump, adaptation, and pandemic spread of Staphylococcus aureus. Proc Natl Acad Sci U S A2009;106:19545-50.

38   Holden MTG, Hsu L-Y, Kurt K, et al. A genomic portrait of the emergence, evolution, and global spread of a methicillin-resistant Staphylococcus aureus pandemic. Genome Res2013;23:653-64.

39   Okoro CK, Kingsley RA, Quail MA, et al. High-resolution single nucleotide polymorphism analysis distinguishes recrudescence and reinfection in recurrent invasive nontyphoidal Salmonella typhimurium disease. Clin Infect Dis2012;54:955-63.

40   Chewapreecha C, Harris SR, Croucher NJ, et al. Dense genomic sampling identifies highways of pneumococcal recombinations. Nat Genet2014;46:305-9.

41   Howden BP, Holt KE, Lam MMC, et al. Genomic insights to control the emergence of vancomycin-resistant enterococci. mBio2013;4:e00412-13.

42   Somboonna N, Wan R, Ojcius DM, et al. Hypervirulent Chlamydia trachomatis clinical strains is a recombinant between Lymphogranuloma venereum (L2) and D lineages. mBio2011;2:e00045-11.

43   Harris SR, Clarke IN, Seth-Smith HMB, et al. Whole genome analysis of diverse Chlamydia trachomatis strains identifies phylogenetic relationships masked by current clinical typing. Nat Genet2012;44:413-9.

44   Bryant JM, Harris SR, Parkhill J, et al. Whole-genome sequencing to establish relapse or re-infection with Mycobacterium tuberculosis: a retrospective observational study. Lancet Respir Med2013;1:786-92.

45   Walker TM, Lalor MK, Broda A, et al. Assessment of Mycobacterium tuberculosis transmission in Oxfordshire, UK, 2007-12, with whole pathogen genome sequences: an observational study. Lancet Respir Med2014;2:285-92.

46   Creamer E, Shore AC, Rossney AS, et al. Transmission of endemic ST22-MRSA-IV on four acute hospital wards investigated using a combination of spa, dru and pulsed-field gel electrophoresis typing. Eur J Clin Microbiol Infect Dis2012;31:3151-61.

47   Turner CE, Dryden M, Holden MTG, et al. Molecular analysis of an outbreak of lethal postpartum sepsis caused by Streptococcus pyogenes. J Clin Microbiol2013;51:2089-95.

48   Wright MS, Haft DH, Harkins DM, et al. New insights into dissemination and variation of the health care-associated pathogen Acinetobacter baumannii from genomic analysis. mBio2014;5:e00963-13.

49   Lewis T, Loman NJ, Bingle L, et al. High-throughput whole-genome sequencing to dissect the epidemiology of Acinetobacter baumannii isolates from a hospital outbreak. J Hosp Infect2010;75:37-41.

50   McAdam PR, Templeton KE, Edwards GF, et al. Molecular tracing of the emergence, adaptation, and transmission of hospital-associated methicillin-resistant Staphylococcus aureus. Proc Natl Acad Sci U SA2012;109:9107-12.

51   Underwood AP, Dallman T, Thomson NR, et al. Public health value of next-generation DNA sequencing of enterohaemorrhagic Escherichia colifrom an outbreak. J Clin Microbiol2013;51:232-7.

52   Sherry NL, Porter JL, Seemann T, et al. Outbreak investigation using high-throughput genome sequencing within a diagnostic microbiology laboratory. J Clin Microbiol2013;51:1396-401.

53   Eyre DW, Golubchik T, Gordon NC, et al. A pilot study of rapid benchtop sequencing of Staphylococcus aureus and Clostridium difficile for outbreak detection and surveillance. BMJ Open2012;2:e001124.

54   Eyre DW, Cule M, Griffiths D, et al. Detection of mixed infection from bacterial whole genome sequence data allows assessment of its role in Clostridium difficile transmission. PLoS Comput Biol2013;9:e1003059.

55   Eyre DW, Griffiths D, Vaughan A, et al. Asymptomatic Clostridium difficile colonisation and onward transmission. PLoS One2013;8:e78445.

56   Harris SR, Cartwright EJP, Török ME, et al. Whole-genome sequencing for analysis of an outbreak of methicillin-resistant Staphylococcus aureus: a descriptive study. Lancet Infect Dis2013;13:130-6.

57   Nübel U, Nachtnebel M, Falkenhorst G, et al. MRSA transmission on a neonatal intensive care unit: epidemiological and genome-based phylogenetic analyses. PLoS One2013;8:e54898.

58   Price J, Gordon NC, Crook D, et al. The usefulness of whole genome sequencing in the management of Staphylococcus aureus infections. Clin Microbiol Infect2013;19:784-9.

59   Price JR, Golubchik T, Cole K, et al. Whole-genome sequencing shows that patient-to-patient transmission rarely accounts for acquisition of Staphylococcus aureus in an intensive care unit. Clin Infect Dis2014;58:609-18.

60   Didelot X, Eyre DW, Cule M, et al. Microevolutionary analysis of Clostridium difficile genomes to investigate transmission. Genome Biol2012;13:R118.

61   Snitkin ES, Zelazny AM, Thomas PJ, et al. Tracking a hospital outbreak of carbapenem-resistant Klebsiella pneumoniae with whole-genome sequencing. Sci Transl Med2012;4:148ra116.

62   Prosperi M, Veras N, Azarian T, et al. Molecular epidemiology of community-associated methicillin-resistant Staphylococcus aureus in the genomic era. Sci Rep2013;3:1902.

63   Xia XY, Ge M, Hsi JH, et al. High-accuracy identification of incident HIV-1 infections using a sequence clustering based diversity measure. PLoS One2014;9:e100081.

64   Bull RA, Eden JS, Luciani F, et al. Contribution of intra- and interhost dynamics to norovirus evolution. J Virol 2012;86:3219-29.

65   Ypma RJ, Jonges M, Bataille A, et al. Genetic data provide evidence to wind-mediated transmission of highly pathogenic avian influenza. J Infect Dis2013;207:730-5.

66   Jolley KA, Hill DMC, Bratcher HB, et al. Resolution of a meningococcal disease outbreak from whole-genome sequence data with rapid web-based analysis methods. J Clin Microbiol2012;50:3046-53.

67   Leekitcharoenphon P, Nielsen EM, Kaas RS, et al. Evaluation of whole genome sequencing for outbreak detection of Salmonella enterica. PLoS One2014;9:e87991.

68   Mellmann A, Harmsen D, Cummings CA, et al. Prospective genomic characterization of the German enterohemorrhagic Escherichia coli O124:H4 outbreak by rapid sequencing. PLoS One2011;6:e22751.

69   Schürch AC, Kremer K, Kiers A, et al. The tempo and mode of molecular evolution of Mycobacterium tuberculosis at patient-to-patient scale. Infect Genet Evol2010;10:108-14.

70   Gardy JL, Johnston JC, Sui SJH, et al. Whole-genome sequencing and social-network analysis of a tuberculosis outbreak. N Engl J Med2011;364:730-9.

71   Gire SK, Goba A, Andersen KG, et al. Genomic surveillance elucidates Ebola virus origin and transmission during the 2014 outbreak. Science2014;345:1369-72.

72   Wright CF, Knowles NJ, Di Nardo A, et al. Reconstructing the origin and transmission dynamics of the 1967-68 foot-and-mouth disease epidemic in the United Kingdom. Infect Genet Evol2013;20:230-8.

73   Rashed SM, Azman AS, Alam M, et al. Genetic variation of Vibrio cholerae during outbreaks, Bangladesh, 2010-2011. Emerg Infect Dis2014;20:54-60.

74   Chin C-S, Sorenson J, Harris JB, et al. The origin of the Haitian cholera outbreak strain. N Engl J Med2011;364:33-42.

75   Bryant JM, Schürch AC, Van Deutekom H, et al. Inferring patient to patient transmission of Mycobacterium tuberculosis from whole genome sequencing data. BMC Infect Dis2013;13:110.

76   Roetzer A, Diel R, Kohl TA, et al. Whole genome sequencing versus traditional genotyping for investigation of a Mycobacterium tuberculosis outbreak: a longitudinal molecular epidemiological study. PLoS Med 2013;10:e1001387.

77   Pérez-Lago L, Comas I, Navarro Y, et al. Whole genome sequencing analysis of inpatient microevolution in Mycobacterium tuberculosis: potential impact on the inference of tuberculosis transmission. J Infect Dis2014;209:98-108.

78   Pérez-Lago L, Navarro Y, Herranz M, et al. Genetic features shared by Mycobacterium tuberculosis strains involved in microevolution events. Infect Genet Evol2013;16:326-9.

79   Fittipaldi N, Beres SB, Olsen RJ, et al. Full-genome dissection of an epidemic of severe invasive disease caused by a hypervirulent, recently emerged clone of Group A streptococcus. Am J Pat hol2012;180:1522-34.

80   Beres SB, Carroll RK, Shea PR, et al. Molecular complexity of successive bacterial epidemics deconvoluted by comparative pathogenomics. Proc Natl Acad Sci U S A2010;107:4371-6.

81   Holt KE, Baker S, Weill FX, et al. Shigella sonnei genome sequencing and phylogenetic analysis indicate recent global dissemination from Europe. Nat Genet2012;44:1056-9.

82   McDonnell J, Dallman T, Atkin S, et al. Retrospective analysis of whole genome sequencing compared to prospective typing data in further informing the epidemiological investigation of an outbreak of Shigella sonnei in the UK. Epidemiol Infect2013;141:2568-75.

83   Zhang N, Lan R, Sun Q, et al. Genomic portrait of the evolution and epidemic spread of a recently emerged multidrug-resistant Shigella flexneri clone in China. J Clin Microbiol2014;52:1119-26.

84   Reuter S, Harrison TG, Kőser CU, et al. A pilot study of rapid whole-genome sequencing for the investigation of a legionella outbreak. BMJ Open2013;3:e002175.

85   Cotten M, Watson SJ, Kellam P, et al. Transmission and evolution of the Middle East respiratory syndrome coronavirus in Saudi Arabia: a descriptive genomic study. Lancet 2013;382:1993-2002.

86   Eyre DW, Cule ML, Wilson DJ, et al. Diverse sources of C difficile infection identified on whole-genome sequencing. N Engl J Med2013;369(13):1195-205.

87   Cruz-Rivera M, Carplo-Pedroza JC, Escobar-Gutiérrez A, et al. Rapid hepatitis C virus divergence among chronically infected individuals. J Clin Microbiol2013;51:629-32.

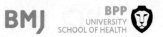

88 Li H, Stoddard MB, Wang S, et al. Elucidation of hepatitis C virus transmission and early diversification by single genome sequencing. PLoS Pathog2012;8:e1002880.

89 Reeves PR, Liu B, Zhou Z, et al. Rates of mutation and host transmission for an Escherichia coli clone over 3 years. PLoS One2011;6:e26907.

90 Didelot X, Nell S, Yang I, et al. Genomic evolution and transmission of Helicobacter pylori in two South African families. Proc Natl Acad Sci U S A2013;110:13880-5.

91 Harris SR, Feil EJ, Holden MT, et al. Evolution of MRSA during hospital transmission and intercontinental spread. Science2010;327:469-74.

92 Mather AE, et al. Distinguishable epidemics of multidrug-resistant Salmonella typhimurium DT104 in different hosts. Science2013;341:1514-7.

93 Dorigatti I, Cauchemez S, Ferguson NM. Increased transmissibility explains the third wave of infection by the 2009 H1N1 pandemic virus in England. Proc Natl Acad Sci U S A2013;110:13422-7.

94 Engelthaler DM, Hicks ND, Gillece JD, et al. Cryptococcus gattii in North American Pacific northwest: whole-population genome analysis provides insights into species evolution and dispersal. mBio2014;5:e01464-14.

95 Cody AJ, McCarthy ND, Jansen van Rensburg M, et al. Real-time genomic epidemiological evaluation of human campylobacter isolates by use of whole-genome multilocus sequence typing. J Clin Microbiol2013;51:2526-34.

96 Croucher NJ, Finkelstein JA, Pelton SI, et al. Population genomics of post-vaccine changes in pneumococcal epidemiology. Nat Genet2013;45:656-63.

97 Jolley KA, Hill DMC, Bratcher HB, et al. Resolution of a meningococcal disease outbreak from whole-genome sequence data with rapid web-based analysis methods. J Clin Microbiol2012;50:3046-53.

98 Coffey LL, Page BL, Greninger AL, et al. Enhanced arbovirus surveillance the deep sequencing: identification of novel rhabdoviruses and bunyaviruses in Australian mosquitoes. Virology2014;448:146-58.

99 Dash PK, Sharma S, Soni M, et al. Complete genome sequencing and evolutionary phylogeography analysis of Indian isolates of dengue virus type 1. Virus Res2015;195:124-34.

100 Parrish CR, Holmes EC, Morens DM, et al. Cross-species viral transmission and the emergence of new epidemic diseases. Microbiol Mol Biol Rev 2008;72:457-70.

101 Futse JE, Brayton KA, Dark MJ, et al. Superinfection as a driver of genomic diversification in antigenically variant pathogens. Proc Natl Acad Sci U S A 2008;105:2123-7.

102 Ågren J, Finn M, Bengtsson B, et al. Microevolution during an anthrax outbreak leading to clonal heterogeneity and penicillin resistance. PLoS One2014;9:e89112.

103 Bull RA, Luciani F, McElroy K, et al. Sequential bottlenecks drive viral evolution in early acute hepatitis C virus infection. PLoS Pathog2011;7:e1002243.

104 Keele BF, Giorgi EE, Salazar-Gonzalez JF, et al.Identification and characterization of transmitted and early founder virus envelopes in primary HIV-1 infection. Proc Natl Acad Sci U S A 2008;105:7552-7.

105 Ghedin E, Fitch A, Boyne A, et al. Mixed infection and the genesis of influenza diversity. J Virol2009;83:8832-41.

106 Wright CF, Morelli MG, Thébaud G, et al. Beyond the consensus: dissecting within-host viral population diversity of foot-and-mouth disease virus by using next-generation genome sequencing. J Virol2011;85:2266-75.

107 Young BC, Golubchik T, Batty EM, et al. Evolutionary dynamics of Staphylococcus aureus during progression from carriage to disease. Proc Natl Acad Sci U S A2012;109:4550-5.

108 Vaughan G, Xia G, Forbli JC, et al. Genetic relatedness among hepatitis A virus strains associated with food-borne outbreaks. PLoS One2013;8:e74546.

109 Octavia S, Wang Q, Tanaka MM, et al. Delineating community outbreaks of Salmonella enterica serovar Typhimurium using whole genome sequencing: insights into genome variability within an outbreak. J Clin Microbiol2015; published online 21 Jan.

110 Nübel U, Strommenger B, Layer F, et al. From types to trees: reconstructing the spatial spread of Staphylococcus aureus based on DNA variation. Int J Med Microbiol2011;301:614-8.

111 Lindsay JA. Evolution of Staphylococcus aureus and MRSA during outbreaks. Infect Genet Evol2014;21:548-53.

112 Ahmed N, Dobrindt U, Kacker J, et al. Genomic fluidity and pathogenic bacteria: applications in diagnostics, epidemiology and intervention. Nat Rev Microbiol2008;6:387-94.

113 Köser CU, Holden MTG, Ellington MJ, et al. Rapid whole-genome sequencing for investigation of a neonatal MRSA outbreak. N England J Med2012;366:2267-75.

114 Le Hello S, Hendriksen RS, Doublet B, et al. International spread of an epidemic population of Salmonella enterica serotype Kentucky ST198 resistant to ciprofloxacin. J Infect Dis2011;204:675-84.

115 Le Hello S, Bekhit A, Granier SA, et al. The global establishment of a highly-fluoroquinolone resistant Salmonella enterica serotype Kentucky ST198 strain. Front Microbiol2013;4:395.

116 Dagan T. Phylogenomic networks. Trends Microbiol2011;19:483-91.

117 Bertels F, Silander OK, Pachkov M, et al. Automated reconstruction of whole-genome phylogenies from short-sequence reads. Mol Biol Evol2014;31:1077-88.

118 Didelot X, Gardy J, Colijn C. Bayesian inference of infectious disease transmission from whole-genome sequence data. Mol Biol Evol2014;31:1869-79.

119 Ypma RJF, van Ballegooijen WM, Wallinga J. Relating phylogenetic trees to transmission trees of infectious disease outbreaks. Genetics2013;195:1055-62.

120 Colijn C, Gardy J. Phylogenetic tree shapes resolve disease transmission patterns. Evol Med Public Health2014;2014:96-108.

121 Robinson ER, Walker TM, Pallen MJ. Genomic and outbreak investigation: from sequence to consequence. Genome Med2013;5:36.

122 Parkhill J, Wren BW. Bacterial epidemiology and biology - lessons from genome sequencing. Genome Biol2011;12:230.

123 Kohl TA, Diel R, Harmsen D, et al. Whole genome based Mycobacterium tuberculosis surveillance: a standardized, portable and expandable approach. J Clin Microbiol2014;52:2479-86.

124 González-Candelas F, Bracho MA, et al. Molecular evolution in court: analysis of a large hepatitis C virus outbreak from an evolving source. BMC Biol2013;11:76.

125 Knobloch JKM, Niemann S, Kohl TA, et al. Whole-genome sequencing for risk assessment of long-term Shiga toxin-producing Escherichia coli. Emerg Infect Dis2014;20:732-3.

126 Conlan S, Thomas PJ, Deming C, et al. Single-molecule sequencing to track plasmid diversity of hospital-associated carbapenemase-producing Enterobacteriaceae. Science Transl Med2014;6:254ra126.

127 Doudna JA, Charpentier E. The new frontier of genome engineering with CRISPR-Cas9. Science2014;346:1077-86.

128 Jombart T, Cori A, Didelot X, et al. Bayesian reconstruction of disease outbreaks by combining epidemiologic and genomic data. PLoS Comput Biol2014;10:e1003457.

129 Ladner JT, Beitzel B, Chain PS, et al. Standards for sequencing viral genomes in the era of high-throughput sequencing. mBio2014;5:e01360-14.

130 Aziz N, Zhao Q, Bry L, et al. College of American Pathologists' laboratory standards for next-generation sequencing clinical tests. Arch Pathol Lab Med2014; published online 25 Aug.

131 Jünemann S, Prior K, Albersmeier A, et al. GABenchToB: a genome assembly benchmark tuned to bacteria and benchtop sequencers. PLoS One2014;9:e107014.

132 Aarestrup FM, Brown EW, Detter C, et al. Integrating genome-based informatics to modernize global disease monitoring, information sharing, and response. Emerg Infect Dis2012;18:e1.

133 Grenfell BT, Pybus OG, Gog JR, et al. Unifying the epidemiological and evolutionary dynamics of pathogens. Science2004;303:327-32.

134 Barabasi A-L, Gulbance N, Loscalzo J. Network medicine: a network-based approach to human disease. Nat Rev Genet2011;12:56-68.

135 Little SJ, Kosakovsky-Pond SL, Anderson CM, et al. Using HIV networks to inform real time prevention interventions. PLoS One2014;9:e98443.

136 Sintchenko V, Roper MPV. Pathogen genome bioinformatics. In: Trent RJA, ed. Clinical bioinformatics, methods in molecular biology. Vol 1168, 2nd ed. Humana Press, Springer Science 2014:173-93.

137 Dutilh BE, Backus L, Edwards RA, et al. Explaining microbial phenotypes on a genomic scale: GWAS for microbes. Brief Funct Genom2013;12:366-80.

138 Vinatzer BA, Monteil CL, Clarke CR. Harnessing population genomics to understand how bacterial pathogens emerge, adapt to crop hosts, and disseminate. Annu Rev Phytopathol2014;52:19-43.

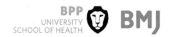

Manifestation, diagnosis, and management of foodborne trematodiasis

Thomas Fürst, research fellow[1][2], Somphou Sayasone, research fellow[3], Peter Odermatt, associate professor and research group leader[1][2], Jennifer Keiser, professor and head of the helminth drug development unit[2][4], Jürg Utzinger, professor and head of the ecosystem health sciences unit[1][2]

[1]Department of Epidemiology and Public Health, Swiss Tropical and Public Health Institute, PO Box, CH-4002 Basel, Switzerland

[2]University of Basel, Basel, Switzerland

[3]National Institute of Public Health, Ministry of Health, Vientiane, Lao People's Democratic Republic

[4]Department of Medical Parasitology and Infection Biology, Swiss Tropical and Public Health Institute, Basel, Switzerland

Correspondence to: J Utzinger juerg.utzinger@unibas.ch

Cite this as: BMJ 2012;344:e4093

DOI: 10.1136/bmj.e4093

http://www.bmj.com/content/344/bmj.e4093

Foodborne trematodiasis is a cluster of zoonotic infections caused by parasitic worms (class: trematoda; also known as flukes), which are transmitted via the ingestion of contaminated, mainly aquatic, food. More than one billion people are at risk of infection according to a systematic review from 2005.[1] Another systematic review and meta-analysis suggests that 56 million people were infected in 2005, mainly in Asia and Latin America, with a global burden of 665 000 disability adjusted life years.[2]

Depending on the fluke species, foodborne trematodiasis is associated with a variety of signs, symptoms, and pathological consequences. The non-specificity of the clinical manifestations, the wide range of fluke species, and shortcomings in current diagnostic techniques are some of the reasons why foodborne trematodiasis is underestimated.[3][4]

This review introduces the most important foodborne trematode species and describes their geographical distribution. It also discusses pathological consequences, clinical manifestations, diagnosis, treatment, and control of foodborne trematodiasis. Our review is based on the limited evidence obtained from the peer reviewed literature, textbooks, reports, and international guidelines.

What causes foodborne trematodiasis?

A recent systematic review listed more than 80 different trematode species that have been identified from human infections.[2] According to the target organ in the definitive host, they are grouped as liver, lung, or intestinal flukes. However, on the basis of recent biomedical reviews and still incomplete national prevalence data, only a dozen species are of public health importance (box 1).[2][5][6][7][8]

The life cycles of the foodborne trematodes are species specific, with distinct snail species being first intermediate hosts, and fish, mollusc, crustacean, amphibian, and insect species being second intermediate hosts (fig 1). Notable exceptions are *Fasciola* spp and *F buski*, which do not need a second intermediate host, as their infectious stages (so called metacercariae) adhere directly to aquatic plants.[3] A detailed list of known first and second intermediate hosts can be found in the annex of a comprehensive technical report published by the World Health Organization.[9]

Humans usually acquire an infection through the ingestion of second intermediate hosts or, in the case of *Fasciola* spp and *F buski*, aquatic plants that contain viable metacercariae. With the exception of *Fasciola* spp and *F buski*, metacercariae are not released from their intermediate hosts into water, so the risk of infection from drinking untreated water is small.[9][10] It is unclear which aspects of food processing (such as heating, freezing, smoking, acidification, salting, drying, washing, disinfection, irradiation, and pressure treatment) inhibit the infectivity of metacercariae, but properly cooked or deeply frozen food is considered safe.[9][11] In the duodenum of an infected human, hermaphroditic juvenile flukes develop from the metacercariae, migrate to their target organ, mature, mate, and start producing eggs. Parasite eggs are then released via the human host's faeces (all foodborne trematodes, including coughed up and swallowed eggs of *Paragonimus* spp) or sputum (only coughed up eggs of *Paragonimus* spp) and have to reach appropriate water bodies with suitable intermediate hosts to complete their life cycles.[3][12]

Where does foodborne trematodiasis occur?

Foodborne trematodiasis is commonly classified as a tropical disease, even though the endemic area is not limited to the tropics.[9][11] *C sinensis* is endemic in East and South East Asia; *O viverrini* in South East Asia; and *O felineus* in central, northern, and western Eurasia. *Fasciola* spp exist worldwide, but most endemic areas are in the Andean region, North Africa, and the Caspian Sea region. *Paragonimus* spp occur in parts of the Andean region, West and Central Africa, East and South East Asia, and North America. Intestinal flukes are found worldwide, with most endemic areas in East and South East Asia. A comprehensive literature review identified allochthonous cases (diagnosed in countries where disease transmission does not naturally occur) all over the world, probably as a result of increasing international travel, human migration, and the food trade.[13] A series of recent reviews suggests that human foodborne trematodiasis is increasing, mainly because of the exponential growth of inland fish production (aquaculture).[1][2][9][11][W1][W2]

SUMMARY POINTS

- Foodborne trematodiasis is a cluster of zoonotic infections caused by parasitic trematodes ingested in undercooked, mainly aquatic, food

- Prevalence is increasing because of the growth of inland fish production; most cases are in Asia and Latin America, but infections in migrants and returning travellers are reported elsewhere, including Europe and North America

- Foodborne trematodes are grouped as liver, lung, and intestinal flukes and—depending on the species, the duration and intensity of infection, and host susceptibility—inflammatory lesions and damage to tissues and organs occur with various clinical manifestations

- The most serious clinical consequences are cancer of the bile duct (in clonorchiasis and opisthorchiasis) and ectopic infections (mainly in paragonimiasis, but also in fascioliasis and intestinal fluke infections)

- Direct parasitological diagnosis via the detection of eggs in faeces (all flukes) and sputum (lung flukes only) is the most common approach

- Praziquantel and triclabendazole are safe and efficacious treatments but other drugs are being investigated

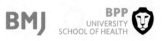

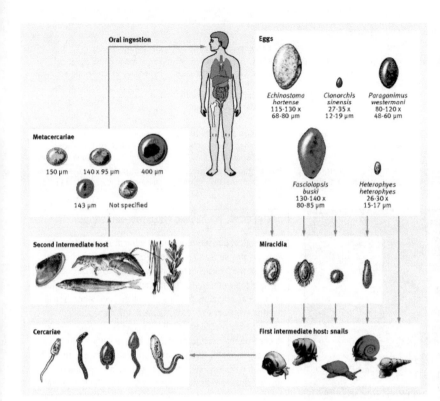

Fig 1 Representative life cycles of five foodborne trematodes—a liver fluke (*Clonorchis sinensis*), a lung fluke (*Paragonimus westermani*), and three intestinal flukes (*Echinostoma hortense, Fasciolopsis buski, and Heterophyes heterophyes*). Adapted from Keiser and Utzinger,[3] with permission from the American Society for Microbiology

At a regional level, foodborne trematodiasis usually shows a focal distribution, which is governed by social-ecological contexts (such as specific eating habits and environmental conditions that favour maintaining the parasites' life cycles).[3][11] At the individual level, a meta-analysis of the proportion of infected humans shedding high numbers of eggs indicates that distribution is highly aggregated: a few people harbour most of the parasites.[2] Hospital based and community based cross sectional surveys in endemic areas show that infection with multiple species of foodborne trematodes is common because they are all acquired through consumption of raw food.[14][W3][W4]

What are the pathological consequences and clinical manifestations?

Morbidity depends on the species involved and also the host's susceptibility, duration of infection, and the number of worms harboured (infection intensity). These parameters govern the occurrence and severity of inflammatory lesions and damage to tissues and target organs. The severity of infection is usually determined by the number of parasite eggs per gram of faeces or per 5 mL of sputum in paragonimiasis.[3][4][5][6][7][8][9][11][15][16][17][W5-W19] Because the egg laying capacity of foodborne trematodes varies greatly—from fewer than 100 eggs per day per worm (*Haplorchis taichui*)[18] to 13 000-26 000 (*F buski*)[19]—species specific thresholds are used to differentiate between light, moderate, and heavy infections. However, these thresholds have never been standardised. Furthermore, some studies challenge a direct association between egg counts and worm burden because crowding effects may lower egg production, obstructions in the hosts' organs may affect the excretion of eggs, and the distribution of eggs in faeces can be uneven.[15][16][20][W20-W24]

BOX 2 LIVER FLUKE INDUCED CHOLANGIOCARCINOMA

Pathological consequences and clinical manifestations
Cholangiocarcinoma is a malignant tumour of the bile duct epithelium. Although the exact mechanism of liver fluke induced carcinogenesis is unclear, chronic biliary infection increases the susceptibility of the bile ducts to the action of carcinogens. Patients usually present with non-specific symptoms, which are similar to those of liver fluke infections. Liver fluke induced cholangiocarcinoma cannot be differentiated from other forms of cholangiocarcinoma. Timely diagnosis is rare and prognosis is poor, even when patients receive appropriate treatment.

Diagnosis
The diagnosis, localisation, and staging of cholangiocarcinoma are challenging and require a combination of imaging, biochemical investigations, and cytological techniques (ultrasonography, cholangiography, choledochoscopy, computed tomography, positron emission tomography, magnetic resonance imaging, biopsy and cytological analysis, and laboratory analysis of serum tumour markers).

Management
Consultation with an infectious disease specialist, hepatologist, and oncologist is recommended. Response to chemotherapy is poor. Complete resection with negative histological margins or transplantation are the only curative interventions. Currently, no effective adjuvant treatment exists, but radiotherapy may be indicated postoperatively. Often, only palliative treatment remains.

Clonorchiasis and opisthorchiasis
The pathological consequences and clinical manifestations of infection with *C sinensis* and *Opisthorchis* spp are similar. After ingestion by the host, the metacercariae excyst in gastric juice and migrate via the duodenum, the ampulla of Vater, and the extrahepatic biliary system to the intrahepatic bile ducts.[11] Pathological changes are mainly confined to the bile duct, liver, and gallbladder.[7] Tissue damage is caused directly by the parasite via mechanical and chemical irritation and indirectly via the immune response, and it can lead to cancer of the bile duct (cholangiocarcinoma; box 2).[11][21] Hepatomegaly, gallbladder enlargement, gallstones, sludge, and periductal fibrosis along the intrahepatic biliary

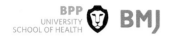

Table 1 Clinical features of main foodborne trematodiases

Parasitosis	Tropism	Start	Symptoms and signs	Complications
Clonorchiasis and opisthorchiasis	Hepatobiliary tract	Insidious for several years: non-specific abdominal pain	Biliary colic, jaundice, cholestasis, cholelithiasis, recurrent pyogenic cholangitis, cholecystitis, hepatic abscess, rarely hepatitis	Pancreatitis, cirrhosis, portal hypertension, cholangiocarcinoma
Fascioliasis		Abrupt start: 1-4 weeks after infection high fever, weakness, weight loss, urticaria, right hypochondrial pain		Pancreatitis, cirrhosis, portal hypertension, rarely ectopic infection
Paragonimiasis	Pulmonary tract	Insidious: anorexia, moderate weight loss, rarely fever	Chronic cough, chest pain, dyspnoea, haemoptysis, rusty sputum	Bronchiectasis, pulmonary consolidation, cyst formation, pleural effusion, ectopic infection
Intestinal fluke infections	Intestinal tract	Insidious: unspecific gastrointestinal problems	Ulceration of intestinal mucosa, malabsorption	Malnutrition, anaemia, oedema or anasarca, rarely ectopic infection

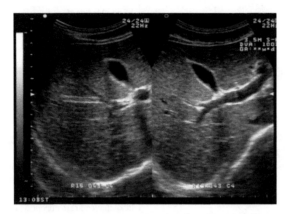

Fig 2 Ultrasonographic image showing highly echogenic pipestem fibrosis around the periportal veins, with echoes seen in two or three segments of the liver, in a man with opisthorchiasis

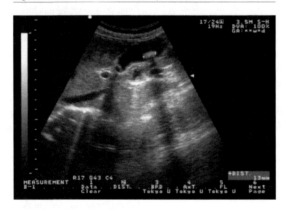

Fig 3 Ultrasonographic image showing echogenic posterior acoustic shadowing or biliary duct stone formation without bile duct dilation in a woman with opisthorchiasis

tree and periportal vein are often seen with ultrasonography (figs 2 and 3).[4]

Acute and light infections are mostly asymptomatic,[3 9 11 21] but an acute onset with hepatitis-like symptoms, including high fever and chills, has been reported, particularly for infection with *O felineus*.[3 7 11 w25] Some moderately infected people may have mild symptoms,[3 21 w8] but even chronic infections may remain asymptomatic, and often only heavily infected people have symptoms, signs, and complications (table 1).[3 7 9 11 21]

Fascioliasis

Unlike other liver flukes, after ingestion and excystment in the duodenum *Fasciola* spp migrate through the intestinal wall into the body cavity and then through the liver into the bile ducts.[11 15] Major pathological changes are associated with migration and the related destruction, focal bleeding,

BOX 3 ECTOPIC FOODBORNE TREMATODE INFECTIONS

Pathological consequences and clinical manifestations
Paragonimus spp, and less often *Fasciola* spp and intestinal flukes of the families heterophyidae and microphallidae, can cause ectopic infections. The reasons for incomplete migration are unclear. Migratory tracks and cavities filled with trapped dead parasites or eggs often cause tissue damage with inflammatory reactions and fibrosis. Clinical manifestations depend on the exact location, and such infections can even cause death. *Paragonimus* spp have been reported in the central nervous system, eyes, skin, heart, abdominal organs, and reproductive organs; *Fasciola* spp in the central nervous system, orbit, subcutaneous tissue, abdominal wall, heart, genitals, spleen, muscles, gastrointestinal tract, blood vessels, lungs, and pleural cavity; and heterophyidae and microphallidae in the central nervous system and heart.

Diagnosis
Suspect ectopic foodborne trematodiasis in a patient with a diagnosis of foodborne trematode infection and unexplained, often severe, manifestations (such as neurological disorders, abscesses) that could result from damage in ectopic locations mentioned above. To confirm the diagnosis, a combination of ultrasonography, radiography, endoscopy, computed tomography, positron emission tomography, magnetic resonance imaging, and biopsy is needed.

Management
Consultation with infectious disease specialists and other relevant specialists is recommended. Treatment with praziquantel or triclabendazole may help in the early phases of infection but should be used with care. Parasite death may lead to antigen release and increased risk of inflammation. Anti-inflammatory drugs (such as corticosteroids) may help to reduce oedema and inflammation during treatment. Parasites, eggs, and lesions may need to be surgically removed. Adjuvant therapy should be used as appropriate.

and inflammation in the host's body (acute phase). Some migrating flukes may die on their way, leaving cavities filled with necrotic debris, or deviate from their usual route to cause ectopic infections (box 3). In the bile ducts (latent phase), the parasites may cause inflammation, resulting in thickening and expansion of the ducts and fibrosis. Imaging may depict these lesions as "tunnels and caves" in peripheral parts of the liver.[4]

Early acute manifestations are typical (table 1).[8 11 15] Although some infected people are asymptomatic in the latent phase, others may experience repeated relapses of the acute manifestations.[8 11 15] When the irritation in the biliary system is severe enough, a permanent obstructive phase, which has additional symptoms, signs, and complications (table 1), may develop.[3 4 8 9 11 15] Rarely, fascioliasis can be fatal.[15 w26]

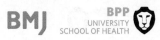

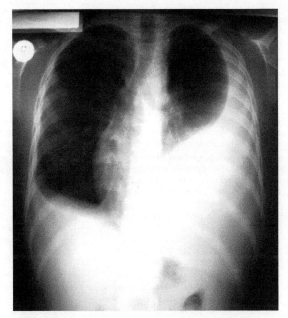

Fig 4 Chest radiograph of a 14 year old boy with paragonimiasis and a bilateral pleural effusion. He had chronic cough, chest pain (>12 months), and haemoptysis. Aspiration showed a thick chylous-like fluid containing 16% eosinophils and 20 typical trematode operculated eggs per mL. *Paragonimus* eggs were found in sputum and stool samples. He admitted that he often ate raw river crabs.[w52] Courtesy of the Institut de la Francophonie pour la Médecine Tropicale (IFMT), Lao People's Democratic Republic

Paragonimiasis

In the classic natural course of pleuropulmonary paragonimiasis, swallowed metacercariae of *Paragonimus* spp excyst in the duodenum, penetrate the intestinal wall, and migrate over several days to the pleural cavity and into the lungs where they mature. After several weeks, adults become encapsulated in fibrotic tissue, where they mate or reproduce parthenogenetically. Eggs pass via the bronchioles into the sputum or, if swallowed, the faeces, and then into the environment. Some of the eggs may be trapped in tissue and, together with aberrantly migrating flukes, provoke further irritation and ectopic infections (box 3).[6 9 11 22] A recent cross sectional study from India found cavity and cyst formations, nodular lesions, fibrotic infiltrates, calcifications, bronchiectasis, pulmonary consolidations, pleural thickening and effusion, mediastinal lymphadenopathy, and patchy ground glass opacity as pleuropulmonary radiological features in paragonimiasis (fig 4).[23]

Unless the patient is heavily infected, early stages of pleuropulmonary infection tend to be asymptomatic. Heavy pleuropulmonary infections may present with many different bronchitis-like, asthma-like, and tuberculosis-like symptoms and signs (table 1). The similarity of the clinical manifestations often result in pleuropulmonary paragonimiasis being misdiagnosed as bronchitis, asthma, or (non-responsive) tuberculosis,[3 6 9 11 22] even though patients with paragonimiasis usually present in comparatively better general health.

Intestinal fluke infection

More than 70 species of intestinal flukes are implicated in human infection.[2 5] The morphology of these flukes is diverse, and their life cycles and geographical distributions not well studied. After ingestion of viable metacercariae, flukes excyst and adhere to the intestinal wall, where mechanical irritation and inflammation may lead to the

manifestations described in table 1.[3 5 9 11] Similar to other foodborne trematode infections, mild intestinal fluke infections are mainly asymptomatic, but heavy infections can be severe.[3 5 9 11 w27]

What are the other complications of foodborne trematodiasis?

Recent reviews have summarised the association between infection with *C sinensis* and *O viverrini* and cholangiocarcinoma, as well as the mechanisms of carcinogenesis, diagnosis, and management (box 2).[21 24 25 w8 w27-w33] On the basis of the epidemiological, experimental, and pathological evidence, these two trematodes have been classified as definite carcinogens (group 1) by the International Agency for Research on Cancer (IARC).[26 27] There is still insufficient evidence of the oncogenic potential of *O felineus* and *Fasciola* spp for them to be classified.[26 27 w28 w34]

Ectopic infections are severe and potentially fatal complications of foodborne trematodiasis (box 3). As highlighted in other reviews, *Paragonimus* spp,[6 9 11 22 w5 w11 w35-w39] and more rarely *Fasciola* spp and intestinal flukes of the heterophyidae and microphallidae families,[9 11 15 w26 w27] do not always enter their usual target organs in the host's body, but continue to migrate to ectopic locations.

How can foodborne trematodiasis be diagnosed?

Accurate diagnosis of foodborne trematodiasis remains a challenge. The three main diagnostic approaches are direct parasitological diagnosis, immunodiagnosis, and molecular diagnosis. Direct parasitological diagnosis is facilitated by the detection of eggs in faeces (all flukes), sputum (only lung flukes), and, more rarely, other biofluids such as bile or duodenal content. Egg detection in faecal samples is the most common approach, and methods include Kato-Katz thick smear, formalin-ethyl-acetate technique, Stoll's dilution egg count method, and sedimentation techniques. However, differential diagnosis is difficult because parasite eggs from different species resemble each other.[3 4 5 6 7 8 11] Furthermore, the small number of eggs discharged by some fluke species, crowding effects, obstructions in the patients' organs, heterogeneous distribution of eggs in the patients' faeces (or sputum in *Paragonimus* spp), and light infections are additional challenges for an accurate diagnosis and require multiple sampling and testing. Occasionally, it is possible to demonstrate adult parasites—for example, when the flukes are excreted in the faeces, coughed up (lung flukes), or removed during surgery.[5 7 8 9 11] The website of the US Centers for Disease Control and Prevention features photographs of parasite eggs, which might help in the diagnosis of foodborne trematode infections.

Immunodiagnostic methods such as intradermal tests, indirect haemagglutination assays, indirect fluorescent antibody tests, and indirect enzyme linked immunosorbent assays (ELISAs) aim to detect specific antibodies.[3 6 7 8 11] Immunodiagnosis is especially useful during the prepatent phase and ectopic infections, or if direct parasitological diagnosis is ambiguous. However, false positive results after the infection has resolved, cross reactivity, high costs, and lack of availability at the point of care in remote rural areas are important problems that need to be tackled.[3 6 7]

Molecular diagnosis—the detection of trematode DNA in samples using the polymerase chain reaction—has a high sensitivity and specificity.[3 6 7 8 11] However, for the

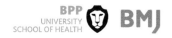

Table 2 Oral drugs and dosages for human foodborne trematodiasis.[11 28 29 W40-W42] The first choice treatment is the first one listed, but alternative drugs or dosages are also given

Parasite	Drug	Dosage	Adverse events (AE)	Limitations to use and main contraindication(s)
Clonorchis sinensis	Praziquantel*‡	25 mg/kg 3 times a day for 2 days (40 mg/kg single dose in preventive chemotherapy)	Common AE include mild and transient insomnia, nausea, headache, dizziness, vomiting, and abdominal pain; less common AE include rash, hypotension, and sudden expulsion of worms aggravating obstruction	Restrained use in pregnant or breastfeeding women and children ‹4 years. Main contraindications are hypersensitivity and cysticercosis
	Albendazole†§	10 mg/kg single dose for 7 days	Occasional AE include abdominal pain, reversible alopecia, and increased serum transaminases; rare AE include leucopenia, rash, and renal toxicity	Restrained use in pregnant women and children ‹1 year. Main contraindications are hypersensitivity and cirrhosis
Opisthorchis spp	Praziquantel*‡	25 mg/kg 3 times a day for 2 days (40 mg/kg single dose in preventive chemotherapy)	Common AE include mild and transient insomnia, nausea, headache, dizziness, vomiting, and abdominal pain; less common AE include rash, hypotension, and sudden expulsion of worms aggravating obstruction	Restrained use in pregnant or breastfeeding women and children ‹4 years. Main contraindications are hypersensitivity and cysticercosis
Fasciola spp	Triclabendazole*¶	10 mg/kg single dose (which may be repeated after 12-24 h in heavy infections)	Common AE include mild and transient abdominal and epigastric pain, sweating, and eosinophilia; less common AE include nausea, vomiting, headache, dizziness, cough, fever, urticaria, pruritus, and skin rash	Restrained use in pregnant or breastfeeding women, people with ectopic infections, and children ‹6 years. Main contraindication is hypersensitivity
	Bithionol**	30-50 mg/kg 10-15 doses on alternate days	Common AE include photosensitivity reactions, vomiting, diarrhoea, abdominal pain, and urticaria; rare AE include leucopenia and toxic hepatitis	Use with caution in people with ectopic infections and children ‹8 years
Paragonimus spp	Praziquantel*‡	25 mg/kg 3 times a day for 2 days	Common AE include mild and transient insomnia, nausea, headache, dizziness, vomiting, and abdominal pain; less common AE include rash and hypotension	Restrained use in pregnant or breastfeeding women, people with ectopic infections, and children ‹4 years. Main contraindications are hypersensitivity and cysticercosis
	Bithionol**	30-50 mg/kg 10-15 doses on alternate days	Common AE include photosensitivity reactions, vomiting, diarrhoea, abdominal pain, and urticaria; rare AE include leucopenia and toxic hepatitis	Use with caution in people with ectopic infections and children ‹8 years
	Triclabendazole*¶	10 mg/kg single dose (which may be repeated after 12-24 h in heavy infections)	Common AE include mild and transient abdominal and epigastric pain, sweating, and eosinophilia; less common AE include nausea, vomiting, headache, dizziness, cough, fever, urticaria, pruritus, and skin rash	Restrained use in pregnant or breastfeeding women, people with ectopic infections, and children ‹6 years. Main contraindication is hypersensitivity
Intestinal flukes	Praziquantel*‡	10-20 mg/kg single dose or 25 mg/kg 3 times a day	Common AE include mild and transient insomnia, nausea, headache, dizziness, vomiting, abdominal pain, and diarrhoea; less common AE include rash, hypotension, and sudden expulsion of worms aggravating obstruction	Restrained use in pregnant or breast feeding women, people with ectopic infections, and children ‹4 years. Main contraindications are hypersensitivity and cysticercosis

*Take with liquids during a meal.
†Take with liquids during a meal; a fatty meal increases bioavailability.
‡Manufacturers: Bayer (Biltricide), Shin Poong (Distocide).
§Manufacturer: GlaxoSmithKline (Albenza).
¶Manufacturer: Novartis (Egaten).
**Manufacturer: Tanabe Japan (Bitin).

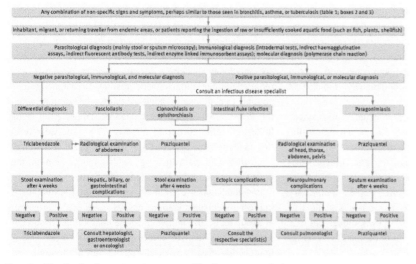

Fig 5 Algorithm for the diagnosis and treatment of foodborne trematodiasis

foreseeable future, molecular diagnosis is unlikely to be used at the point of care in endemic areas.[3 6]

Radiological methods such as ultrasound, computer tomography, and magnetic resonance imaging are complementary tools for an accurate diagnosis. Although these techniques might be available in well equipped laboratories in the developed world and undoubtedly help characterise pathological changes caused by foodborne trematodiasis, they are currently out of reach in resource constrained areas.[3 6 7 8 9 11]

How can foodborne trematodiasis be treated?

Praziquantel and triclabendazole are the two drugs of choice; however, triclabendazole is currently registered for human use in only four countries. Various treatment regimens are suggested for the treatment of foodborne trematodiasis.[3 5 6 7 8 11 28 W40] For clonorchiasis and opisthorchiasis, the recommended treatment schedule is praziquantel 25 mg/kg three times a day for two consecutive days.[3 7 11 28] The same treatment regimen has been successfully used in paragonimiasis.[3 6 11 28] The first choice treatment against intestinal fluke infections is also praziquantel, and a single dose of 10-20 mg/kg is efficacious against all intestinal fluke species,[29] but higher dosages of three times 25 mg/kg in one day have also been proposed.[3 5 8 11 28] The drug of choice against fascioliasis is a single (10 mg/kg) or double dose (two times 10 mg/kg) of triclabendazole.[3 8 11 28] Triclabendazole (single dose of 10 mg/kg, or two doses of 10 mg/kg each within 12-24 hours) is also efficacious against paragonimiasis.[3] In general, all treatments are safe with no serious adverse events. Table 2 summarises the dosages

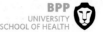

BMJ · BPP UNIVERSITY SCHOOL OF HEALTH

SOURCES AND SELECTION CRITERIA

Information for this clinical review was obtained from a database that we established for a project to estimate the global burden of foodborne trematodiasis.[2] The database originated from a systematic review of 11 electronic datasources: PubMed, WHOLIS, FAOBIB, Embase, CAB Abstracts, LILACS, ISI Web of Science, BIOSIS Preview, Science Direct, African Journals Online, and SIGLE. It included all available literature from 1 January 1980 to 31 December 2008 and had no language restrictions. Details on the initial search strategy and database have been presented elsewhere.[2] For this review, the database was updated to include all available information until 30 September 2011. The data were complemented by personal reference archives and the authors' experience.

A PATIENT'S PERSPECTIVE: OPISTHORCHIASIS IN LAO PEOPLE'S DEMOCRATIC REPUBLIC

I am a 46 year old teacher and often go fishing in the Mekong River with friends. We eat the caught fish uncooked.

For more than a year I felt unwell—tired and without energy. I had many gastritis-like symptoms, such as abdominal pain, bowel rumbling, nausea, and bloating. I also had itchy rashes on my arms, stomach, and legs. I lost about 5 kg in weight but always felt hungry. After meals, particularly dinner, I often had stomach cramps and sometimes vomiting.

After repeated visits to different health services, I went to the hospital and had an abdominal ultrasound scan, in addition to blood and stool tests. The ultrasound results were normal and my blood was negative for hepatitis. However, liver fluke eggs were detected in my stool. I learnt that this parasite is acquired by consumption of raw fish and that after treatment I could be reinfected if I continue to eat undercooked fish. I received medicine called praziquantel. The rash on my arms, legs, and abdomen disappeared two weeks after treatment and I generally felt better. One month later my stool was free of parasite eggs. However, the abdominal discomfort disappeared only slowly. Three months after treatment, I occasionally have bowel rumbling, nausea, and abdominal bloating. My doctor assures me that the cure takes time and that it is most important not to eat raw fish.

ADDITIONAL EDUCATIONAL RESOURCES FOR PATIENTS AND HEALTHCARE PROFESSIONALS

US Centers for Disease Control and Prevention (www.cdc.gov/parasites/clonorchis; www.dpd.cdc.gov/dpdx/html/clonorchiasis.htm; www.cdc.gov/parasites/opisthorchis; www.dpd.cdc.gov/dpdx/html/opisthorchiasis.htm; www.cdc.gov/parasites/fasciola; www.dpd.cdc.gov/dpdx/html/fascioliasis.htm; www.cdc.gov/parasites/paragonimus; www.dpd.cdc.gov/dpdx/html/paragonimiasis.htm; www.cdc.gov/parasites/fasciolopsis; www.dpd.cdc.gov/dpdx/html/fasciolopsiasis.htm; www.dpd.cdc.gov/dpdx/html/echinostomiasis.htm; www.dpd.cdc.gov/dpdx/html/heterophyiasis.htm; www.dpd.cdc.gov/dpdx/html/metagonimiasis.htm)—One of the few fully functional, up to date, open access sources of information. It contains a wealth of data on the most important foodborne trematode infections and is suitable for healthcare professionals and patients

AREAS FOR FUTURE RESEARCH

- More precise data on the extent of the human and veterinary disease burden of foodborne trematode infections (geographical distribution, prevalence, infection intensity, coinfection, subtle morbidity, and societal impact) are needed to increase awareness (in patients and clinicians) and raise political commitment to foster control and elimination efforts
- Additional studies should verify the taxonomy of foodborne trematodes and associated intermediate, reservoir, and definitive hosts
- New diagnostic methods with a high sensitivity and specificity that are inexpensive and can be used at point of contact are needed
- New trematocidal drugs and alternative treatment regimens (for example, multiple dosing, combination treatment) that are safe and efficacious need to be developed
- Molecular research on the antigenic structure and immunology of foodborne trematodes and research into the immune mechanisms of infected humans and animals may be useful for vaccine development
- A better knowledge of liver fluke induced carcinogenesis may improve the diagnosis, treatment, and prevention of cholangiocarcinoma and provide fundamental insights into carcinogenesis in general
- Mechanisms of ectopic foodborne trematode infections should be further explored to improve diagnosis, treatment, and prevention of severe complications
- Improved knowledge on physical and chemical parameters to inhibit infectivity of metacercariae could help to advance safe food processing methods and guidelines
- The cost effectiveness of integrated control programmes for foodborne trematodes—which include different stakeholders, a variety of interventions (such as chemotherapy, improved sanitation, food inspections, information, education and communication campaigns, and control of non-human parasite life cycles), and that take advantage of synergy between different sectors (public health, livestock production, food industry, water and sanitation, socioeconomic development, education)—should be determined

of praziquantel, triclabendazole, and alternative drugs, including reported adverse events and contraindications. Figure 5 shows a diagnostic and treatment algorithm.

Towards control and elimination: challenges and opportunities

New diagnostic techniques that have a high sensitivity and specificity and are simple and inexpensive are key to understanding the extent of the problem.[2] Improved point of care diagnostics could conceivably improve the management of cases and avoid severe sequelae.

The development of new drugs is a low priority for drug companies.[28] The treatment of foodborne trematodiasis currently relies on two drugs, and two small drug intervention studies reported unexpectedly low cure rates against clonorchiasis and fascioliasis.[30][31] A recent review recommended pursuing promising drug candidates (such as tribendimidine, the artemisinins, and synthetic trioxolanes) and combination treatments.[32] The development of vaccines for animals against infections with Fasciola spp is at an advanced stage. Vaccination of animals and humans may become an important means of interrupting transmission.[33][W43]

Drugs are currently the main method of controlling the morbidity associated with foodborne trematodiasis, but integrated programmes are vital for sustainable disease control and eventual elimination.[11][15][19][W22][W27][W44][W45] Several follow-up studies highlighted the complexity of the epidemiological settings and showed high reinfection rates after drug based interventions.[W21][W46-W51] Hence, integrated control strategies should also include improved sanitation, food inspections, information, education, and communication campaigns (also for travellers) and, as far as feasible, control of intermediate, reservoir, and non-human definitive hosts. These additional interventions aim to change human behaviour and interrupt disease transmission.[3][6][7][8][9][11][21][W2][W30] However, considering deeply rooted eating habits in humans and the myriad non-human hosts these aims pose formidable challenges. Only a few endemic countries have embarked on national control programmes against foodborne trematodiasis. Integration with control programmes targeting other infectious diseases as well as collaborations beyond the health sector (such as with the agricultural, environmental, and educational sectors) may offer largely untapped opportunities for prevention and control.[9][34][W2]

We thank P Steinmann, H Zhou, M Tsai, P Ayé Soukhathammavong, K Phongluxa, G Casagrande, H Immler, R Hirsbrunner, M Hellstern, R Gutknecht, and H Walter (all Swiss Tropical and Public Health Institute, Basel, Switzerland) for their invaluable help in obtaining and translating foreign language literature. Sincere thanks to P Ayé Soukhathammavong for providing figs 2 and 3 and M Strobel for providing fig 4. We are also grateful to S Becker and S Odermatt-Biays for carefully checking the signs, symptoms, and pathological implications of foodborne trematodiasis.

Contributors: TF, JK, and JU conceived and wrote the first draft. SS and PO provided the patient perspective, organised figs 2-4, and revised the manuscript. All authors had access to all data. TF and JU are guarantors.

Funding: TF is associated to the National Centre of Competence in Research (NCCR) North-South and received financial support through a Pro*Doc Research Module from the Swiss National Science Foundation (SNSF; project number PDFMP3-123185). JK acknowledges a personal career development grant from SNSF (projects no PP00A3-114941 and PP00P3_135170). The donors had no influence on study design, data collection, analysis, interpretation, writing, or submission.

Competing interests: All authors have completed the ICMJE uniform disclosure form at www.icmje.org/coi_disclosure.pdf (available on request from the corresponding author) and declare: all authors completely disclosed their funding for the submitted work in the funding statement above; no financial relationships with any

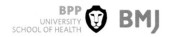

organisations that might have an interest in the submitted work in the previous three years; no other relationships or activities that could appear to have influenced the submitted work.

Provenance and peer review: Not commissioned, externally peer reviewed.

Patient consent obtained.

1 Keiser J, Utzinger J. Emerging foodborne trematodiasis. *Emerg Infect Dis* 2005;11:1507-14.
2 Fürst T, Keiser J, Utzinger J. Global burden of human food-borne trematodiasis: a systematic review and meta-analysis. *Lancet Infect Dis* 2012;12:210-21.
3 Keiser J, Utzinger J. Food-borne trematodiases. *Clin Microbiol Rev* 2009;22:466-83.
4 Sripa B, Kaewkes S, Intapan PM, Maleewong W, Brindley PJ. Food-borne trematodiases in Southeast Asia: epidemiology, pathology, clinical manifestation and control. *Adv Parasitol* 2010;72:305-50.
5 Chai JY. Intestinal flukes. In: Murrell KD, Fried B, eds. *World class parasites*. Vol 11. Springer, 2007:53-115.
6 Blair D, Agatsuma T, Wang W. Paragonimiasis. In: Murrell KD, Fried B, eds. *World class parasites*. Vol 11. Springer, 2007:117-50.
7 Sithithaworn P, Yongvanit P, Tesana S, Pairojkul C. Liver flukes. In: Murrell KD, Fried B, eds. *World class parasites*. Vol 11. Springer, 2007:3-52.
8 Mas-Coma S, Bargues MD, Valero MA. Plant-borne trematode zoonoses: fascioliasis and fasciolopsiasis. In: Murrell KD, Fried B, eds. *World class parasites*. Vol 11. Springer, 2007:293-334.
9 WHO. Control of foodborne trematode infections. Report of a WHO study group. *WHO Tech Rep Ser* 1995;849:1-157.
10 Graczyk TK, Fried B. Human water-borne trematode and protozoan infections. *Adv Parasitol* 2007;64:111-60.
11 Sithithaworn P, Sripa B, Kaewkes S, Haswell-Elkins MR. Food-borne trematodes. In: Cook GC, Zumla AI, eds. *Manson's tropical diseases*. WB Saunders, 2009:1461-76.
12 Chen MG, Chang ZS, Shao XY, Liu MD, Blair D, Chen SH,et al. Paragonimiasis in Yongjia county, Zhejiang province, China: clinical, parasitological and karyotypic studies on Paragonimus westermani. *Southeast Asian J Trop Med Public Health* 2001;32:760-9.
13 Fürst T, Duthaler U, Sripa B, Utzinger J, Keiser J. Trematode infections: liver and lung flukes. *Infect Dis Clin North Am* 2012;26:399-419.
14 Sayasone S, Vonghajack Y, Vanmany M, Rasphone O, Tesana S, Utzinger J,et al. Diversity of human intestinal helminthiasis in Lao PDR. *Trans R Soc Trop Med Hyg* 2009;103:247-54.
15 Mas-Coma S, Bargues MD, Esteban JG. Human fasciolosis. In: Dalton JP, ed. *Fasciolosis* . CAB International, 1999:411-34.
16 Elkins DB, Sithithaworn P, Haswell-Elkins MR, Kaewkes S, Awacharagan P, Wongratanacheewin S. Opisthorchis viverrini: relationships between egg counts, worms recovered and antibody-levels within an endemic community in northeast Thailand. *Parasitology* 1991;102:283-8.
17 Yu SH, Mott KE. Epidemiology and morbidity of food-borne intestinal trematode infections. WHO (WHO/SCHISTO/94.108). 1994:1-26.
18 Sato M, Sanguankiat S, Pubampen S, Kusolsuk T, Maipanich W, Waikagul J. Egg laying capacity of Haplorchis taichui (Digenea: Heterophyidae) in humans. *Korean J Parasitol* 2009;47:315-8.
19 Mas-Coma S, Bargues MD, Valero MA. Fascioliasis and other plant-borne trematode zoonoses. *Int J Parasitol* 2005;35:1255-78.
20 Valero MA, De Renzi M, Panova M, Garcia-Bodelon MA, Periago MV, Ordonez D,et al. Crowding effect on adult growth, pre-patent period and egg shedding of Fasciola hepatica. *Parasitology* 2006;133:453-63.
21 Rim HJ. Clonorchiasis: an update. *J Helminthol* 2005;79:269-81.
22 Yang JS, Chen MG, Zheng F, Blair D. Paragonimus and paragonimiasis in China: a review of the literature. *Chin J Parasitol Parasit Dis* 2000;18:1-78.
23 Devi KR, Narain K, Bhattacharya S, Negmu K, Agatsuma T, Blair D,et al. Pleuropulmonary paragonimiasis due to Paragonimus heterotremus: molecular diagnosis, prevalence of infection and clinicoradiological features in an endemic area of northeastern India. *Trans R Soc Trop Med Hyg* 2007;101:786-92.
24 Sripa B, Kaewkes S, Sithithaworn P, Mairiang E, Laha T, Smout M,et al. Liver fluke induces cholangiocarcinoma. *PLoS Med* 2007;4:e201.
25 Khan SA, Thomas HC, Davidson BR, Taylor-Robinson SD. Cholangiocarcinoma. *Lancet* 2005;366:1303-14.
26 International Agency for Research on Cancer. Infection with liver flukes (Opisthorchis viverrini, Opisthorchis felineus and Clonorchis sinensis). *IARC Monogr Eval Carcinog Risks Hum* 1994;61:121-75.
27 Bouvard V, Baan R, Straif K, Grosse Y, Secretan B, El-Ghissassi F,et al. A review of human carcinogens. Part B: biological agents. *Lancet Oncol* 2009;10:321-2.
28 Keiser J, Utzinger J. Chemotherapy for major food-borne trematodes: a review. *Expert Opin Pharmacother* 2004;5:1711-26.
29 Chai JY, Shin EH, Lee SH, Rim HJ. Foodborne intestinal flukes in Southeast Asia. *Korean J Parasitol* 2009;47:S69-102.
30 Tinga N, De N, Vien HV, Chau L, Toan ND, Kager PA,et al. Little effect of praziquantel or artemisinin on clonorchiasis in northern Vietnam. A pilot study. *Trop Med Int Health* 1999;4:814-8.
31 Mansour-Ghanaei F, Shafaghi A, Fallah M. The effect of metronidazole in treating human fascioliasis. *Med Sci Monit* 2003;9:PI127-30.
32 Keiser J, Utzinger J. The drugs we have and the drugs we need against major helminth infections. *Adv Parasitol* 2010;73:197-230.
33 Bergquist R, Lustigman S. Control of important helminthic infections: vaccine development as part of the solution. *Adv Parasitol* 2010;73:297-326.
34 Montresor A, Cong DT, Sinuon M, Tsuyuoka R, Chanthavisouk C, Strandgaard H,et al. Large-scale preventive chemotherapy for the control of helminth infection in western Pacific countries: six years later. *PLoS Negl Trop Dis* 2008;2:e278.

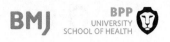

Strongyloides stercoralis infection

Daniel Greaves, registrar in infectious diseases and microbiology[1], Sian Coggle, registrar in infectious diseases and microbiology[1], Christopher Pollard, visiting fellow/research physician[2], Sani H Aliyu, consultant in infectious diseases and microbiology[3], Elinor M Moore, consultant in infectious diseases[1]

[1]Department of Infectious Diseases, Addenbrooke's Hospital, Cambridge CB2 0QQ, UK

[2]Mahidol-Oxford Tropical Medicine Research Unit, Faculty of Tropical Medicine, Mahidol University, Bangkok, Thailand

[3]Department of Microbiology, Addenbrooke's Hospital, Cambridge, UK

Correspondence to: D Greaves greaves@doctors.org.uk

Cite this as: BMJ 2013;347:f4610

DOI: 10.1136/bmj.e4093

http://www.bmj.com/content/347/bmj.f4610

Strongyloides stercoralis is an intestinal helminth that infects humans through contact with soil containing the larvae. Between 30 and 100 million people are infected worldwide.[1] In the United Kingdom, strongyloidiasis is seen predominantly in migrants and returning travellers from endemic areas in the tropics and subtropics. Strongyloidiasis may present with cutaneous or gastrointestinal symptoms but is asymptomatic in over 60% of cases and only indicated by a raised blood eosinophil count.[2] Diagnosis is important as the infection may persist for decades.[3] Immunosuppressed patients with chronic strongyloidiasis are at high risk of developing strongyloides hyperinfection syndrome, a life threatening complication whereby larval proliferation leads to systemic sepsis and multiorgan failure. If strongyloidiasis is diagnosed early, however, it is easily treatable with oral antihelmintic drugs. In this article we review the epidemiology and common symptoms of strongyloidiasis and strongyloides hyperinfection syndrome, discuss the appropriate investigations, and summarise the evidence on treatment.

What is the lifecycle of strongyloides?

S stercoralis larvae are most likely to be present in rural areas with poor sanitation, resulting in faecal soil contamination. The infection starts when the host walks barefoot on contaminated soil and infectious filariform larvae penetrate the skin (figure). The larvae enter the venous circulation and migrate to the lungs from where they are expectorated to the pharynx and swallowed. In the small intestine the larvae develop into adult females, which reproduce asexually and release eggs into the gastrointestinal tract. The eggs then hatch into non-infectious rhabditiform larvae and are excreted in stool. Outside of the human host the free-living rhabditiform larvae either mature into male and female adult worms, which reproduce sexually, or transform directly into filariform larvae ready to invade another host.

S stercoralis can be distinguished from most other intestinal parasites by its ability to reinfect the host through the wall of the gastrointestinal tract. This phenomenon is called autoinfection and occurs when some of the rhabditiform larvae in the faeces transform into infectious filariform larvae in the host's gastrointestinal tract. These larvae then penetrate the gut wall and re-enter the circulation back to the lungs to begin the cycle again. This is the key to the persistence of strongyloides infection and explains why it has been detected decades after initial exposure, up to 75 years later in one case report.[3]

Who gets strongyloidiasis?

Strongyloidiasis is most commonly encountered in sub-Saharan Africa, South America, and South East Asia, where prevalence may exceed 20%.[4] The disease is also encountered in resident populations of the south eastern United States and in parts of southern Europe, in particular Spain and Italy.

In the United Kingdom, strongyloidiasis is primarily seen in immigrants or returning travellers from endemic areas. An estimated 499 780 non-European Union citizens arrived to live in the United Kingdom in the year to March 2013, representing a population at risk.[5] Although no UK data on the prevalence of strongyloidiasis in these populations has been published, several studies from other countries have shown that the burden of disease in immigrants may be considerable. Studies from North America and Canada have shown the presence of serum antibodies to S stercoralis in 23-65% of immigrants from Africa and South East Asia.[6] [7]

Strongyloidiasis can also be transmitted sexually through oro-anal contact. This is most commonly seen in men who have sex with men.[8] Case reports also exist of strongyloidiasis in recipients of solid organ transplants, derived from the donor organ.[9] Infection with S stercoralis through the faecal-oral route may also be possible, as larvae have been identified in contaminated water used to wash vegetables in endemic areas.[10]

What are the symptoms of strongyloidiasis?

Infection with S stercoralis is often mild or asymptomatic. Two case series of 33 and 70 patients with strongyloidiasis found that 51% and 64%, respectively, had no symptoms.[2] [11] In such cases the only sign of infection is an increased peripheral blood eosinophil count.

Acute infection may give a characteristic cutaneous reaction as the larvae penetrate the skin, known as ground itch. The foot is the most commonly affected site and can result in serpiginous or urticarial tracts with severe pruritus lasting for several days. The rash may be difficult to distinguish from cutaneous larva migrans, a condition caused by animal species of hookworm that penetrate human skin but are unable to migrate further than the epidermis. In chronic infection S stercoralis larvae can also migrate intradermally, giving a different appearance from that of cutaneous larva migrans owing to the rapid speed of migration, progressing at around 5-15 cm per hour. This results in intensely itchy red tracts, usually on the perianal area and upper thighs, known as larva currens (literally "running larvae"), which are pathognomonic for strongyloidiasis.

SUMMARY POINTS

- Strongyloidiasis is endemic in the tropics and subtropics and anyone who has travelled to, or lived in, these areas is at risk
- Unlike most other intestinal parasite infections, strongyloidiasis may be life long
- The infection is often asymptomatic and may only be indicated by a peripheral blood eosinophilia
- Diagnosis is important as immunosuppression in patients with chronic infection can precipitate a life threatening hyperinfection syndrome
- Serology is the investigation of choice for diagnosis and follow-up, as stool microscopy has a low sensitivity
- Treatment is with 2×200 µg/kg doses of oral ivermectin given two weeks apart

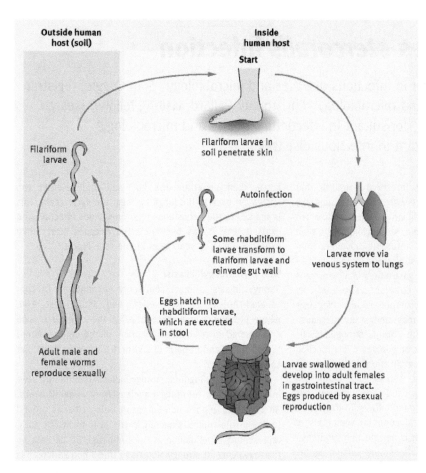

Life cycle of *Strongyloides stercoralis*

As the larvae migrate through the lungs they can produce respiratory symptoms, such as a dry cough or wheeze. A Loeffler's-like syndrome, characterised by fever, dyspnoea, wheeze, pulmonary infiltrates on chest radiographs, and accompanying blood eosinophilia is rarely seen. Chronic strongyloidiasis can lead to recurrent pulmonary symptoms, such as repeated mild pneumonitis with fever or restrictive pulmonary disease.

Once the adult worms reach the small intestine they can stimulate vague gastrointestinal symptoms such as diarrhoea, anorexia, and vomiting, and epigastric pain worsened by eating. In one recent case series of 70 patients, gastrointestinal symptoms were present in 23%.[2]

How is strongyloidiasis diagnosed?
As strongyloidiasis is most commonly asymptomatic, or presents with vague symptoms, diagnostic investigations are key. Blood eosinophilia should always be investigated further, in the first instance by repeating the test to confirm the result. The commonest causes of eosinophilia are parasitic infections, atopy, and drugs (see box for other common causes). A careful history should therefore be taken, including the patient's travel record, the presence of allergic symptoms, and a drug review. The degree of eosinophilia with each of these conditions is highly variable and so cannot be reliably used for differentiation, although it is uncommon for atopy to give rise to an eosinophil count of $>2\times10^9$/L.[12]

Patients with a history of travel to an area where strongyloidiasis is endemic and either compatible symptoms or a blood eosinophilia should be investigated further, with three stool samples for microscopy (collected on separate days) and a blood test for *S stercoralis* serology.

Standard stool microscopy for ova, cysts, and parasites is available at all National Health Service hospitals in the United Kingdom with a microbiology laboratory. Although it is a standard test for many intestinal protozoa and helminth infections, stool microscopy has low sensitivity for detecting *S stercoralis* (around 50%) because of intermittent larval excretion and low infectious burden.[13][14] Certain stool concentration techniques performed in the laboratory, such as the Baermann technique and modified agar plate method, can be used to improve the sensitivity. Despite the low sensitivity, stool microscopy should still be routinely performed, as it is the gold standard for diagnosis. It can take 3-4 weeks for larvae to appear in the stool after dermal penetration.

Serological testing, which consists of an enzyme linked immunosorbent assay to detect IgG to a filariform larval antigen, is generally considered to be a superior investigation. Commercially available assays have a sensitivity between 83% and 89% and a specificity of 97.2%.[15] In the presence of other helmintic infections there is a risk of a false positive result owing to cross reactivity. This is particularly true for filariasis, where up to 60% of patients may have false positive *S stercoralis* serology.[15] In the United Kingdom the serology test is only performed at large parasitology reference laboratories. All samples received by local hospitals are forwarded to these laboratories.

When should patients with strongyloidiasis be referred?
The diagnosis of strongyloidiasis can be made in primary care by stool microscopy and serology. In the event of a proved case, it is reasonable to refer the patient to an infectious diseases doctor, as commonly used treatments may be difficult to attain for many pharmacies outside of hospital.

Several other important parasitic infections may present with asymptomatic eosinophilia, particularly filariasis and schistosomiasis. As cross reactivity may occur between serological assays, this can complicate the diagnostic process. Therefore, if patients with unexplained eosinophilia have travelled to an area where strongyloidiasis, filariasis, and schistosomiasis are endemic, particularly sub-Saharan Africa, it is also advisable to refer them to a specialist.

Patients with a definite diagnosis of strongyloidiasis for whom immunosuppression is planned should also be referred, as the risk of developing strongyloides hyperinfection syndrome must be assessed and appropriate counselling provided.

What is strongyloides hyperinfection syndrome?
Strongyloides hyperinfection syndrome occurs when patients chronically infected with *S stercoralis* become immunosuppressed, such as those receiving treatment for autoimmune disease or malignancy, or if immunosuppressed patients develop acute strongyloidiasis. This results in uncontrolled over-proliferation of larvae with dissemination to end organs, including the lungs, liver, and brain. Systemic sepsis is a common complication owing to translocation of enteric bacteria accompanying larval invasion of the gut wall.

The strongest risk factor seems to be administered corticosteroids. Case reports exist of strongyloides hyperinfection syndrome after courses of steroid as short as six days[16] and with a dose of oral prednisolone as low as 20 mg per day.[17] Individual cases linked with other steroid sparing immunosuppressants and chemotherapeutics have also been described,[18] as well as strongyloides

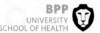
SOURCES AND SELECTION CRITERIA

We performed a search of PubMed using the search term *"Strongyloides stercoralis"*, and included English language studies only. There is a paucity of randomised controlled trails investigating the treatment of strongyloides infection, and no Cochrane reviews have been published. Likewise there are no national or globally recognised guidelines for the investigation and management of this condition. We therefore relied on the studies from our literature search and clinical experience.

OTHER COMMON CAUSES OF EOSINOPHILIA

- Allergy
- Asthma
- Atopic dermatitis
- Acute urticaria
- Parasitic infection
- Schistosomiasis
- Filariasis
- Hookworm
- *Toxocara canis*
- Fungal infection
- Allergic bronchopulmonary aspergillosis
- Coccidioidomycosis
- HIV
- Churg-Strauss syndrome
- Haematological disorders
- Eosinophilic leukaemia
- Hypereosinophilic syndrome
- Adrenocortical insufficiency

ADDITIONAL EDUCATIONAL RESOURCES

- Checkley AM, Chiodini PL, Dockrell DH, Bates I, Thwaites GE, Booth HL, et al. Eosinophilia in returning travellers and migrants from the tropics: UK recommendations for investigation and initial management. *J Infect* 2010;60:1-20. (Subscription required)
- Sims H, Erber WN. Investigation of an incidental finding of eosinophilia. *BMJ* 2011;342:2670

EXPERIENCE OF TREATING STRONGYLOIDES INFECTION IN THE TROPICS

In Thailand the prevalence of strongyloidiasis is estimated to be between 15.9% and 20.6% in certain rural areas. Furthermore, the Foreign and Commonwealth Office states that over 800 000 British nationals visit Thailand every year,[41] so UK based clinicians should be vigilant.

Although the incidence of strongyloides hyperinfection syndrome is low, around 12-24 cases per year are seen at the Hospital for Tropical Diseases in Bangkok. The diagnosis of strongyloidiasis in this environment can be challenging, although clinicians have a low threshold for routine stool examination. Serological testing is also available but is used less often.

In Thailand the first line treatment for adults and children remains albendazole. Ivermectin is not available in all centres so is considered second line treatment despite superior efficacy. Cases of strongyloides hyperinfection syndrome are treated with monthly cycles of albendazole (once daily for five days) followed by ivermectin (single dose) every month for as long as *Strongyloides stercoralis* larvae are detectable in stool.

Patients with intestinal infection alone (that is, non-strongyloides hyperinfection syndrome) have a stool microscopy follow-up a week, one month, and two months after treatment. Serology follow-up occurs in some cases 3-6 months after treatment, at the clinician's discretion. Ongoing serial follow-up occurs if the patient remains positive.

TIPS FOR NON-SPECIALISTS

Patients who should be investigated for strongyloidiasis
- People who travel to, or migrate from, an endemic area and develop the following within 3-4 weeks of travel:
- Persistent unexplained eosinophilia
- Gastrointestinal symptoms: nausea, vomiting, abdominal pain, bloating
- Pulmonary symptoms: fever, wheeze, persistent cough
- Cutaneous symptoms: larva currens, hives, or pustules

Patients in whom strongyloides hyperinfection should be suspected
- Risk factors for strongyloides as above plus:
- Immunosuppressive drug therapy (particularly with steroids)
- Bone marrow allograft
- Solid organ transplantation
- HTLV-I infection

QUESTIONS FOR FUTURE RESEARCH
- What is the UK prevalence of strongyloidiasis among immigrant populations from endemic areas?
- Is ivermectin the best drug for treatment of strongyloidiasis and what is the optimal dosing regimen?
- What is the optimum treatment regime for strongyloides hyperinfection syndrome?
- Can serological testing be improved to allow more accurate post-treatment evaluation of the likelihood of cure?

The initial symptoms of strongyloides hyperinfection syndrome may include fever, haemoptysis, and wheeze. A chest radiograph may reveal pulmonary infiltrates, which can represent a combination of oedema, haemorrhage, and pneumonitis. Gastrointestinal disturbance is common and may progress to paralytic ileus or frank bleeding. Hyponatraemia as a result of the syndrome of inappropriate antidiuretic hormone secretion (SIADH) has also been reported but is less common.[25] Septicaemia and multiorgan failure secondary to translocated gut flora may follow, along with Gram negative meningitis due to bacterial invasion of the cerebrospinal fluid.

Filariform larvae may be found in bodily fluids such as sputum or pleural or peritoneal fluid. Because of the effects of immunosuppression, eosinophilia is often absent.[25]

How is strongyloidiasis treated?

Studies investigating the efficacy of drug treatment for *S stercoralis* have the drawback of being small open label clinical trials. None the less, ivermectin has consistently been shown to be the drug of choice to achieve parasitological cure (that is, the absence of larvae on stool examination) with few side effects.

Ivermectin is a semisynthetic antihelmintic drug derived from avermectin B1. It has a different mechanism of action to the benzimidazoles, such as albendazole, which are also commonly prescribed for intestinal helminth infections. The drug works by binding to glutamate gated chloride ion channels, resulting in hyperpolarisation of neuronal cells and death of the parasite due to paralysis. This effect is not found in humans as ivermectin does not cross the blood-brain barrier.

Ivermectin is currently unlicensed for the treatment of strongyloidiasis in the United Kingdom and hence is only available from "special order" manufacturers and importing companies. The drug is most commonly administered as an oral preparation.

hyperinfection syndrome in both solid organ and bone marrow transplant recipients.[19] [20] Infection with human T cell leukaemia/lymphoma virus type I (HTLV-I) is also a major risk factor for strongyloides hyperinfection syndrome.[21] Observational studies have reported treatment failure of chronic strongyloidiasis in patients infected with HTLV-I[22] along with strongyloides hyperinfection syndrome in the absence of immunosuppression.[23] By contrast, HIV infection does not seem to predispose to strongyloides hyperinfection syndrome, although a greater prevalence of strongyloidiasis was seen in this group than in non-HIV infected people in one cross sectional study.[24]

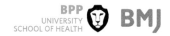

Four studies have compared the efficacy of a single oral dose of 200 µg/kg of ivermectin with two oral doses of 200 µg/kg given either on consecutive days or two weeks apart.[26] [27] [28] [29] Only one study showed a greater efficacy of two doses over a single dose (100% v 77% cure, respectively[28]) whereas the other three showed comparative efficacy (>93%) for both regimens.[26] [27] [29] However, as an autoinfection cycle takes 3-4 weeks to complete[27] and the activity of ivermectin on the extraintestinal stages of the parasite remains uncertain, our local practise is to give two doses two weeks apart.

From our experience, ivermectin is generally well tolerated with few side effects. Two studies have noted a transient increase in alanine aminotransferase levels with ivermectin treatment in a small number of patients,[26] [30] while abdominal distension and chest tightness have also been reported.[31]

Ivermectin also has activity against parasites other than S stercoralis, which may result in unintended harmful treatment effects. This is particularly important for Loa loa, an insect-borne filarial infection characterised by migration of large adult worms through subcutaneous tissues of the body. This manifests as transient localised subcutaneous swellings (Calabar swellings) and occasional visible passage of worms beneath the conjunctiva. Epidemiological evidence shows that patients coinfected with L loa show an increased incidence of encephalopathy in association with ivermectin treatment.[32] It is therefore advisable that patients who have travelled to west and central Africa, where both conditions are endemic, are screened for L loa microfilaraemia with a blood film before treatment with ivermectin. We recommend referral of such patients to an infectious diseases doctor.

In patients who are unable to tolerate ivermectin, albendazole is a reasonable alternative, although cure rates in clinical trials were inferior.[26] [30] [31] [33] In one recent study a course of 400 mg twice daily for seven days produced a cure rate of 63.3%.[26]

How is strongyloides hyperinfection syndrome treated?

Strongyloides hyperinfection syndrome is a difficult condition to treat and is associated with a high mortality. Management involves a combination of antibiotic treatment for systemic Gram negative bacterial sepsis, antihelmintic treatment of S stercoralis itself, multiple organ support during the critical phase of the illness, and reduction of immunosuppression where possible.[18] [34] Ivermectin is still considered the drug of choice,[18] although this is based only on case report evidence. Due to the high burden of larvae in strongyloides hyperinfection syndrome compared with chronic strongyloidiasis, stool microscopy is used to determine treatment efficacy. Daily dosing with ivermectin should therefore continue until two weeks after the last positive stool sample to cover a complete autoinfection cycle.[34] Parenteral ivermectin has been shown to be effective in cases complicated by paralytic ileus or gastrointestinal bleeding where the oral route is not suitable.[35] [36] It should be noted, however, that parenteral ivermectin is currently only available as a veterinary preparation and therefore is not licensed for use in humans. We recommend that expert advice should be sought in such cases.

How is treatment efficacy assessed?

As strongyloidiasis is often asymptomatic, resolution of symptoms is a poor indicator of treatment efficacy. Stool microscopy is also inadequate owing to low sensitivity.

Repeat serological testing after treatment seems to be the best way to test for cure. If the antibody titre has decreased at 6-12 months after treatment this is indicative of eradication of the parasite.[37] It has been suggested that a post-treatment to pre-treatment titre ratio of <0.6 is a good indicator of treatment success,[38] and this has been observed in 65-90% of patients at six months after treatment.[37] [39] Monitoring of blood eosinophil count may also be an effective tool, as a significant decrease in count was seen at an average of 96 days after treatment in one retrospective study.[40] Patients who fail to clear the parasite after two doses of ivermectin should be tested for HTLV-I infection.[22] A concerted effort to look for other causes of eosinophilia is recommended if it persists after three months despite a serological response to ivermectin treatment.

We thank Dorn Watthanakulpanich (Helminthology Department, Mahidol University, Thailand) for his time, knowledge, and expertise.

Contributors: DG had the idea for the article. DG, SC, and CP performed the literature search and wrote the article. SHA and EMM reviewed the manuscript and contributed to the final version of the article. DG is the guarantor.

Competing interests: All authors have completed the ICMJE uniform disclosure form at www.icmje.org/coi_disclosure.pdf and declare: no support from any organisation for the submitted work; no financial relationships with any organisations that might have an interest in the submitted work in the previous three years; no other relationships or activities that could appear to have influenced the submitted work.

Provenance and peer review: Unsolicited; externally peer reviewed.

1   World Health Organization. Neglected tropical diseases—strongyloidiasis. 2013. www.who.int/neglected_diseases/diseases/strongyloidiasis/en/.
2   Valerio L, Roure S, Fernandez-Rivas G, Basile L, Martinez-Cuevas O, Ballesteros AL, et al. Strongyloides stercoralis, the hidden worm. Epidemiological and clinical characteristics of 70 cases diagnosed in the North Metropolitan Area of Barcelona, Spain, 2003-2012. Trans R Soc Trop Med Hyg 2013;107:465-70.
3   Prendki V, Fenaux P, Durand R, Thellier M, Bouchaud O. Strongyloidiasis in man 75 years after initial exposure. Emerg Infect Dis 2011;17:931-2.
4   Siddiqui AA, Berk SL. Diagnosis of Strongyloides stercoralis infection. Clin Infect Dis 2001;33:1040-7.
5   HM Government. Home Office immigration statistics January to March 2013. www.gov.uk/government/publications/immigration-statistics-january-to-march-2013/immigration-statistics-january-to-march-2013.
6   Gyorkos TW, Genta RM, Viens P, MacLean JD. Seroepidemiology of Strongyloides infection in the Southeast Asian refugee population in Canada. Am J Epidemiol 1990;132:257-64.
7   Posey DL, Blackburn BG, Weinberg M, Flagg EW, Ortega L, Wilson M, et al. High prevalence and presumptive treatment of schistosomiasis and strongyloidiasis among African refugees. Clin Infect Dis 2007;45:1310-5.
8   Sorvillo F, Mori K, Sewake W, Fishman L. Sexual transmission of Strongyloides stercoralis among homosexual men. Br J Vener Dis 1983;59:342.
9   Hamilton KW, Abt PL, Rosenbach MA, Bleicher MB, Levine MS, Mehta J, et al. Donor-derived Strongyloides stercoralis infections in renal transplant recipients. Transplantation 2011;91:1019-24.
10 Zeehaida M, Zairi NZ, Rahmah N, Maimunah A, Madihah B. Strongyloides stercoralis in common vegetables and herbs in Kota Bharu, Kelantan, Malaysia. Trop Biomed 2011;28:188-93.
11 Gonzalez A, Gallo M, Valls ME, Munoz J, Puyol L, Pinazo MJ, et al. Clinical and epidemiological features of 33 imported Strongyloides stercoralis infections. Trans R Soc Trop Med Hyg 2010;104:613-6.
12 Sims H, Erber WN. Investigation of an incidental finding of eosinophilia. BMJ 2011;342:d2670.
13 Jones CA, Abadie SH. Studies in human strongyloidiasis. II. A comparison of the efficiency of diagnosis by examination of feces and duodenal fluid. Am J Clin Pathol 1954;24:1154-8.
14 Boulware DR, Stauffer WM 3rd, Walker PF. Hypereosinophilic syndrome and mepolizumab. N Engl J Med 2008;358:2839; author reply 39-40.
15 Van Doorn HR, Koelewijn R, Hofwegen H, Gilis H, Wetsteyn JC, Wismans PJ, et al. Use of enzyme-linked immunosorbent assay and dipstick assay for detection of Strongyloides stercoralis infection in humans. J Clin Microbiol 2007;45:438-42.
16 Ghosh K. Strongyloides stercoralis septicaemia following steroid therapy for eosinophilia: report of three cases. Trans R Soc Trop Med Hyg 2007;101:1163-5.
17 Wurtz R, Mirot M, Fronda G, Peters C, Kocka F. Short report: gastric infection by Strongyloides stercoralis. Am J Trop Med Hyg 1994;51:339-40.

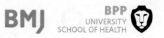

18 Keiser PB, Nutman TB. Strongyloides stercoralis in the immunocompromised population. *Clin Microbiol Rev* 2004;17:208-17.

19 Roxby AC, Gottlieb GS, Limaye AP. Strongyloidiasis in transplant patients. *Clin Infect Dis* 2009;49:1411-23.

20 Dulley FL, Costa S, Cosentino R, Gamba C, Saboya R. Strongyloides stercoralis hyperinfection after allogeneic stem cell transplantation. *Bone Marrow Transplant* 2009;43:741-2.

21 Verdonck K, Gonzalez E, Van Dooren S, Vandamme AM, Vanham G, Gotuzzo E. Human T-lymphotropic virus 1: recent knowledge about an ancient infection. *Lancet Infect Dis* 2007;7:266-81.

22 Terashima A, Alvarez H, Tello R, Infante R, Freedman DO, Gotuzzo E. Treatment failure in intestinal strongyloidiasis: an indicator of HTLV-I infection. *Int J Infect Dis* 2002;6:28-30.

23 Gotuzzo E, Terashima A, Alvarez H, Tello R, Infante R, Watts DM, et al. Strongyloides stercoralis hyperinfection associated with human T cell lymphotropic virus type-1 infection in Peru. *Am J Trop Med Hyg* 1999;60:146-9.

24 Assefa S, Erko B, Medhin G, Assefa Z, Shimelis T. Intestinal parasitic infections in relation to HIV/AIDS status, diarrhea and CD4 T-cell count. *BMC Infect Dis* 2009;9:155.

25 Greaves D, Gouliouris T, O'Donovan M, Craig JI, Torok ME. Strongyloides stercoralis hyperinfection in a patient treated for multiple myeloma. *Br J Haematol* 2012;158:2.

26 Suputtamongkol Y, Premasathian N, Bhumimuang K, Waywa D, Nilganuwong S, Karuphong E, et al. Efficacy and safety of single and double doses of ivermectin versus 7-day high dose albendazole for chronic strongyloidiasis. *PLoS Negl Trop Dis* 2011;5:e1044.

27 Zaha O, Hirata T, Uchima N, Kinjo F, Saito A. Comparison of anthelmintic effects of two doses of ivermectin on intestinal strongyloidiasis in patients negative or positive for anti-HTLV-1 antibody. *J Infect Chemother* 2004;10:348-51.

28 Igual-Adell R, Oltra-Alcaraz C, Soler-Company E, Sanchez-Sanchez P, Matogo-Oyana J, Rodriguez-Calabuig D. Efficacy and safety of ivermectin and thiabendazole in the treatment of strongyloidiasis. *Expert Opin Pharmacother* 2004;5:2615-9.

29 Gann PH, Neva FA, Gam AA. A randomized trial of single- and two-dose ivermectin versus thiabendazole for treatment of strongyloidiasis. *J Infect Dis* 1994;169:1076-9.

30 Datry A, Hilmarsdottir I, Mayorga-Sagastume R, Lyagoubi M, Gaxotte P, Biligui S, et al. Treatment of Strongyloides stercoralis infection with ivermectin compared with albendazole: results of an open study of 60 cases. *Trans R Soc Trop Med Hyg* 1994;88:344-5.

31 Marti H, Haji HJ, Savioli L, Chwaya HM, Mgeni AF, Ameir JS, et al. A comparative trial of a single-dose ivermectin versus three days of albendazole for treatment of Strongyloides stercoralis and other soil-transmitted helminth infections in children. *Am J Trop Med Hyg* 1996;55:477-81.

32 Gardon J, Gardon-Wendel N, Demanga N, Kamgno J, Chippaux JP, Boussinesq M. Serious reactions after mass treatment of onchocerciasis with ivermectin in an area endemic for Loa loa infection. *Lancet* 1997;350:18-22.

33 Nontasut P, Muennoo C, Sa-nguankiat S, Fongsri S, Vichit A. Prevalence of strongyloides in Northern Thailand and treatment with ivermectin vs albendazole. *Southeast Asian J Trop Med Public Health* 2005;36:442-4.

34 Mejia R, Nutman TB. Screening, prevention, and treatment for hyperinfection syndrome and disseminated infections caused by Strongyloides stercoralis. *Curr Opin Infect Dis* 2012;25:458-63.

35 Chiodini PL, Reid AJ, Wiselka MJ, Firmin R, Foweraker J. Parenteral ivermectin in Strongyloides hyperinfection. *Lancet* 2000;355:43-4.

36 Lichtenberger P, Rosa-Cunha I, Morris M, Nishida S, Akpinar E, Gaitan J, et al. Hyperinfection strongyloidiasis in a liver transplant recipient treated with parenteral ivermectin. *Transpl Infect Dis* 2009;11:137-42.

37 Biggs BA, Caruana S, Mihrshahi S, Jolley D, Leydon J, Chea L, et al. Management of chronic strongyloidiasis in immigrants and refugees: is serologic testing useful? *Am J Trop Med Hyg* 2009;80:788-91.

38 Kobayashi J, Sato Y, Toma H, Takara M, Shiroma Y. Application of enzyme immunoassay for postchemotherapy evaluation of human strongyloidiasis. *Diagn Microbiol Infect Dis* 1994;18:19-23.

39 Loutfy MR, Wilson M, Keystone JS, Kain KC. Serology and eosinophil count in the diagnosis and management of strongyloidiasis in a non-endemic area. *Am J Trop Med Hyg* 2002;66:749-52.

40 Nuesch R, Zimmerli L, Stockli R, Gyr N, Christoph Hatz FR. Imported strongyloidosis: a longitudinal analysis of 31 cases. *J Travel Med* 2005;12:80-4.

41 HM Government. Foreign and Commonwealth Office. Travel advice by country—Thailand. 2013. www.fco.gov.uk/en/travel-and-living-abroad/travel-advice-by-country/asia-oceania/thailand/.

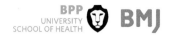

Management of adolescents and adults with febrile illness in resource limited areas

John A Crump, associate professor of medicine and pathology[1 2 3 4], Sandy Gove, team leader[5], Christopher M Parry, senior clinical consultant[6 7]

[1]Division of Infectious Diseases and International Health, Department of Medicine, and Department of Pathology, Duke University, Durham, NC 27710, USA

[2]Duke Global Health Institute, Duke University, Durham, NC, USA

[3]Kilimanjaro Christian Medical Centre, Moshi, Tanzania

[4]Kilimanjaro Christian Medical College, Tumaini University, Moshi, Tanzania

[5]Integrated Management of Adolescent and Adult Illness (IMAI), World Health Organization, Department of HIV/AIDS, Geneva, Switzerland

[6]Wellcome Trust Major Overseas Programme, Mahidol Oxford Tropical Medicine Research Unit, Bangkok, Thailand

[7]Angkor Hospital for Children, Siem Reap, Cambodia

Correspondence to: J A Crump john. crump@duke.edu

Cite this as: BMJ 2011;343:d4847

DOI: 10.1136/bmj.d4847

http://www.bmj.com/content/343/bmj.d4847

Fever is common among adolescents and adults seeking healthcare in low income countries; in this setting, case fatality rates are often high and the range of potential infectious and non-infectious causes is broad (table 1).[1][2] These differences, combined with limited resources, mean that management guidelines developed for high income countries cannot readily be adapted to resource limited areas. It is often difficult to establish a diagnosis from the clinical history and physical examination alone because a range of diseases share similar clinical features. The diagnostic problem may be compounded by limited laboratory capacity for diagnostic testing.[3] There may be limited or no laboratory services available; laboratory services may be prohibitively expensive for users; concerns may exist regarding the quality of results; and practical reliable diagnostic tests may not have been developed for some infections of local importance. When clinical and laboratory evaluations do not identify a specific cause for fever, healthcare providers may treat empirically according to the "syndrome" of clinical features that the patient presents with, often guided by management guidelines that recommend approaches to treatment based on syndromes. World Health Organization algorithms for the management of infants and children with a range of clinical syndromes have been developed for primary healthcare providers and district hospital clinicians in low income countries.[4][5] Similar guidelines for adolescents and adults were published in 2004 and updated in 2009 for primary healthcare providers at first level health facilities.[6] A WHO manual to guide district hospital clinicians is in development. Ideally, guidelines should be validated, adapted to local conditions, and improved on the basis of the results of locally or nationally available surveillance or sentinel hospital studies.

We review the approach to the management of adolescents and adults with febrile illness—which we define as having a history of fever in the past 48 hours, feeling hot, or having an axillary temperature of 37.5°C or more—in low income areas. Focusing on infectious causes, we will draw on international guidelines and evidence from systematic reviews and take into account resources currently available to most clinicians.

How should febrile adults be managed at the first level health facility?

Rapid triage and emergency management

The WHO acute care guideline on integrated management of adolescent and adult illness (IMAI) recommends that the patient be rapidly assessed for the presence of emergency signs.[6] Patients with airway obstruction, central cyanosis, severe respiratory distress, or circulatory failure (weak or fast pulse, or slow capillary refill) require urgent management, and referral to a hospital is recommended. Fever from a life threatening cause is defined as fever that is associated with neck stiffness, extreme weakness or inability to stand, lethargy, unconsciousness, convulsions, severe abdominal pain, or respiratory distress. For those with fever from a life threatening cause, the guideline recommends assessment of temperature and blood pressure and quick establishment of intravenous access, so that fluids and antimicrobial agents can be given if the patient is in shock or if sepsis is suspected. For patients with life threatening febrile illness, such as severe sepsis as a result of bacteraemia and meningitis, the guidelines recommend administering parenteral antibacterials, antimalarials, and glucose; patients should then be urgently referred to hospital.[6] Selection of the parenteral antibacterial agent should ideally be based on knowledge of patterns of antimicrobial susceptibility among relevant organisms in the area. However, because of widespread resistance to traditional first line antimicrobials, such as penicillins, and invasive *Salmonella* making aminoglycoside monotherapy a poor choice in many areas, extended spectrum cephalosporins such as ceftriaxone are commonly used (boxes 1 and 2).

Assessment, classification, and management of acute illness

The updated IMAI acute care guidelines, based on current WHO malaria guidelines,[7] recommend that once emergency conditions are identified and managed, assessment of the acute illness should focus on classifying the patient's health problem on the basis of the presenting symptoms. For patients who give a history of fever in the past 48 hours, feel hot, or have an axillary temperature of 37.5°C or more, the history and physical examination focus on trying to identify a source for the fever and on stratifying their malaria risk. Risk of malaria is based on age, malaria transmission in the area of residence, travel history, pregnancy, and HIV infection status. A malaria rapid diagnostic test or malaria smear is indicated if the patient is considered to be at high risk of malaria, or if no obvious source of the fever can be found in a patient at low risk of malaria. Further management depends on the presence or absence of specific signs of illness. Among those without severe disease, especially if

SUMMARY POINTS

- Overlap in the clinical features of febrile illnesses and limited laboratory services make the management of febrile patients in resource limited settings challenging
- WHO guidelines for managing febrile adolescents and adults in resource limited settings are available for first level health facilities and are forthcoming for district hospitals
- First level health facility guidelines recommend antimalarials for those with a positive malaria diagnostic test, antibacterials for those with signs of severe illness or specific bacterial infections, and hospital referral of those with severe illness or no apparent diagnosis
- Management guidelines should be validated, locally adapted, and improved on the basis of local or national surveillance data and sentinel hospital studies
- Malaria, tuberculosis, and HIV diagnostic tests can enhance management by ruling out a specific illness or by directing towards a particular diagnosis
- Clinical trials of empirical treatment strategies and advocacy for better clinical laboratory services could help improve management guidelines and patient outcomes

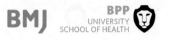

Table 1 Differential diagnosis for fever without obvious cause at the district hospital level

Syndrome	Differential diagnosis
Fever <7 days without clinically obvious focus or site	Malaria
	Bacteraemic sepsis
	Meningococcal disease
	Typhoid and paratyphoid fever
	Rickettsial disease
	Dengue fever
	Chikungunya
	Influenza
	Yellow fever
	Primary HIV infection
	Acute strongyloidiasis
	Relapsing fever (tick or louse borne borreliosis)
	Acute schistosomiasis
	Immune reconstitution inflammatory syndrome
	Drug induced fever
	Rheumatic fever
	Mononucleosis caused by Epstein-Barr virus or cytomegalovirus
	Toxoplasmosis
	Q fever
	Leptospirosis
Fever ≥7 days without clinically obvious focus or site	Tuberculosis
	Typhoid and paratyphoid fever
	Malaria
	Osteomyelitis
	Infective endocarditis
	Liver abscess
	Brucellosis
	Yellow fever
	Plague
	Cryptococcosis
	Non-tuberculous mycobacterial infection
	Lymphoma
	Deep fungal infections, such as histoplasmosis, penicilliosis, coccidiomycosis, paracoccidiomycosis
	Cytomegalovirus
	Toxoplasmosis
	Human African trypanosomiasis (sleeping sickness)
	American trypanosomiasis (Chagas disease)
	Visceral leishmaniasis (kala azar)

the malaria test is negative, other causes of fever should be considered using the full IMAI acute care algorithm.[6] Other causes include upper respiratory tract infections such as sinusitis, pneumonia, gastroenteritis, urinary tract infection, pelvic inflammatory disease, tuberculosis, HIV related illness, antiretroviral drug reactions, and severe soft tissue or muscle infection. Very severe illness in patients not at risk for malaria is managed with parenteral antibacterials and glucose. Artesunate, artemether, or quinine is suggested for treatment of severe malaria. However, when illness persists for at least seven days, it is recommended that the apparent cause be treated, that tuberculosis and other HIV related conditions be considered, and that patients with no apparent cause be referred for assessment at the district hospital. Simple fevers in patients with no malaria risk are managed by treating the apparent cause and evaluating after one week (box 1).

Quality of evidence
The IMAI acute care algorithms incorporate elements of other WHO guidelines such as those for lung health, HIV counselling and testing, tuberculosis, sexually transmitted infections, and malaria, and they have been developed from expert group meetings and review of the published literature. The algorithms have been refined by validation studies in low income countries through the country's own experience with adaptation and use.[6] Although interventions

BOX 1 PRACTICAL EXAMPLES OF THE USE OF THE INTEGRATED MANAGEMENT OF ADOLESCENT AND ADULT ILLNESS ALGORITHM IN FEBRILE PATIENTS

Severe illness

At first level health facility

- Clinical features: Triage assessment shows patient weak and unable to stand; weak fast pulse, and capillary refill >3 seconds. Oral temperature 39.5°C, pulse 126 beats/min, and blood pressure 85/40 mm Hg. Conscious; no neck stiffness, abdominal pain, or signs of respiratory distress
- Epidemiological context: Area of low malaria transmission intensity
- Rapid diagnostic tests: Negative for malaria and HIV
- Syndromic diagnosis: Very severe febrile disease or suspected sepsis with shock
- Management: Pre-referral intramuscular antimicrobial (extended spectrum cephalosporin, or ampicillin plus gentamicin) and glucose given; urgent referral to district hospital

At district hospital level

- Clinical features: Triage assessment by the nurse confirmed the patient is in shock with systolic blood pressure of 85 mm Hg
- Management: Initially in emergency section for septic shock: intravenous fluids; extended spectrum cephalosporin, or ampicillin plus gentamicin; supplemental oxygen titrated to oxygen saturation of 90% by pulse oximetry
- Laboratory investigations: Peripheral blood smear preparation and microscopy negative for malaria parasites; haemoglobin concentration 80 g/L; serum glucose concentration normal
- Further management: Clinical assessment and investigations to identify the source of infection while continuing resuscitation with close monitoring

Non-severe illness

- Location: First level health facility
- Clinical features: Fever for three days; patient fully ambulatory; pulse normal character and rate, capillary refill <2 seconds. Oral temperature 38.0°C, pulse 90 beats/min, and blood pressure 124/82 mm Hg. Conscious; no neck stiffness, abdominal pain, or signs of respiratory distress
- Epidemiological context: Area of high malaria transmission intensity
- Rapid diagnostic tests: Positive for malaria; negative for HIV
- Syndromic diagnosis: Malaria, non-severe
- Management: Oral artemisinin combination treatment; follow-up at three days if still febrile; took blood for culture
- Clinical course: Patient remained febrile after seven days; sent sputum for tuberculosis and referred to district hospital

BOX 2 RECOMMENDATIONS FOR FIRST LEVEL HEALTH PROVIDERS

- Perform a rapid assessment for the presence of emergency signs and manage emergency conditions
- Identify patients with fever from a life threatening cause: fever with stiff neck, extreme weakness or inability to stand, lethargy, unconsciousness, convulsions, severe abdominal pain, or respiratory distress
- Use intravenous fluids for patients with shock and start appropriate parenteral antibacterials, antimalarials, and the administration of glucose; refer urgently to hospital
- Routinely offer HIV testing
- Assess the severity of the acute illness; treat and refer patients who have severe illness or no apparent diagnosis to hospital

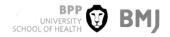

Table 2 Laboratory tests at the district hospital*

Category	Test type
General	Full blood count and differential
	Blood collection and crossmatching for transfusion
HIV	Rapid HIV antibody tests: first, second, and third tests
	CD4 absolute count and percentage: on site or sent out
	Early infant diagnosis preparation of dried blood spot: sent out for virological testing
Tuberculosis	Acid fast stain and microscopy
Malaria (endemic areas)	Peripheral blood smear preparation and microscopy
	Rapid test to detect and discriminate between *Plasmodium falciparum* and mixed *Plasmodium* species
Other laboratory evaluations	Rapid syphilis test
	Syphilis: rapid plasma reagin
	Urine dipstick for sugar, protein, leucocytes, ketones
	Gram stain
	Microscopy and chemistry for cerebrospinal fluid, urine, thoracentesis, and paracentesis
	Saline wet mount and potassium hydroxide for bacterial vaginosis and *Trichomonas vaginalis*
	Blood and sputum cultures: sent out
	Cryptococcal antigen or India ink stain (or both)
	Lactic acid
	Stool microscopy for ova and parasites: on site or sent out
	Rapid hepatitis B test
	Hepatitis B enzyme linked immunosorbent assay
Other investigations	Electrolytes, urea, creatinine, glucose
	Oxygen saturation by pulse oximetry
	Radiography: chest, plain film abdomen, cervical spine, bone
	Ultrasound examination
Additional investigations that may be available at regional or central laboratories as send-out tests	Serum and cerebrospinal fluid total protein
	Liver enzymes
	Mycobacterial culture and susceptibility testing
	Nucleic acid amplification tests for *Mycobacterium tuberculosis*
	Cryptococcal antigen testing of serum and cerebrospinal fluid
	Measurement of HIV-1 RNA
	Fungal stains
	Blood culture
	Urine culture
	Stool culture
	Toxoplasma serology
	Cytology: for example, cerebrospinal fluid, cervical
	Silver stain or direct fluorescent antibody test for *Pneumocystis jirovecii*
	Fungal cultures, including of blood
	Nucleic acid amplification tests for respiratory viruses including influenza
	Histopathology: for example, cervical, lymph node, skin biopsy
	Serological tests, nucleic acid amplification tests, other investigations or special cultures may be available at a central laboratory to diagnose brucellosis, dengue, fascioliasis, leishmaniasis, cysticercosis, strongyloidiasis, trypanosomiasis, and other infections

*Prioritisation and availability of tests will vary according to geographical location and epidemiology.

for specific infections such as malaria have been evaluated in randomised, controlled trials, trial data are not available from low income countries for some syndrome based interventions, such as those for very severe illness.

What are the challenges for clinicians at the district hospital level?

WHO is developing resources to guide the management of adolescent and adult illness at the district hospital level, including the assessment, classification, and management of febrile illness.[8] This manual, which will be available soon, will be analogous to the currently available pocket book of hospital care for children.[5] As at the first referral level, clear processes for rapid triage and emergency management of patients must be in place at the district hospital.

Inadequate facilities for diagnosis

The IMAI guidance for first level health facilities anticipates that the hospital to which the severely ill febrile adult or adolescent is referred will have enhanced facilities for diagnosis and management, but this is not always the case. Table 2 lists tests that are valuable for managing febrile

patients and that should be made available at the district hospital level, according to expert consensus and the IMAI second level learning programme.[9] If these capacities are not already in place, it is recommended that they be prioritised for development. However, district clinicians need to be prepared to form a differential diagnosis of fever based on a wider range of main symptoms; to recognise diseases presenting with symptoms in multiple organ systems such as endocarditis, dengue, typhoid, and paratyphoid fever; and to have an approach to the diagnostic challenge presented by fever with no obvious clinical cause that uses both clinical assessment and limited laboratory tests.[10] Table 1 lists the differential diagnoses for fever without an obvious cause according to whether the fever lasts for less than seven days or seven days or more.

Few point of care tests

At present, no rapid point of care tests exist for the detection of most of the micro-organisms that cause bloodstream infections. Reliable, inexpensive, simple, and rapid point of case tests are useful in situations where it is not feasible to establish a conventional clinical laboratory. Despite

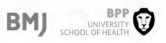

considerable attention and resources having been directed towards developing such tests in recent years, only a few have become widely used in routine practice. Rapid tests that are in widespread use include those for HIV, malaria, and syphilis. Others have been hampered by inadequate test performance characteristics (for example, typhoid rapid antibody tests[11]) or prohibitive cost (for example, tests detecting urine pneumococcal antigen[12]). Use of rapid diagnostic tests with poor performance characteristics has the potential to harm patients by directing clinicians towards incorrect diagnoses. A rapid tuberculosis nucleic acid amplification test suitable for use at the district hospital level has recently been endorsed by WHO, but is not yet in widespread use.[13] Because of the wide range of potential causes of fever, integration of tests on single platforms is an important goal.

Barriers to changing clinicians' behaviour

In settings where empirical management supported by few diagnostic tests is the established norm, it can be difficult to change the behaviour of clinicians so that they respond to additional diagnostic information. Clinicians may fail to use available laboratory services because they think that results are unreliable. When a new diagnostic test is introduced, the results may not necessarily change the way that patients are managed and the degree of adherence to management guidelines may be limited. The introduction of malaria rapid diagnostic tests in some settings, for example, may not reduce the overtreatment of malaria.[14]

Why is ruling out malaria important?

In some areas most patients treated empirically for malaria do not have malaria when rigorously assessed.[15] Consequently, WHO recommends that the diagnosis of malaria be confirmed by a malaria diagnostic test.[7] In areas with any malaria risk, the ability to rule out malaria by malaria film or by use of a malaria rapid diagnostic test can prevent unnecessary use of antimalarial drugs and direct clinical thinking towards alternative diagnoses (such as bacterial infection) and treatment options. Furthermore, in areas of high malaria transmission intensity, a positive malaria film may be an incidental finding, and other causes for the current febrile illness, such as bacteraemia, may be present. Clinicians need to be reminded that the overdiagnosis of malaria may lead to poor outcomes for febrile patients with non-malaria infections who are subsequently treated inappropriately with antimalarial drugs.[15]

Is it strictly necessary to diagnose HIV infection?

WHO/Joint United Nations Programme on HIV/AIDS guidance recommends that providers initiate HIV diagnostic testing for all patients, including those with fever. The results of HIV counselling and testing in turn provides a risk assessment for HIV coinfections.[16] A recent observational study of febrile inpatients in Tanzania showed that the population with fever had a much higher prevalence of HIV infection than the general population from which it was drawn, because people infected with HIV have increased risk for a range of febrile illnesses.[17] Furthermore, acute HIV infection may be a cause of febrile illness in its own right but is not reliably detected by antibody testing.[18] The diagnosis of HIV in a febrile inpatient greatly raises the probability of particular coinfections, such as cryptococcal disease; tuberculosis

(including disseminated forms of the disease that may not localise to the lung[19]); invasive non-typhoidal *Salmonella* infection; pneumococcal disease[20]; and, in southeast Asia, penicilliosis.[21] [22] Furthermore, clinical staging or staging based on immunological status using the CD4 positive T cell count supports risk stratification for specific HIV coinfections.[23]

Why is it important to know the local causes of fever?

Limitations of empirical treatment

A diverse range of invasive bacterial and fungal infections may occur in developing countries, often with high case fatality rates. These may not respond to standard empirical antimicrobials.[20] The range of potential causative agents of fever are too numerous to cover comprehensively in this review, but table 1 lists some of the main ones. Aggregate data on invasive infections and anticipated patterns of antimicrobial resistance can provide useful local epidemiological data to inform and validate empirical management recommendations.

Multidrug resistant bacterial infections—such as typhoid, extended spectrum β lactamase producing Gram negative infections, and infections with meticillin resistant *Staphylococcus aureus*—and difficult to treat infections, such as melioidosis caused by *Burkholderia pseudomallei*, may be common in some areas.[24] [25] [26] Leptospirosis, Q fever, and rickettsial infections may be common but under-appreciated in many resource limited settings.[27] [28] [29] Arthropod borne infections, including arboviruses, other viral diseases, parasitic infections, such as leishmaniasis and trypanosomiasis, and other conditions of local importance should be considered on the basis of clinical features, risk factors, and local epidemiological data.

Limited diagnostic testing

Diagnostic tests such as blood culture or other techniques for identifying invasive infections (such as cryptococcal antigen testing, urine antigen testing for pneumococcal disease), along with the results of antimicrobial susceptibility testing, if available, will help in the subsequent rationalisation or discontinuation of initial antimicrobial treatment. However, reliable diagnostic tests for many infections are often not available at the hospital level or even at the national reference laboratory in resource limited settings. Although *Leptospira* spp are susceptible to antimicrobial agents usually used in the empirical management of febrile adolescents and adults, *Coxiella burnetii* and *Rickettsia* spp are not. Thus, a tetracycline should be considered for patients in whom Q fever or rickettsial infection is highly likely, and in those patients who do not respond to initial empirical treatment.

How can local epidemiological data be acquired?

Systematic surveillance or sentinel site studies of the causes of febrile illness may identify a mismatch between treatment strategies and local causative agents associated with poor patient outcomes.[17]

Local and national surveillance

If a local clinical laboratory is used systematically by clinicians and can provide quality controlled diagnostic tests for patients with febrile illness, data on invasive infections and patterns of antimicrobial resistance can be aggregated

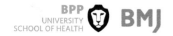

SOURCES AND SELECTION CRITERIA

We searched for papers that were published between 1990 and January 2011 using the following MeSH terms: "(developing countries and guideline) and (fever, bacter(a)emia, HIV, hospital laboratories, malaria, tuberculosis)" in the National Library of Medicine's computerised search service PubMed. We sought Cochrane database systematic reviews. We reviewed relevant articles and sought online resources.

QUESTIONS FOR FUTURE RESEARCH

- How can choice, dose, and duration of empirical treatment be improved so that it better matches local causative agents and avoids overuse of antimicrobials?
- Can our understanding of local causes of febrile illness be improved by expanding the use of sentinel hospital studies or enhanced national surveillance?
- Do randomised controlled trials have a role in identifying the best empirical management strategies for febrile illness in resource poor settings?
- How can diagnostic services be improved in clinical laboratories and at the point of care in low income countries?
- Can rapid, practical and reliable point of care diagnostic tests be designed for common causes of fever other than malaria, tuberculosis, and HIV?
- What determines the behaviour of clinicians managing febrile patients?

ADDITIONAL EDUCATIONAL RESOURCES

Resources for healthcare professionals

- Malaria Atlas Project (www.map.ox.ac.uk/)—Uses a spatial database of linked information based on medical intelligence and satellite derived climate data to constrain and map the limits of malaria transmission and to provide an archive of community based estimates of prevalence of the malaria parasite
- WHO. Guidelines for the treatment of malaria. 2nd ed. 2010. www.who.int/malaria/publications/atoz/9789241547925/en/index.html
- WHO. Guidance on provider-initiated HIV testing and counselling in health facilities. 2007. www.who.int/hiv/pub/vct/pitc/en/index.html
- WHO. International standards for tuberculosis care. 2006. http://whqlibdoc.who.int/publications/2006/istc_report_eng.pdf

Resources for patients and the community

- WHO (www.who.int/hiv/topics/capacity/en/index.html)—Integrated management of adolescent and adult illness (IMAI) resources for patients
- WHO patient self management booklet (www.who.int/hiv/pub/imai/patient_self/en/index.html)—Designed to be used by patients, treatment supporters, and caregivers in resource poor settings; focused on HIV/AIDS
- WHO caregiver booklet (www.who.int/hiv/pub/imai/patient_caregiver/en/index.html)—Designed to be used by health workers to educate family members and other caregivers and then be used by patients as a reference in the home based care of serious long term illness

A PATIENT'S STORY FROM EAST AFRICA

On the first day of illness, I awoke with headache, fever, chills, nausea, vomiting, somnolence, and fatigue. These symptoms worsened over the course of the day. A malaria smear was performed at a private hospital; it was negative. I was very unwell so I was brought to a large referral hospital. Two more malaria slides were performed; both were negative. Nevertheless, I was started on a quinine drip for treatment of malaria. I was also given an intravenous injection of ceftriaxone. No blood was drawn for culture. The next morning I felt much better. I was discharged and told to continue with a five day course of oral antimalarials. I received ceftriaxone injections for two days. Three days after discharge and one day after stopping ceftriaxone my initial symptoms recurred. Although I was still taking artemisinin combination treatment for presumed malaria, when my symptoms relapsed the doctor insisted on starting a quinine drip. A colleague recommended that ceftriaxone be restarted. The next morning, my symptoms had again resolved and I was discharged. The doctor advised me to continue oral antimalarials and ceftriaxone injections for five days. I took only ceftriaxone and experienced no recurrence. The cause of my fever was never identified.

to provide useful local epidemiological information and to validate and guide recommendations for empirical management. When available, reliable national surveillance data for specific infections (such as malaria, dengue) can help to establish background rates of endemic infections and to identify disease outbreaks.

Sentinel hospital studies

In instances where routinely collected data on causes of febrile illness are not available, sentinel hospital studies are a useful means of improving local recommendations on empirical management.[17 20 24 25 27 30] Such studies are typically conducted over a year or more, enrol participants who meet the eligibility criteria for the syndrome of interest, collect data that match symptoms and signs in management guidelines, and provide an expanded range of diagnostic tests for the period of the study. The findings are used to validate and improve local management recommendations.

Future directions

The development and implementation of hospital level guidelines for the management of adolescents and adults, complementing those already available for children, will provide an important framework for improving the management of febrile illness in low income countries. Validation, local adaptation, and improvement of these guidelines using studies incorporating both patient outcomes and laboratory end points will be needed. The evidence base for interventions could be strengthened by clinical trials that evaluate empirical treatment strategies for severely ill patients. Support and advocacy for excellent clinical laboratory services in resource poor settings is warranted. High quality laboratory data can inform the selection and rational use of antimicrobial treatment and provide local data on the epidemiology of infectious causes of febrile illness. This effort should be supplemented by evaluation and implementation of reliable, inexpensive, simple, and rapid point of case tests that influence patient management decisions and improve patient outcomes.

Thanks to Valérie D'Acremont of the Global Malaria Programme, WHO, Geneva, Switzerland, and the Swiss Tropical and Public Health Institute, Basel, Switzerland, for her comments and suggestions on this manuscript.

Contributors: JAC did the literature and database search, sought online resources, prepared the initial draft of the paper, and is guarantor. All authors framed the content of the paper and made critical revisions. SG ensured that content was consistent with available WHO documents.

Funding: JAC received support from United States National Institutes of Health (NIH) funded programs International Studies on AIDS Associated Co-infections (U01 AI062563); AIDS International Training and Research Program (D43 PA-03-018); the Duke Clinical Trials Unit and Clinical Research Sites (U01 AI069484); the Duke Center for AIDS Research (P30 AI 64518); and the Center for HIV/AIDS Vaccine Immunology (U01 AI067854). CMP received support from the Wellcome Trust and the Li Ka Shing Foundation.

Competing interests: All authors have completed the Unified Competing Interest form at www.icmje.org/coi_disclosure.pdf (available on request from the corresponding author) and declare JAC had support from the US National Institutes of Health for the submitted work; no financial relationships with any organisations that might have an interest in the submitted work in the previous three years; no other relationships or activities that could appear to have influenced the submitted work.

Provenance and peer review: Commissioned; externally peer reviewed.

Patient consent obtained.

1 Petit PL, van Ginneken JK. Analysis of hospital records in four African countries, 1975-1990, with emphasis on infectious diseases. J Trop Med Hyg 1995;98:217-27.
2 Cheng AC, West TE, Limmathurotsakul D, Peacock SJ. Strategies to reduce mortality from bacterial sepsis in adults in developing countries. PLoS Med 2008;5:e175.
3 Petti CA, Polage CR, Quinn TC, Ronald AR, Sande MA. Laboratory medicine in Africa: a barrier to effective health care. Clin Infect Dis 2006;42:377-82.
4 World Health Organisation Division of Diarrhoea and Acute Respiratory Disease Control, United Nations Children's Fund. Integrated management of the sick child. Bull World Health Organ 1995;73:735-40.

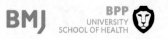

5   WHO. Pocket book of hospital care for children: guidelines for the management of common illnesses with limited resources. 2005. http://whqlibdoc.who.int/publications/2005/9241546700.pdf.

6   WHO. IMAI acute care: guidelines for first-level facility health workers at health centre and district outpatient clinic. 2009. www.who.int/hiv/pub/imai/acute_care.pdf.

7   WHO. Guidelines for the treatment of malaria. 2nd ed. 2010. http://whqlibdoc.who.int/publications/2010/9789241547925_eng.pdf.

8   WHO. IMAI district clinician manual: hospital care for adolescents and adults – guidelines for the management of illnesses with limited resources. 2011 [forthcoming]. www.who.int/hiv/topics/capacity/en/.

9   WHO, WHO African Regional Office, US Centers for Disease Control and Prevention, American Society for Clinical Pathology. Consultation on technical and operational recommendations for clinical laboratory testing harmonization and standardization. 2008:20. www.who.int/hiv/amds/amds_cons_tech_oper_lab_test.pdf.

10 Mundy CJ, Bates I, Nkhoma W, Floyd K, Kadewele G, Ngwira M, et al. The operation, quality and costs of a district hospital laboratory service in Malawi. Trans R Soc Trop Med Hyg 2003;97:403-8.

11 Olsen SJ, Pruckler J, Bibb W, Thanh NT, Trinh TM, Minh NT, et al. Evaluation of rapid diagnostic tests for typhoid fever. J Clin Microbiol 2004;42:1885-9.

12 Smith MD, Derrington P, Evans R, Creek M, Morris R, Dance DA, et al. Rapid diagnosis of bacteremic pneumococcal infections in adults by using the Binax NOW Streptococcus pneumoniae urinary antigen test: a prospective, controlled clinical evaluation. J Clin Microbiol 2003;41:2810-3.

13 Boehme CC, Nabeta P, Hillemann D, Nicol MP, Shenai S, Krapp F, et al. Rapid molecular detection of tuberculosis and rifiampicin resistance. N Engl J Med 2010;363:1005-15.

14 Reyburn H, Mbakilwa H, Mwangi R, Mwerinde O, Olomi R, Drakeley C, et al. Rapid diagnostic tests compared with malaria microscopy for guiding outpatient treatment of febrile illness in Tanzania: randomised trial. BMJ 2007;334:403.

15 Reyburn H, Mbatia R, Drakeley C, Carneiro I, Mwakasungula E, Mwerinde O, et al. Overdiagnosis of malaria in patients with severe febrile illness in Tanzania: a prospective study. BMJ 2004;329:1212-5.

16 WHO/UNAIDS. Guidance on provider-initiated HIV testing and counselling in healthcare facilities. 2007. www.who.int/hiv/pub/guidelines/9789241595568_en.pdf.

17 Crump JA, Ramadhani HO, Morrissey AB, Saganda W, Mwako MS, Yang L-Y, et al. Invasive bacterial and fungal infections among hospitalized HIV-infected and HIV-uninfected adults and adolescents in northern Tanzania. Clin Infect Dis 2011;52:341-8.

18 Sanders EJ, Wahome E, Mwangome M, Thiong'o AN, Okuku HS, Price MA, et al. Most adults seek urgent healthcare when acquiring HIV-1 and are frequently treated for malaria in coastal Kenya. AIDS 2011;25:1219-24.

19 Archibald LK, den Dulk MO, Pallangyo KJ, Reller LB. Fatal Mycobacterium tuberculosis bloodstream infections in febrile hospitalized adults in Dar es Salaam, Tanzania. Clin Infect Dis 1998;26:290-6.

20 Reddy EA, Shaw AV, Crump JA. Community acquired bloodstream infections in Africa: a systematic review and meta-analysis. Lancet Infect Dis 2010;10:417-32.

21 Louie JK, Chi NH, Thao LTT, Quang VM, Campbell J, Chau NV, et al. Opportunistic infections in hospitalized HIV-infected adults in Ho Chi Minh City, Vietnam: a cross-sectional study. Int J STD AIDS 2004;15:758-61.

22 Chierakul W, Rajanuwong A, Wuthiekanun V, Teerawattanasook N, Gasiprong M, Simpson A, et al. The changing pattern of bloodstream infections associated with the rise in HIV prevalence in northeastern Thailand. Trans R Soc Trop Med Hyg 2004;98:678-86.

23 Grant AD, Djomand G, Smets P, Kadio A, Coulibaly M, Kakou A, et al. Profound immunosuppression across the spectrum of opportunistic disease among hospitalized HIV-infected adults in Abidjan, Cote d'Ivoire. AIDS 1997;11:1357-64.

24 Chaowagul W, White NJ, Dance DA, Wattanagoon Y, Naigowit P, Davis TM, et al. Melioidosis: a major cause of community-acquired septicemia in northeastern Thailand. J Infect Dis 1989;159:890-9.

25 Phetsouvanh R, Phongmany S, Soukaloun D, Rasachak B, Soukhaseum V, Soukhaseum S, et al. Causes of community-acquired bacteremia and patterns of antimicrobial resistance in Vientiane, Laos. Am J Trop Med Hyg 2006;75:978-85.

26 Chheng K, Tarquinio S, Wuthiekanun V, Sin L, Thaipadungpanit J, Amornchai P, et al. Emergence of community-associated methicillin-resistant Staphylococcus aureus associated with pediatric infection in Cambodia. PLoS One 2009;4:e6630.

27 Murdoch DR, Woods CW, Zimmerman MD, Dull PM, Belbase RH, Keenan AJ, et al. The etiology of febrile illness in adults presenting to Patan Hospital in Kathmandu, Nepal. Am J Trop Med Hyg 2004;70:670-5.

28 Biggs HM, Bui DM, Galloway RL, Stoddard RA, Shadomy SV, Morrissey AB, et al. Leptospirosis among hospitalized febrile patients in northern Tanzania. Am J Trop Med Hyg 2011;85:275-81.

29 Prabhu M, Nicholson WL, Roche AJ, Kersh GJ, Fitzpatrick KA, Oliver LD, et al. Q fever, spotted fever group and typhus group rickettsioses among hospitalized febrile patients in northern Tanzania. Clin Infect Dis 2011;53:e8-15.

30 Archibald LK, Reller LB. Clinical microbiology in developing countries. Emerg Infect Dis 2001;7:302-5.

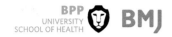

Tick bite prevention and tick removal

Christina Due, research scientist[1][2], Wendy Fox, founder of Borreliosis and Associated Diseases Awareness UK[2], Jolyon M Medlock, head of medical entomology[3], Maaike Pietzsch, senior project scientist, medical entomology and zoonoses ecology[3], James G Logan, senior lecturer in medical entomology[1][2]

[1]Department of Disease Control, London School of Hygiene and Tropical Medicine, London, UK

[2]Borreliosis and Associated Diseases Awareness UK (BADA-UK), Wath upon Dearne, Rotherham, UK

[3]Public Health England, Porton Down, Salisbury, UK

Correspondence to: J G Logan James.Logan@lshtm.ac.uk

Cite this as: BMJ 2013;347:f7123

DOI: 10.1136/bmj.f7123

http://www.bmj.com/content/347/bmj.f7123

Ticks are small blood feeding ectoparasites with a global distribution. They are important vectors of disease pathogens including rickettsiae, spirochaetes, and viruses. Prevention of tick attachment and rapid removal reduce the risk of contracting tickborne diseases, and there are many recommendations on how to achieve this. This article aims to review the evidence base for tick bite prevention and tick removal strategies.

What is a tick?

Ticks are arachnids and can be divided into two families known as Ixodidae (hard ticks) and Argasidae (soft ticks). Hard ticks have a shield-like scutum on their dorsal side and visible mouthparts that protrude forward. Soft ticks lack a scutum and their mouthparts are located on the underside and are therefore not visible. Hard ticks have a three stage life cycle, comprising larval, nymph, and adult stages, whereas soft ticks have two or more additional nymph stages. Larval hard ticks are typically 0.5 mm long (the size of a poppy seed) and have six legs. Nymphal ticks are about 1.5 mm long and adult unfed ticks are about 3 mm long, although once fed they can enlarge to 11 mm in length (fig 1). Both nymphs and adults have eight legs. Tick coloration varies between species, sexes, and different stages of engorgement. Unfed ticks can range from black to a red-brown colour, but once engorged they can appear light pink, purple, dark red, or grey-blue.[1] Each life stage requires a blood meal and feeding may occur in spring, summer, or autumn. The soft ticks feed for up to several hours, whereas adult hard ticks, if left undisturbed, can feed for up to one week until engorgement is reached. They then detach and moult to the next lifecycle stage.[2]

What diseases are spread by ticks?

The most widespread human tickborne disease is Lyme borreliosis, which is commonly transmitted to humans by *Ixodes ricinus*, known as the deer/sheep/castor bean tick. In the United Kingdom, Public Health England (PHE) reported 959 laboratory confirmed cases in 2011 (incidence of 1.73/100 000), compared with 268 cases in 2005 (incidence of 0.50/100 000). In the United States, the Centers for Disease Control and Prevention estimated that 30 000 people were diagnosed as having the disease in 2012.[3]

Several other diseases are caused by tickborne pathogens. Tickborne encephalitis is a viral disease (Flaviviridae virus family) that causes 10 000 cases annually across Europe.[4] Rickettsioses are another group of emerging tickborne diseases caused by obligate intracellular bacteria. They include Rocky Mountain spotted fever (*Rickettsia rickettsii* found in the US), Mediterranean spotted fever (*R conorii* found in the Mediterranean), and African tick bite fever (*R africae* found in sub-Saharan Africa and the Caribbean). Since the 1980s, 12 new rickettsial species and subspecies have been described. Furthermore, a new study showed that pathogenic rickettsiae now occur in British ticks.[5][6] Another emerging tickborne disease is babesiosis, which is caused by haematotropic parasites that infect red blood cells. Several species of babesia can cause disease, including *Babesia divergens*, which causes most European cases,[7] although *B microti* is the most prevalent and is found mainly in the US. Furthermore, a new subspecies of *Borrelia* has recently emerged in the UK (*Borrelia miyamotoi*).

How can tick bites be prevented?

The first step to preventing tick bites is to educate people about ticks and the risks of tick infested areas. One theory based educational randomised controlled trial showed that borrelia infections are reduced in people who receive education about ticks.[8] Other randomised controlled trials that assessed the impact of education and prevention concluded that people who receive education about ticks have greater understanding and change their attitude and behaviour to reflect this.[9][10] Therefore, we recommend that medical practitioners, local authorities, and land owners and managers inform the public through appropriate means, such as information leaflets, posters, websites, and signs.

Which repellents are effective against ticks?

Trans-p-methane-3,8-diol (PMD)
Lemon eucalyptus oil, with the active ingredient *trans*-p-methane-3,8-diol (PMD), is highly repellent against ticks, varying from 100% protection five minutes after application to 85-91% after 48 hours (laboratory studies with rabbits' ears).[11][12] Field studies that compared untreated material and material treated with *Corymbia citriodora* oil and a commercial repellent (MyggA Natural)—both of which contain PMD—found a repellency of 74-85% when dragged over a tick infested area. Repellency lasted for several days, although protection was reduced to 42-45% after three to six days.[12][13] A prospective crossover clinical trial that tested Citriodiol (*cis*-and-*trans*-p-methane-3,8-diol) on volunteers found that the mean number of *I ricinus* ticks attached to each person

SUMMARY POINTS (ADVICE FOR PATIENTS)

- When outdoors check for ticks every 2-3 hours and promptly remove them; self examine the body after being in a tick infested area
- Wear appropriate clothing—long trousers with socks tucked in and shirts tucked into trousers
- Use permethrin treated clothing and a repellent containing PMD or DEET in tick infested areas
- Use fine tipped forceps to remove ticks, grasping the tick close to the skin and pulling steadily without twisting
- If bitten, report symptoms such as rash, unexplained headache, facial palsy, or arthralgia to your GP
- If bitten in a Lyme disease endemic area, consult your GP to discuss antibiotic prophylaxis

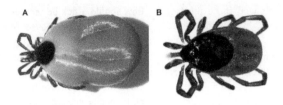

Fig 1 (A) Engorged and (B) unfed female adult *Ixodes ricinus* (hard bodied) tick. Reproduced with permission from Public Health England

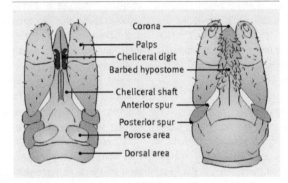

Corona
Palps
Cheliceral digit
Barbed hypostome
Cheliceral shaft
Anterior spur
Posterior spur
Porose area
Dorsal area

Fig 2 Diagram of the mouthparts of a hard bodied tick

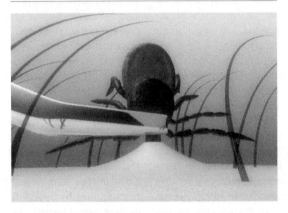

Fig 3 Correct tick removal with fine tipped forceps; reproduced with permission from Sebastian Kaulitzki

was 0.5 to people wearing the repellent compared with 1.5 for controls.[14] PMD is recommended and has the advantage that it can be reapplied as often as necessary because it has little to no demonstrated toxicity. One review suggested that PMD should not be used in children under the age of 3 years, but this was largely because of lack of data on younger patients rather than evidence of toxic effects.[15]

N,N-diethyl-3-methylbenzamide and other synthetic repellents

N,N-diethyl-3-methylbenzamide (DEET) is an effective and widely used insect repellent.[16] However, other than laboratory studies, there is little robust evidence for its efficacy against tick attachment. Laboratory studies that tested DEET against several tick species found that DEET can be effective when used in high concentrations (30%), with a repellency of 80-100%; however, the duration was short and varied from two to five hours.[17 18 19 20 21]

Other synthetic repellents, such as Picaridin and IR3535, that have been tested in laboratory trials generally show a lower efficacy than DEET.[20 22] One exception is Ai3-37220 (a piperdine derivative), which had greater repellency than DEET over a six hour test period in a laboratory study.[21]

Laboratory studies show that DEET can be effective at preventing tick attachment, but efficacy is variable and short. These factors should be considered when using DEET. There has been some public concern over the safety of DEET, but those concerns are largely unfounded. Although toxic effects have been seen when DEET is ingested,[15] there is little evidence of risk associated with the use of topically applied DEET. The use of DEET has been implicated in causing seizures in a small number of children under 8 years,[14] but the US Environmental Protection Agency states that the available data do not support a link between DEET and seizures.[23] A double blind randomised therapeutic trial asked pregnant women in their second and third trimesters to apply DEET on a daily basis and found no adverse neurological, gastrointestinal, or dermatological effects. Furthermore, there were no adverse effects on survival, growth, or development of the fetus at birth and one year later.[24] Patients should follow the recommendations of use stated on the label with regard to application rates.

Does protective clothing prevent tick bites?

A simple preventive measure is to wear protective clothing, although this does not guarantee full protection. This includes wearing boots, long trousers tucked into socks, and long sleeved shirts tucked into trousers.[25] Clothing should be checked for ticks every two to three hours during a trip to tick infested areas and for up to one week after returning home because ticks can remain hidden within clothing and attach later.

How effective is permethrin or DEET impregnated clothing?

The use of topically applied repellents is unlikely to achieve 100% coverage because ticks may still attach and move to unprotected skin. Additional protection can be given through the use of clothing impregnated with a toxic active ingredient. Permethrin is a synthetic pyrethroid insecticide commonly used for clothing, tents, and sleeping bags. It has low toxicity, some repellency, and other physiological effects on ticks including "hot feet" and knockdown (where the arthropod is rendered immobile).[26] In two field studies, clothing that had been dipped or sprayed with permethrin provided 100% protection against all life stages (tick species tested included *I dammini* and *Amblyomma americanum*), whereas DEET provided 86-92% protection. Dipping or spraying can be recommended to protect against ticks. Clothing must be retreated every 20 washes to achieve 100% knockdown after 15 minutes of contact time or more often to achieve 100% knockdown in under 15 minutes.[26 27 28]

The safest and most efficient method is thought to be polymerisation of permethrin into the fibre surface of clothing in the factory.[26] Field studies of clothing treated in this way showed high repellency against ticks, ranging from 93-98%, whereas clothing treated with DEET gave a repellency of 60%. Furthermore, it has a longlasting effect on the fabric and is resistant to washing. In one study, in which impregnated fabric was washed 100 times, 100% knockdown was still achieved with 15 minutes of exposure to *I ricinus* nymphs.[27] One non-randomised open label pilot study that asked outdoor workers to wear permethrin treated clothing for seven months found a 93% reduction in tick bites compared with controls.[29] Permethrin impregnated

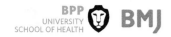

clothing is recommended for people who spend prolonged periods of time in tick infested areas.

How do ticks attach and why is removal important?

To begin feeding, ticks cut through the skin using chelicerae and insert a feeding tube, called a hypostome, into the opening (fig 2). The hypostome is covered with backward facing projections, known as denticles, which anchor the tick on to the host. Some species also secrete a cement-like substance from the salivary glands, which hardens around the mouthparts to form a collar that allows the tick to remain firmly in place. Any cement that is left in the skin may cause an allergic reaction or infection.[30] Tick removal is important to prevent the transmission of infectious agents and localised infection from the tick bite.

How quickly should a tick be removed?

Borrelia burgdorferi sensu lato spirochaetes, which cause Lyme disease, reside and replicate in the midgut epithelium of the tick. When a tick attaches, the spirochaetes migrate to the salivary glands and are then transmitted to the host. Laboratory studies have shown that the risk of contracting Lyme disease is low if a tick has been attached for less that 24-36 hours, the time needed for the bacteria to migrate from the midgut to the salivary glands, and that this time frame is crucial in preventing transmission.[31] [32] The longer the tick feeds the higher the risk of contracting Lyme disease. However, a laboratory transmission study that gave rodents nymph infected feeds found that transmission occurred within 16 hours.[33] Furthermore, this study showed that ticks infected with *B afzelii* start to transmit infection earlier than ticks infected with *B burgdorferi* sensu stricto, suggesting that there is variation within the species complex. Although the evidence for removing a tick within a specific timeframe is not clear, ticks should be removed sooner rather than later. We strongly recommend the use of an appropriate tool for removal. During prolonged travel in known tick infested areas, it is strongly recommended that people always carry a tick removal tool.

Which methods of removal don't work?

Several methods for tick removal have been proposed that supposedly induce the tick to detach itself from the skin owing to lack of oxygen. These include rubbing petroleum jelly, gasoline, fingernail polish, or 70% isopropyl alcohol over the tick's mouthparts, or placing a lit match next to the tick. None of these methods is effective because ticks have a low respiratory rate.[34] Furthermore, using a lighted match could burn the skin or cause the tick to burst and spread potentially infectious fluids. One state-wide cross sectional study in the US investigated risk factors for *B burgdorferi* antibodies and found evidence that the use of gasoline to remove ticks may increase the risk of *B burgdorferi* infection (odds ratio 4.5, 95% confidence interval 1.2 to 17.6).[35] Some studies argue that the method of tick removal does not influence the risk of transmission of *B burgdorferi*. A laboratory study that used various methods for removal saw no difference in squeezing the tick before removing it and pulling steadily.[31] Another laboratory study found that crushing or gently pulling the tick were both equally effective at stopping transmission within a certain time.[36] These methods are not recommended because they do not promptly detach the tick and may increase the chance of the tick regurgitating its stomach contents, thereby facilitating transmission of pathogens.[37]

How should a tick be removed correctly?

Ticks should be removed using fine forceps by steadily pulling the tick upwards (fig 3). PHE, the NHS, and studies that have examined different methods of tick removal all recommend that fine tipped forceps should be used to grasp the tick as close to the skin as possible and then to pull steadily upwards with an even pressure. They do not recommend twisting or jerking the tick because this may break the mouthparts.[38] [39] [40] [41] Furthermore, one study that compared the use of forceps with other methods of tick removal found that forceps protected against *B burgdorferi* and *Rickettsia conorii*. Patients were also protected against infection and complications.[42]

Although forceps are considered the best removal method, some specially designed tick removal tools are also available. However, these tools have been studied only in animals and not yet in humans. One study recruited pet owners through veterinarians and asked them to remove ticks from their pets using four different tick removal tools that were randomly assigned using an intervention grid. A total of 236 ticks were removed by both pet owners and veterinarians. The study concluded that people removing the ticks preferred the tick remover tool (O'Tom Tick Twister) over fine tipped forceps because the ticks were easier to grab and quicker to remove. The tool also used less force for extraction and caused less damage to the ticks mouthparts. Another animal study compared three commercially available tick removal tools (Ticked Off, Pro-Tick Remedy, and Tick Plier) against medium tipped forceps. They concluded that the commercially available tools removed nymphs better than forceps because they removed more cement and caused less damage to tick mouthparts. However, nymphs were still more difficult to remove than adults. The authors of this study recommended commercially available tools over medium tipped forceps because they removed nymphs better.[43] More studies assessing the use of these tools in humans are needed before commercial tick removal tools can be recommended in humans. If a person is inexperienced in removing ticks, tools such as these may be an option for ease of use, but we recommend the use of fine tipped tweezers for tick removal until more evidence is available.[44]

What to do after a tick bite?

People who have been bitten by a tick or spent time outdoors in tick infested areas should look for symptoms associated with Lyme disease. About 60% of patients will experience erythema migrans, a localised bull's eye rash. Other symptoms are unexplained headaches and neck stiffness, flu-like symptoms, facial palsy, arthralgia, heart palpitations, or dizziness within weeks of the tick bite or exposure.[45] [46] People who develop any of these symptoms should notify their general practitioner for a diagnosis and possible treatment. In highly endemic areas, the use of antibiotics can be used as a prophylaxis. A randomised double blind placebo controlled trial found that a 200 mg dose of doxycycline prevented Lyme disease if given within 72 hours of a tick bite.[47]

PHE conducts surveillance of ticks in the UK, and all patients presenting with a tick bite are encouraged to submit the tick to the medical entomology group for identification. It is crucial that tick awareness materials are available within GP surgeries and in nature reserves in areas where ticks are problematic and where Lyme borreliosis is endemic. Understanding the incidence rate of tick bites and

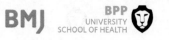

erythema migrans across the UK, and how this is changing over time, is now a priority for PHE.

SOURCES AND SELECTION CRITERIA

We used PubMed and Google Scholar as search engines. Keywords included ticks, *Ixodes ricinus*, tick removal, tick prevention, tick control, impregnated clothing ticks, repellent ticks, natural repellents ticks, DEET ticks, and DEET *Ixodes ricinus*. We aimed to use papers published in the past 20 years but did not exclude older ones if relevant.

ADDITIONAL EDUCATIONAL RESOURCES

Resources for healthcare professionals

• Public Health England (www.hpa.org.uk/Topics/ InfectiousDiseases/InfectionsAZ/LymeDisease/ GeneralInformation/lymoo5GeneralInformation/)—Clear information on Lyme disease and links to other useful websites

• Public Health England (www.hpa.org.uk/Topics/ InfectiousDiseases/InfectionsAZ/LymeDisease/)—Information on Lyme disease, epidemiological data, and Lyme disease diagnostic services in the UK. Patient leaflets and recommendations for diagnosis and treatment across Europe and North America also available

• Public Health England (www.hpa.org.uk/ Topics/InfectiousDiseases/InfectionsAZ/Ticks/ TickPreventionAndRemoval/)—Advice on how to prevent tick bites and minimise ticks in gardens

• US Centers for Disease Control and Prevention (www. cdc.gov/ticks/removing_a_tick.html)—Instructions on tick removal, with a diagram

Resources for patients

• Borreliosis and Associated Diseases Awareness UK (www. bada-uk.org/)—Clear information on many tickborne diseases found in Europe. All of the information is gathered from scientific resources or research

• Patient.co.uk (www.patient.co.uk/health/lyme-disease)— Information on Lyme disease and links to patient support groups and recent articles

---

QUESTIONS FOR FUTURE RESEARCH

• Do different tick species have different sensitivities to repellents or insecticides (such as DEET and permethrin)?

• How effective are DEET and other repellents in field studies when used on human skin?

• How well do commercial tick removal tools work?

Contributors: JGL and WF put forward the topic for this review. CD searched the literature and all authors helped write the review. JGL is guarantor.

Funding: This paper received no funding.

Competing interests: We have read and understood the BMJ Group policy on declaration of interests and declare the following interests: None.

Provenance and peer review: Not commissioned; externally peer reviewed.

1 Hillyard PD. Ticks of north-west Europe. Barnes RSK, Crothers JH, eds. Field Studies Council in association with the Natural History Museum, 1996.

2 Jongejan F, Uilenberg G. The global importance of ticks. *Parasitology* 2004;129:S3-14.

3 Centers for Disease Control and Prevention. Reported cases of Lyme disease by year, United States, 2003-2012. 2013 www.cdc.gov/lyme/ stats/chartstables/casesbyyear.html.

4 Bonnefoy X, Kampen H, Sweeney K. Public health significance of urban pests. WHO, 2008. www.euro.who.int/__data/assets/pdf_ file/0011/98426/E91435.pdf.

5 Tijsse-Klasen E, Hansford KM, Jahfari S, Phipps P, Sprong H, Medlock JM. Spotted fever group rickettsiae in Dermacentor reticulatus and Haemaphysalis punctata ticks in the UK. *Parasit Vectors* 2013;6:212.

6 Parola P. Tick-borne rickettsial diseases: emerging risks in Europe. *Comp Immunol Microbiol Infect Dis* 2004;27:297-304.

7 Homer MJ, Aguilar-Delfin I, Telford SR 3rd, Krause PJ, Persing DH. Babesiosis. *Clin Microbiol Rev* 2000;13:451-69.

8 Daltroy LH, Phillips C, Lew R, Wright E, Shadick NA, Liang MH. A controlled trial of a novel primary prevention program for Lyme disease and other tick-borne illnesses. *Health Educ Behav* 2007;34:531-42.

9 Malouin R, Winch P, Leontsini E, Glass G, Simon D, Hayes EB, et al. Longitudinal evaluation of an educational intervention for preventing tick bites in an area with endemic Lyme disease in Baltimore County, Maryland. *Am J Epidemiol* 2003;157:1039-51.

10 Mowbray F, Richard A, Rubin GJ. Ticking all the boxes? A systematic review on education and communication intervention to prevent tick-borne diseases. *Vector Borne Zoonotic Dis* 2012;12:817-25.

11 Trigg JK, Hill N. Laboratory evaluation of a eucalyptus-based repellent against four biting arthropods. *Phytother Res* 1996;10:313-6.

12 Jaenson TGT, Garboui S, Pålsson K. Repellency of oils of lemon eucalyptus, geranium, and lavender and the mosquito repellent MyggA Natural to Ixodes ricinus (Acari: Ixodidae) in the laboratory and field. *J Med Entomol* 2006;43:731-6.

13 Garboui S, Jaenson TGT, Palsson K. Repellency of MyggA Natural spray (para-menthane 3,8-diol) and RB86 (neem oil) against the tick Ixodes ricinus (Acari: Ixodidae) in the field in east-central Sweden. *Exp Appl Acarol* 2006;40:271-7.

14 Gardulf A, Wohlfart I, Gustafson R. A prospective cross-over field trial shows protection of lemon eucalyptus extract against tick bites. *J Med Entomol* 2004;41:1064-7.

15 Koren G, Matsui D, Bailey B. DEET-based insect repellents: safety implications for children and pregnant and lactating women. *CMAJ* 2003;169:209-12.

16 Brown M, Hebert AA. Insect repellents: an overview. *J Am Acad Dermatol* 1997;36:243-9.

17 Jensenius M, Pretorius A-M, Clarke F, Myrvang B. Repellent efficacy of four commercial DEET lotions against Amblyomma hebraeum (Acari: Ixodidae), the principal vector of Rickettsia africae in southern Africa. *Trans R Soc Trop Med Hyg* 2005;99:708-11.

18 Staub D, Debrunner M, Amsler L, Steffen R. Effectiveness of a repellent containing DEET and EBAAP for preventing tick bites. *Wilderness Environ Med* 2002;13:12-20.

19 Semmler M, Abdel-Ghaffar F. Comparison of tick repellent efficacy of chemical and biological products originating from Europe and the USA. *Parasitol Res* 2011;108:899-904.

20 Pretorius A-M, Jensenius M, Clarke F, Ringertz SH. Repellent efficacy of DEET and KBR 3023 against Amblyomma hebraeum (Acari: Ixodidae). *J Med Entomol* 2003;40:245-8.

21 Solberg VB, Klein TA, Mcpherson KR, Bradford BA, Burge JR, Wirtz RA. Field evaluation of DEET and Piperdine repellent (AI3-37220) against Amblyomma americanum (Acari: Ixodidae). *J Med Entomol* 1995;32:870-5.

22 Stafford KC. Tick bite prevention and the use of insect repellents. 2005. www.ct.gov/caes/lib/caes/documents/publications/fact_sheets/ tickbiteprevention05.pdf.

23 US Environmental Protection Agency. Reregistration eligibility decision (RED) for DEET. 1998. www.epa.gov/oppsrrd1/REDs/0002red.pdf.

24 McGready R, Hamilton KA, Simpson JA, Cho T, Luxemburger C, Edwards R, et al. Safety of the insect repellent N,N-diethyl-M-toluamide (DEET) in pregnancy. *Am J Trop Med Hyg* 2001;65:285-9.

25 Piesman J, Lars E. Prevention of tick-borne diseases. *Annu Rev Entomol* 2008;53:23-43.

26 Faulde M, Uedelhoven W, Maleruis M, Robbins RG. Factory-based Permethrin impregnation of uniforms: residual activity against Aedes aegypti and Ixodes ricinus in battle dress uniforms worn under field conditions, and cross-contamination during the laundering and storage process. *Milit Med* 2006;171:472-7.

27 Faulde MK, Uedelhoven WM, Robbins RG. Contact toxicity and residual activity of different permethrin-based fabric impregnation methods for Aedes aegypti (Diptera: Culicidae), Ixodes ricinus (Acari: Ixodidae), and Lepisma saccharina (Thysanura: Lepismatidae). *J Med Entomol* 2003;40:935-41.

28 Faulde M, Uedelhoven W. A new clothing impregnation method for personal protection against ticks and biting insects. *Int J Med Microbiol* 2006;296(suppl 1):225-9.

29 Vaughn WK, Meshnick SR. Pilot study assessing the effectiveness of long-lasting permethrin-impregnated clothing for the prevention of tick bites. *Vector Borne Zoonotic Dis* 2011;11:869-75.

30 Pitches DW. Removal of ticks: a review of the literature. *Euro Surveill* 2006;11:E0608174.

31 Kahl O, Janetzki-Mittmann C, Gray JS, Jonas R, Stein J, de Boer R. Risk of infection with Borrelia burgdorferi sense lato for a host in relation to the duration of nymphal Ixodes ricinus feeding and the method of tick removal. *Zentralblatt für Bakteriologie* 1998;287:41-52.

32 Radolf JD, Caimano MJ, Stevenson B, Hu LT. Of ticks, mice and men: understanding the dual-host lifestyle of Lyme disease spirochaetes. *Nat Rev Micro* 2012;10:87-99.

33 Crippa M, Rais O, Gern L. Investigations on the mode and dynamics of transmission and infectivity of Borrelia burgdorferi Sensu Stricto and Borrelia afzelii in Ixodes ricinus ticks. *Vector Borne Zoonotic Dis* 2002;2:3-9.

34 De Boer R, Van den Bogaard AE. Removal of attached nymphs and adults of Ixodes ricinus (Acari: Ixodidae). *J Med Entomol* 1993;30:748-52.

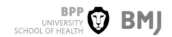

35 Schwartz BS, Goldstein MD. Lyme disease in outdoor workers: risk factors, preventative measures and tick removal methods. *Am J Epidemiol* 1990;131:877-85.

36 Piesman J, Dolan MC. Protection against Lyme disease spirochete transmission provided by prompt removal of nymphal Ixodes scapularis (Acari: Ixodidae). *J Med Entomol* 2002;39:509-12.

37 Connat J-L. Demonstration of regurgitation of gut content during blood meals of the tick Ornithodoros moubata. *Parasitol Res* 1991;77:452-4.

38 NHS Choices. Insect bites and stings. Treatments. 2012. www.nhs.uk/Conditions/Bites-insect/Pages/Treatment.aspx.

39 Centers for Disease Control and Prevention. Tick removal. 2011. www.cdc.gov/lyme/removal/index.html.

40 Needham GR. Evaluation of five popular methods for tick removal. *Pediatrics* 1985;75:997-1002.

41 Bowles DE, McHugh CP, Spraling SL. Evaluation of devices for removing attached Rhipicephalus sanguineus (Acari: Ixodidae). *J Med Entomol* 1992;30:748-52.

42 Oteo JA, Martinez de Artola, V, Gómez-Cadiñanos R, Casas JM, Blanco JR, Rosel L. Evaluation of methods of tick removal in human ixodidiasis. *Rev Clin Esp* 1996;196:584-7.

43 Stewart RL, Burgdorfer W, Needham GR. Evaluation of three commercial tick removal tools. *Wilderness Environment Med* 1998;9:137-42.

44 Zenner L, Drevon-Gaillot E, Callait-Cardinal MP. Evaluation of four manual tick-removal devices for dogs and cats. *Vet Rec* 2006;159:526-9.

45 Centers for Disease Control and Prevention. Signs and symptoms of Lyme disease. 2013. www.cdc.gov/lyme/signs_symptoms/index.html.

46 O'Connell S. Lyme disease in the UK: epidemiology, clinical presentations and diagnosis. *J Med Microbiol* 1994;40:77-8.

47 Nadelman RB, Nowakowski J, Fish D, Falco RC, Freeman K, McKenna D, et al. Prophylaxis with single-dose doxycycline for the prevention of Lyme disease after an Ixodes scapularis tick bite. *N Engl J Med* 2001;345:79-84.

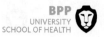

Bed bug infestation

Celine Bernardeschi, dermatologist[1], Laurence Le Cleach, dermatologist[1],
Pascal Delaunay, parasitologist-entomologist[2], Olivier Chosidow, professor of dermatology[1] [3]

[1]AP-HP, Groupe Hospitalier Henri-Mondor, Department of Dermatology, Créteil, France

[2]Laboratoire de Parasitologie-Mycologie, Hôpital de l'Archet, Centre Chospitalier Universitaire de Nice-Université de Nice-Sophia Antipolis/Inserm U1065, Nice, France

[3]UPEC-Université Paris Est-Créteil Val-de-Marne, France

Correspondence to: O Chosidow, Service de Dermatologie, Hôpital Henri-Mondor, 51, avenue du Maréchal-de-Lattre-de-Tassigny, 94010 Créteil Cedex, France olivier.chosidow@hmn.aphp.fr

Cite this as: BMJ 2013;346:f138

DOI: 10.1136/bmj.f138

http://www.bmj.com/content/346/bmj.f138

Bed bugs are bloodfeeding insects that seem to be resurging in developed countries,[1] possibly due to international travel and changes in pest control practices.[2] Diagnosis of bed bug infestation relies on clinical manifestations of bites and direct observation of the arthropod, which is rarely recognised by those who are bitten.[3] Evidence is lacking on the bed bug's capacity to transmit disease, management of eradication, and the economic impact of infestations. This summary of the available evidence on the diagnosis and management of bed bug infestation aims to help general practitioners identify the clinical signs of bed bug bites and help patients identify and manage infestations.

What are bed bugs?

The two main species of bed bugs are *Cimex lectularius* and *Cimex hemipterus*, which are found in temperate areas and tropical zones, respectively. They are brown, wingless, flat, 2-5 mm long insects that resemble apple seeds. If in doubt, contact an entomologist for precise identification. The bugs have a multi-stage developmental life cycle and require a human blood meal every 3-5 days to progress from one stage to another (fig 1).[1] After contamination by a few bed bugs, their number increases exponentially. They can survive for one year without eating.

Where are bed bugs found?

Over the past 10 years, bed bugs—which had almost disappeared after the second world war—have increasingly been found in low budget and upmarket hotels, hostels, bed and breakfasts, private homes, night trains, cruise ships, and even nursing homes.[1] [4]

Bed bugs are usually transported passively, mainly in clothing and luggage, but also on furniture (such as mattresses). Less commonly, they spread actively from room to room in communities, mostly through electric wiring or ventilation ducts. During the day they hide in dark places—such as spaces under baseboards, loose or peeling wallpaper, and crevices in furniture and mattresses—and they feed at night. They fear light and usually avoid smooth or glossy surfaces, such as tiles.[2] Despite being easily visible, most people cannot recognise bed bugs—in a survey conducted in three counties in the United Kingdom, only 10% of 358 people identified them from pictures (fig 2).[3]

SUMMARY POINTS

- Bed bug infestation seems to be re-emerging worldwide
- The diagnosis of bed bug infestation starts with consultation for clinical reactions to bites but symptoms vary greatly
- Suspect bed bug bites whenever a patient consults for papules positioned in groups of three or four bites forming a "breakfast-lunch-dinner" curve or line
- Eradication requires patient education and the help of pest eradication professionals to identify pests and perform non-chemical and chemical interventions

How common are bed bug infestations?

The idea of a resurgence is based on Australian and European observational studies that have shown increases in pest manager interventions (700% increase between 1997-2000 and 2001-04 in Australia, 100% rise from 2002 (383 cases) to 2006 (770 cases) in Sweden). There were also increases in calls received about bed bugs in two London boroughs between 2000 (87 calls) and 2006 (334 calls), and more inquiries about species (nine samples of bed bugs submitted to the Department of Medical Entomology, Institute of Clinical Pathology and Westmead Hospital, Sydney, Australia in 1997 compared with 37 samples in 2000). The identification of bed bugs in Australian laboratories also increased between 2001 and 2004 as did the number of bed bugs intercepted by Australian customs officials between 1999 and 2003.[5] [6] [7]

The reasons for this resurgence are unknown. Contributing factors may include increased domestic and international travel.[8] As a consequence, bed bugs, which were most common among the disadvantaged social classes in the first half of the last century, can now be encountered in all economic contexts. Other factors are enhanced resistance to pyrethroid insecticides,[2] [9] perhaps because of multiple mutations conferring metabolic resistance,[10] and the fact that newer techniques for controlling cockroaches with bait do not kill bed bugs.[11]

What are the symptoms of bed bug infestation?

Because bed bugs feed at night and inject an anaesthetic when biting, the initial bite is not felt and most patients have no reaction; moreover, symptom onset, caused by allergic reactions to saliva, can be delayed.[2] In 2009, an ethics committee approved experiment,[12] conducted by laboratory scientists who volunteered to be bitten by bed bugs placed on their arms, confirmed that reactions to bites manifest up to 11 days later. In a recent questionnaire based study, only 30% of people living in bed bug infested households reported skin reactions.[13]

A 2009 systematic review of 18 articles on clinical reactions to bed bug bites reported the most common reactions to be 2-5 mm pruritic maculopapular lesions with a central haemorrhagic punctum, corresponding to the bite site, that are usually located on uncovered areas of the body.[2] Skin lesions, such as three or four bites forming a curve or line ("breakfast-lunch-dinner alignment," fig 3A), are suggestive of but not specific to bed bugs. Other cutaneous symptoms include isolated pruritis, papules, nodules (fig 3B), and bullous eruptions (fig 3C).[14]

Some isolated case reports have reported systemic reactions, such as diffuse urticaria (fig 3D), asthma, and anaphylaxis.[2] Bed bug infestation is usually looked for after a clinical diagnosis of bed bug bites. Similar symptoms in people sharing a bed, onset of the lesions after travelling or sleeping away from home, detection of bed bug faecal matter (small dark marks) in or around the bed, or disappearance of symptoms after changing sleeping place should trigger suspicion of infestation. However, the discovery of bed bugs on site confirms active infestation.

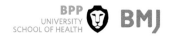

Bed bug bites versus other arthropod bites: main clinical and epidemiological features*

Arthropod	Clinical features on examination	Location	Timing of pruritus	Context
Bed bugs	3-4 bites in a line or curve	Uncovered areas	Morning	Travelling
Fleas	3-4 bites in a line or curve	Legs and buttocks	Daytime	Pet owners or rural living
Mosquitoes	Non-specific urticarial papules	Potentially anywhere	*Anopheles* spp night; *Culex* spp night; *Aedes* spp day	Worldwide distribution
Head lice[32]	Live lice on the head associated with itchy, scratched lesions	Scalp, ears, and neck	Any	Children, parents, or contact with children
Body lice[32]	Excoriated papules and hyperpigmentation; live lice inside clothes	Back	Any	Homeless people, developing countries
Sarcoptes scabiei mites (scabies)[32]	Vesicles, burrows, nodules and non-specific secondary lesions	Interdigital spaces, forearms, breasts, genitalia	Night	Sexually transmitted, households or institutions
Ticks	Erythema migrans or ulcer	Potentially anywhere	Asymptomatic	Pet owners or hikers
Pyemotes ventricosus	Comet sign,[33] a linear erythematous macular tract	Under clothes	Any time when inside habitat	People exposed to woodworm contaminated furniture (*P ventricosus* is a woodworm parasite)
Spiders	Necrosis (uncommon)	Face and arms	Immediate pain, no itching	Rural living

It is difficult to diagnose a bite. Diagnosis relies on an array of arguments, none of which is specific by itself; it is the association of elements that is suggestive. Any arthropod bite can be totally asymptomatic.

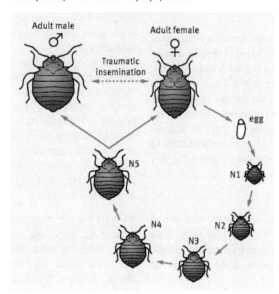

Fig 1 The life cycle of the bed bug (adapted from Delaunay and colleagues[1])

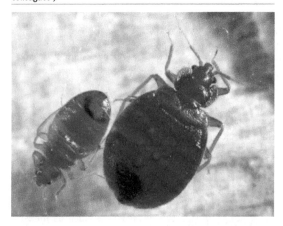

Fig 2 Bed bug nymph (1-4 mm) and adult (5-7 mm): *Cimex lectularius*

What are the differential diagnoses of bed bug bites?

The most common differential diagnoses are other arthropod bites,[15] especially those of fleas, which form similar three or four bite lines or curves. Scabies can be confounding but differs from bed bug bites by the absence of visible puncta and the predominance of scratching in sites such as forearms, nipples, and genitals (table 1).

In addition to arthropod bites, there are several dermatological differential diagnoses.[16] These include erythema multiforme, which is characterised by target lesions on the extremities, and, sometimes, mucous membrane erosions; Sweet's syndrome or acute febrile neutrophilic dermatosis, which includes papulonodular lesions on the extremities associated with general symptoms, such as arthralgias, fever, and leucocytosis; bullous dermatitis, which can affect the mucous cavities and unlike bed bug bites, can be seen on covered areas of the body; and vasculitis, which is characterised by polymorphous lesions, usually on the lower limbs, and sometimes affecting several organs. When such manifestations are seen, refer the patient to a dermatologist for further investigations, including a skin biopsy, if necessary.

What complications can arise from bed bug infestations?

Scratching can cause secondary infection—usually *Staphylococcus aureus* or *Streptococcus* spp—of skin lesions (usually impetigo).[17]

Evidence for disease transmission is less clear. Some pathogens have been detected in or on bed bugs. These include hepatitis B virus, *Trypanosoma cruzi*,[1] hepatitis C virus,[18] HIV,[2] *Aspergillus* spp, and, more recently, meticillin resistant *S aureus*,[19] but no study has yet demonstrated their vectorial role—their capacity to transmit diseases to humans.[1]

The psychological burden of bed bug infestation remains to be evaluated.

Although the economic impact is not known, bed bugs result in loss of productivity and costs include those of pest managers' interventions and replacement of infested furniture.[11]

How are bed bug infestations managed?

Bed bug control is difficult, mainly because of the parasite's hiding behaviour, and also because chemical and non-chemical technologies need to be combined for optimal effect.[1] "Integrated pest management (IPM)" combines detection of the pest with non-chemical and chemical elimination strategies.

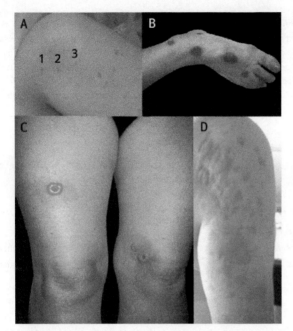

Fig 3 Clinical manifestations of bed bug bites: three or four skin lesions are often seen in a "breakfast (1), lunch (2), dinner (3)" distribution (A) or "wheel" distribution (B). Atypical bullous lesions (C) and urticaria (D)

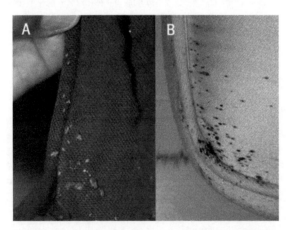

Fig 4 To educate patients to the "search and destroy" strategy, GPs should show them pictures of (A) bed bugs and their typical hideouts and (B) bed bug faecal traces on the mattress

A randomised study conducted in 16 highly infested dwellings, divided into two groups, compared IPM using traps containing a killing agent and chemical treatment with diatomaceous earth dust (D-IPM) versus IPM in which bed bugs were sprayed with chlorfenapyr (S-IPM) but traps were not used.[20] Both groups received patient targeted information provided by a brochure. They were also given advice on searching mattresses for hiding bugs; laundering bed linens weekly; and steaming floors, bed frames, sofas, and other infested furniture and sites. Insecticides were applied every two weeks over 10 weeks. Bed bug counts decreased by 97.6% and 89.7% after the intervention in the S-IPM and D-IPM groups, respectively.

Such eradication strategies were grouped together in documents called "Codes of practice" written by experts in Europe, the United States, and Australia,[21] but their use, although recommended by some municipalities, is not mandatory.

How should bed bug bites be treated?

Guidelines based on expert opinions recommend treating the symptoms of bed bug bites with topical steroids (such as hydrocortisone 1%) once or twice a day for no longer than seven days.[22] Prescribe systemic antihistamines only when pruritis is associated with sleeping difficulties.[22] Antibiotics, either topical (such as mupirocin or fusidic acid three times a day for 7-10 days) or systemic, might be needed for secondary impetigo, depending on its severity.[23]

How can bed bugs be identified and eradicated?

Patient education

Professionals need to educate patients on how to identify bed bugs and prevent spread (box). GPs can educate patients to use a "search and destroy" strategy by providing basic knowledge about the parasite. They should stress that each insect needs to bite a human every three to five days to grow and reproduce but can survive for one year without feeding, and how to detect and identify the arthropod (fig 4A) or its faecal traces (fig 4B) in suspected areas, mostly mattresses and cracks and crevices in wooden furniture. This detection strategy should be applied whenever travelling.

Non-chemical intervention

Small case series suggest that washing at 60°C, tumble drying at 40°C, or dry cleaning is effective against all life stages.[24] A recent trial also suggested that freezing can be used to decontaminate infested clothing.[24] However, because bed bugs can survive for up to one year without feeding, keeping an infested room vacant is not an effective option.[1] Disposal of highly infested items, together with physical removal of bed bugs and mattress covers and vacuuming, are recommended by pest managers' codes of practice,[21] even though scientific evidence of their efficacy is lacking.

The silicates (mostly diatomaceous earth dust) are somewhere between non-chemical and chemical treatments, and require further investigation before being used in pest management programmes.[20]

Chemical treatment

Although insecticides can be bought in supermarkets and on the internet, for efficacy and safety reasons they must be used only by professionals. Clinicians should be aware that misuse of insecticides may have clinical consequences. The Centers for Disease Control and Prevention recently identified 111 cases of illness attributed to insecticide misuse in an attempt to control bed bugs.[25] Pyrethroids were implicated in 89% of those events and caused neurological, respiratory, and gastrointestinal symptoms.

The three main groups of currently used insecticides for bed bug infestations are pyrethroids (the most common),[26] insect growth regulators, and carbamates. The organophosphates, like dichlorvos, are no longer used in Europe except in impregnated strips.[27] Several large well conducted experimental studies have found high levels of bed bug resistance to all available products.[9][28] Moreover, product formulation may influence their efficacy—a laboratory study showed that pyrethroid dusts kill bed bugs more effectively than sprays.[29]

Because of different resistance levels among bed bugs, a combination of insecticides should be applied to all harbourage areas: mattress seams; cracks in furniture, box

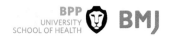

SOURCES AND SELECTION CRITERIA

We focused on articles published since October 2008 to update Goddard and colleagues' systematic review.[2] We searched PubMed and Embase databases until July 2012, using the search terms "bedbugs [Mesh] OR bed bugs OR bed bug OR Cimex". We also manually searched textbooks, newspapers, and websites, mainly those listed by the Centers for Disease Control and Prevention (www.cdc.gov/nceh/ehs/topics/bedbugs.htm). Our selection criteria were case reports on more than five patients, and results related to humans in the field of prevention and elimination of bed bugs or clinical manifestations of their bites.

PATIENT EDUCATION

Detection

- Look for brown insects no bigger than apple seeds on the mattress, sofa, and curtains and in darker places in the room (especially cracks in the walls, crevices in box springs, and furniture)
- Look for black spots on the mattress or blood traces on the sheets

Elimination

- Contact a pest management company
- Wash clothes at 60°C or freeze delicate clothing, vacuum, and clean your home before the pest manager visits
- Collaborate with professionals who are used to dealing with bed bug infestation to increase eradication efficacy

Prevention

- Carefully examine secondhand furniture to assure the absence of bed bugs before purchase so as not to contaminate your home
- When sleeping in a hotel, even an upmarket establishment, lift mattresses to look for bed bugs or black spots
- Do not leave luggage in dark places, near furniture, or close to your bed. Before going to bed, close suitcases and put them in the bathroom—in the bathtub or shower stall

---

TIPS FOR NON-SPECIALISTS

- Inform patients who are about to travel of the resurgence of bed bugs and teach them how to recognise the arthropod
- Suspect bed bug infestations in patients who consult for pruritic linear papules, especially when similar symptoms are found in people sharing a bed, and onset of the lesions after travelling or sleeping away from home Look for atypical skin reactions (blisters, crusts, necrosis) or general symptoms (fever) that may justify skin biopsy or further dermatological investigations
- Encourage infested patients to call a pest manager as soon as the pest has been identified
- Prescribe a mild potency topical steroid treatment once or twice a day for seven days to treat symptomatic bed bug bites

---

ADDITIONAL EDUCATIONAL RESOURCES

Resources for healthcare professionals

- University of Kentucky (www.ca.uky.edu/entomology/entfacts/entfactpdf/ef636.pdf)—Comprehensive lesson on bed bugs
- Centers for Disease Control and Prevention (www.cdc.gov/nceh/ehs/topics/bedbugs.htm)—Link to various articles on bed bugs
- NHS Choices (http://nhs.uk/conditions/bites-insect/pages/introduction.aspx)—Clinical knowledge summary about insect bites

Resources for patients

- Easing bedbug anxiety: what you need to know about the recent bedbug resurgence. *Harvard's Women's Health Watch* 2011;18:7
- Up to Date (www.uptodate.com/contents/bedbugs?source=search_result&search=bedbugs&selectedTitle=1~10)—Provides accurate general knowledge about bed bugs
- Bed-Bugs.co.uk (http://bed-bugs.co.uk/)—Provides an interesting picture gallery of bed bugs and their bites, together with practical tips for eradication
- Pest Control UK (www.pestcontrol-uk.org/pests/bed-bugs)—DIY control of bed bugs

---

QUESTIONS FOR FUTURE RESEARCH

- What are the risk factors for bed bug infestation?
- What are the psychological complications of bed bug bites?
- Can bed bugs transmit diseases to humans?
- What is the best eradication strategy?
- What are the mechanisms of pesticide resistance?
- Are prevention approaches (sniffing dogs, resin strips, traps) effective?

---

springs, and bed frames; peeling wallpaper; and under carpets and floorboards.[21]

It is unclear how often these techniques should be applied, but because insecticides have a limited ovicidal effect, expert guidelines recommend a second look by the pest manager, with eventual retreatment 4-20 days after the first intervention. The length of this waiting time depends on the average temperature of the infested site.

How can infestation be prevented?

Evidence is lacking about the effectiveness of prevention procedures. Experts recommend washing mattress encasement and bed linens at temperatures above 60°C,[21] and advise against purchasing second hand mattresses or furniture. However, it is not recommended that mattresses are pretreated with insecticides or preventive insecticide applications.

Early detection of the bed bugs may be an effective way to prevent their spread. Notably, experimental studies have shown the efficacy of bed bug traps in attracting the parasites, especially when combined with carbon dioxide and heat,[30] but their ability to control infestation without the addition of chemical techniques has not been assessed. Results of a comparative study indicated that canine detection may be an option but is operator dependent,[31] and further evaluation of this method is needed.

Acknowledgments: Thanks to Tu-Anh Duong, Arnaud Canet, Sebastien Larréché, and Pierre Wolkenstein for their collaboration and Janet Jacobson for editorial assistance.

Contributors: OC conceived the project, which was drafted by CB and revised by all authors. OC finally approved the article. All authors are guarantors.

Funding: No special funding received.

Competing interests: All authors have completed the ICMJE uniform disclosure form at www.icmje.org/coi_disclosure.pdf (available on request from the corresponding author) and declare: no support from any organisation for the submitted work; no financial relationships with any organisations that might have an interest in the submitted work in the previous three years; no other relationships or activities that could appear to have influenced the submitted work.

Provenance and peer review: Not commissioned; externally peer reviewed.

1   Delaunay P, Blanc V, Del Giudice P, Levy-Bencheton A, Chosidow O, Marty P, et al. Bedbugs and infectious diseases. *Clin Infect Dis* 2011;52:200-10.
2   Goddard J, deShazo R. Bed bugs (Cimex lectularius) and clinical consequences of their bites. *JAMA* 2009;301:1358-66.
3   Reinhardt K, Harder A, Holland S, Hooper J, Leake-Lyall C. Who knows the bed bug? Knowledge of adult bed bug appearance increases with people's age in three counties of Great Britain. *J Med Entomol* 2008;45:956-8.
4   Delaunay P, Blanc V, Dandine M, Del Giudice P, Franc M, Pomares-Estran C, et al. Bedbugs and healthcare-associated dermatitis, France. *Emerging Infect Dis* 2009;15:989-90.
5   Doggett S, Greary M, Russell R. The resurgence of bed bugs in Australia. *Environ Health* 2004;4:30-8.
6   Richards L, Boase CJ, Gezan S, Cameron MM. Are bed bug infestations on the increase within Greater London. *J Environ Health Res* 2009;9:17-22.
7   Kilpinen O, Vagn Jensen KM, Kristensen M. Bed bug problems in Denmark, with a European perspective. In Robinson WH, Bajomi D, eds. Proceedings of the 6th International Conference on Urban Pests. OOK-Press Kft, 2008:395-9.
8   US Department of Health and Human Services. Joint statement on bed bug control in the United States from the US Centers for Disease Control and Prevention (CDC) and the US Environmental Protection Agency (EPA). 2010. www.cdc.gov/nceh/ehs/publications/bed_bugs_cdc-epa_statement.htm.
9   Tawatsin A, Thavara U, Chompoosri J, Phusup Y, Jonjang N, Khumsawads C, et al. Insecticide resistance in bedbugs in Thailand and laboratory evaluation of insecticides for the control of Cimex hemipterus and Cimex lectularius (Hemiptera: Cimicidae). *J Med Entomol* 2011;48:1023-30.
10 Zhu F, Wigginton J, Romero A, Moore A, Ferguson K, Palli R, et al. Widespread distribution of knockdown resistance mutations in the bed bug, Cimex lectularius (Hemiptera: Cimicidae), populations in the United States. *Arch Insect Biochem Physiol* 2010;73:245-57.
11 Doggett SL, Dwyer DE, Peñas PF, Russell RC. Bed bugs: clinical relevance and control options. *Clin Microbiol Rev* 2012;25:164-92.
12 Reinhardt K, Kempke D, Naylor RA, Siva-Jothy MT. Sensitivity to bites by the bedbug, Cimex lectularius. *Med Vet Entomol* 2009;23:163-6.
13 Potter Mf, Haynes KF, Connelly K. The sensitivity spectrum: human reactions to bed bug bites. *Pest Control Technol* 2010;38:70-4.
14 DeShazo RD, Feldlaufer MF, Mihm MC Jr, Goddard J. Bullous reactions to bedbug bites reflect cutaneous vasculitis. *Am J Med* 2012;125:688-94.
15 Steen CJ, Carbonaro PA, Schwartz RA. Arthropods in dermatology. *J Am Acad Dermatol* 2004;50:819-42.
16 Rook A, Burns T. Rook's textbook of dermatology. Wiley-Blackwell, 2010.
17 Heukelbach J, Hengge UR. Bed bugs, leeches and hookworm larvae in the skin. *Clin Dermatol* 2009;27:285-90.
18 Silverman AL, Qu LH, Blow J, Zitron IM, Gordon SC, Walker ED. Assessment of hepatitis B virus DNA and hepatitis C virus RNA in the common bedbug (Cimex lectularius L.) and kissing bug (Rodnius prolixus). *Am J Gastroenterol* 2001;96:2194-8.
19 Lowe CF, Romney MG. Bedbugs as vectors for drug-resistant bacteria. *Emerging Infect Dis* 2011;17:1132-4.
20 Wang C, Gibb T, Bennett GW. Evaluation of two least toxic integrated pest management programs for managing bed bugs (Heteroptera: Cimicidae) with discussion of a bed bug intercepting device. *J Med Entomol* 2009;46:566-71.
21 Doggett SL; Australian Environmental Pest Managers Association. A code of practice for the control of bed bug infestations in Australia. Westmead Hospital, 2011. www.medent.usyd.edu.au/bedbug/bedbug_cop.htm.
22 Management of simple insect bites: where's the evidence? *Drug Ther Bull* 2012;50:45-8.
23 Koning S, van der Sande R, Verhagen AP, van Suijlekom-Smit LWA, Morris AD, Butler CC, et al. Interventions for impetigo. *Cochrane Database Syst Rev* 2012;1:CD003261.
24 Naylor RA, Boase CJ. Practical solutions for treating laundry infested with Cimex lectularius (Hemiptera: Cimicidae). *J Econ Entomol* 2010;103:136-9.
25 Centers for Disease Control and Prevention (CDC). Acute illnesses associated with insecticides used to control bed bugs-seven states, 2003-2010. *Morb Mortal Wkly Rep* 2011;60:1269-74.
26 Davies TGE, Field LM, Williamson MS. The re-emergence of the bed bug as a nuisance pest: implications of resistance to the pyrethroid insecticides. *Med Vet Entomol* 2012;26:241-54.
27 Lehnert MP, Pereira RM, Koehler PG, Walker W, Lehnert MS. Control of Cimex lectularius using heat combined with dichlorvos resin strips. *Med Vet Entomol* 2011;25:460-4.
28 Kilpinen O, Kristensen M, Jensen K-MV. Resistance differences between chlorpyrifos and synthetic pyrethroids in Cimex lectularius population from Denmark. *Parasitol Res* 2011;109:1461-4.
29 Romero A, Potter MF, Haynes KF. Bed bugs; are dusts the bed bug bullet? *Pest Manag Prof* 2011;77:22-30.
30 Wang C, Gibb T, Bennett GW, McKnight S. Bed bug (Heteroptera: Cimicidae) attraction to pitfall traps baited with carbon dioxide, heat, and chemical lure. *J Econ Entomol* 2009;102:1580-5.
31 Wang C, Cooper R. Detection tools and techniques. *Pest Control Technol* 2011;39:72, 74, 76, 78-9.
32 Chosidow O. Scabies and pediculosis. *Lancet* 2000;355:819-26.
33 Del Giudice P, Blanc-Amrane V, Bahadoran P, Caumes E, Marty P, Lazar M, et al. Pyemotes ventricosus dermatitis, southeastern France. *Emerg Infect Dis* 2008;14:1759-61.

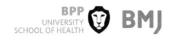

Management of sharps injuries in the healthcare setting

Anna Riddell, specialist registrar in infectious diseases and virology[1], Ioana Kennedy, consultant occupational health physician[2], C Y William Tong, consultant virologist and honorary reader[1][3]

[1]Department of Infection, Barts Health NHS Trust, London E1 2ES, UK

[2]Occupational Health Service, Guy's and St Thomas' NHS Foundation Trust, London, UK

[3]Blizard Institute, Barts and the London School of Medicine and Dentistry, Queen Mary University of London, London, UK

Correspondence to: C Y William Tong
william.tong@nhs.net

Cite this as: BMJ 2015;351:h3733

DOI: 10.1136/bmj.h3733

http://www.bmj.com/content/351/bmj.h3733

Sharps injuries are common in the healthcare setting. Between 2004 and 2013 a total of 4830 healthcare associated occupational exposures to body fluid were reported in the UK, 71% of these for percutaneous injuries.[1] As the reporting system is likely to have recorded only cases with an important exposure, the actual burden of sharps injuries is likely to be much higher. Healthcare workers need to be familiar with immediate management both for themselves if they become injured and for assisting injured colleagues. Many healthcare workers do not know how to manage a sharps injury,[2] particularly if this occurs out of hours. This review presents a summary of the immediate management of sharps injuries and outlines the risk assessment and management strategies to prevent the transmission of HIV, hepatitis B virus, and hepatitis C virus.

What is a sharps injury?

A sharps injury occurs when a sharp object such as a needle, a scalpel, bone fragments, or teeth penetrate(s) the skin. A splash of body fluid to mucous membrane or non-intact skin is another form of exposure to body fluids that could have a similar consequence.

Where do sharps injuries occur?

Healthcare related sharps injuries are not confined to hospitals, with 3-7% occurring outside.[1] The most commonly reported injuries are associated with venepuncture. Injuries to nurses and healthcare assistants accounted for 42% of all reports, whereas doctors and dental professions accounted for 41% and 5%, respectively.[1] Worryingly, ancillary healthcare workers without direct patient contact were also injured by inappropriate disposal of sharps.

What are the risks associated with sharps injuries?

Apart from the trauma of the injury itself, a major concern with sharps injuries is the risk of infection. In Western countries the three most common blood borne infections usually associated with transmission through sharps injuries are HIV, hepatitis B virus, and hepatitis C virus. Rarely, other infections such as malaria,[3] human T cell leukaemia viruses (types I and II),[4] and haemorrhagic fever viruses, such as Ebola virus,[5] may be implicated. The risks of transmission of hepatitis B virus (when positive for HB e antigen), hepatitis C virus, and HIV through sharps injuries are often quoted as 1:3, 1:30, and 1:300, respectively.[6][7] Mucosal exposure to body fluid carries a much lower risk (<1:1000 for HIV).[7]

The actual risk of transmission during an incident depends on several factors, such as the type of injury, the viral load of the source patient, the immune status of the recipient, and risk reduction strategies implemented in the healthcare setting. Since 1997 there has only been one documented case in the UK of HIV seroconversion in a healthcare worker after an occupational exposure.[8] Despite hepatitis B virus being highly infectious, no transmission by sharps injuries has been reported in the UK in the past 10 years. This probably relates to the high percentage of healthcare workers who are immunised against hepatitis B virus. Hepatitis C virus is most commonly associated with sharps injuries, with the virus involved in 50% of all reported cases. Since 1997 a total of 21 hepatitis C virus seroconversions in healthcare workers have been reported in the UK.[1]

As these infections have a relatively long incubation period, of as much as 3-6 months, the psychological impact and associated anxiety of potential infection during the follow-up period should not be underestimated.[9]

What should be done immediately after a sharps injury?

First aid should be performed on-site immediately after a sharps injury (box 1).

How is a risk assessment performed?

Prompt reporting of injuries is necessary so that a risk assessment can be carried out urgently by an appropriately trained individual (other than the exposed worker) who is familiar with the local management pathway. The arrangement for the provision of post-exposure advice varies between hospitals and time of day. All healthcare workers should be familiar with local policy.

The first step in risk assessment is to establish the type of injury (box 2). In the case of bites, it is important to establish whether the source patient has been bleeding from the mouth—for example, from a fight.

The next step is to consider the body fluid involved (box 3). An exposure is considered clinically important if the injury carries a risk and the body fluid is considered high risk. Where the injury does not carry a risk or the body fluid is not high risk, no further action is required other than a review of vaccine history for hepatitis B virus and the offer of vaccination if indicated.[12] The risk of transmission of a blood borne virus is related to the volume of blood transferred; thus hollow bore needles carry more risk than solid instruments. A case-control study identified high risk

THE BOTTOM LINE

- First aid should be undertaken as soon as possible and a risk assessment needs to be carried out urgently by an appropriately trained individual
- If post-exposure prophylaxis is deemed necessary this should begin as soon as possible without waiting for the test results of the source patient
- Post-exposure prophylaxis using antiretroviral drugs within the hour after injury can considerably reduce the risk of HIV transmission
- Hepatitis B vaccine is highly effective in the prevention of hepatitis B; all healthcare workers should be immunised against the virus
- Despite the lack of post-exposure prophylaxis to hepatitis C, such exposure should be followed up vigorously as treatment has a high success rate

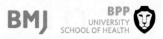

BOX 1 IMMEDIATE FIRST AID AFTER EXPOSURE TO BODY FLUID (BASED ON UK GUIDELINES)[7]

- Gently encourage bleeding in the puncture site
- Wash the injured area with soap and water
- Do not scrub the site or use antiseptic agents
- Cover the wound with an impermeable dressing after cleansing
- In the case of mucosal exposure, wash the exposed area copiously with water or normal saline
- If contact lenses are worn, wash the eyes with water or normal saline both before and after removing the lenses

BOX 2 RISK ASSESSMENT BASED ON INJURY TYPE (ADAPTED FROM UK GUIDELINES[6] AND CASE-CONTROL STUDIES[10 11])

High risk exposures

- Deep percutaneous injury
- Freshly used sharps
- Visible blood on sharps
- Needle used on source's blood vessels

Low risk exposures

- Superficial injury, exposure through broken skin, mucosal exposure
- Old discarded sharps
- No visible blood on sharps
- Needle not used on blood vessels—for example, suturing, subcutaneous injection needles

Exposures with no or minimal risk

- Skin not breached
- Contact of body fluid with intact skin
- Contact with saliva (non-dental), urine, vomit, or faeces that is not visibly blood stained
- Needle not used on a patient before injury

BOX 3 BODY FLUIDS AND RISK FOR TRANSMISSION OF BLOOD BORNE VIRUSES (IN ALPHABETICAL ORDER, BASED ON UK GUIDELINES[6 7])

High risk body fluids

- Amniotic fluid
- Blood
- Cerebrospinal fluid
- Exudative or other tissue fluid from burns or skin lesions
- Human breast milk
- Pericardial fluid
- Peritoneal fluid
- Pleural fluid
- Saliva in association with dentistry (likely to be contaminated with blood, even when not visibly so)
- Semen
- Synovial fluid
- Unfixed human tissues and organs
- Vaginal secretions

Low risk body fluids (unless visibly blood stained)

- Saliva (non-dentistry associated)
- Stool
- Urine
- Vomit

factors for transmission of HIV from an infected source patient after a sharps injury as a device visibly contaminated with blood, a cannula that has been inserted in the source patient's artery or vein, a deep injury, and a source patient with a high plasma viral load (for example, at the time of

seroconversion) or in the advanced stages of untreated HIV infection (box 4).[10]

What blood tests are required for source patients and recipients?

If the risk assessment indicates that a clinically important exposure to body fluid has occurred, the status of the source patient's blood borne viruses should be established. In some cases it may be possible to ascertain this from the source patient's medical records. If the blood borne virus status is not known, appropriate arrangements should be made, with the consent of the source patient, either to test an existing blood sample or to take a fresh sample for testing.[13] Box 5 lists the recommended tests. Immediate management and prophylaxis should be offered based on the initial risk assessment and should not be delayed while waiting the results of blood tests.

A baseline serum sample should be taken from the recipient and stored for potential retrospective testing. If the hepatitis B virus immunity status of the recipient is not already known, the baseline sample can be tested for antihepatitis B surface antibody to guide further immunisation against hepatitis B virus. Further blood borne virus testing of the recipient at this stage is unnecessary, as this only reflects the status of the recipient at the time of testing and not whether transmission has occurred.

What consent is required?

In addition to obtaining the source patient's consent for blood borne virus testing, consent should also be sought for disclosure of the test results to the occupational health service and the injured healthcare worker. If the source patient is deemed not to have capacity to consent, the tests cannot be performed, as this is for the benefit of a third party and not in the patient's own best interests.[13] Next of kin cannot give consent on behalf of a patient, unless the patient is deceased, or a child, in which case the parents or guardians may give consent. The recipient of the sharps injury should not approach the source patient for consent as this may influence the source patient's decision and could invalidate the consent. If the incident happened during a procedure where sedation or anaesthesia was given, the source patient should be given sufficient time to recover capacity. If there are practical obstacles to obtaining consent promptly, the decision for starting post-exposure prophylaxis should be based on the information available at the time.

When should post-exposure prophylaxis for HIV be started?

The evidence for efficacy of post-exposure prophylaxis in preventing transmission of HIV is limited.[15] Transmission of simian immunodeficiency virus in macaques was shown to be prevented by tenofovir when given within 24 hours of inoculation and continued for four weeks.[16] Treatment efficacy was reduced if there was a delay between inoculation and treatment and if the duration of treatment was shortened. The use of post-exposure prophylaxis in an occupational health setting was based on an observational study, which showed that the use of zidovudine reduced the risk of transmission after exposure by 80%.[10] Table 1 summarises the recommended use of post-exposure prophylaxis based on risk assessment.

Although the risk of HIV transmission is increased if patients have a high viral load, it is not clear what the

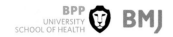

Table 1 Recommendation for HIV post-exposure prophylaxis based on HIV status of source patient and nature of incident (based on UK guidelines[7])

Incident risk and nature of exposure	Status of source patient*	
	No or low risk for HIV	High risk or known to be HIV positive
Minimal risk incident or low risk exposure		
Post-exposure prophylaxis	Not recommended	Not recommended
Follow-up	Not required	Not required
Low risk incident and high risk exposure		
Post-exposure prophylaxis	Not recommended	Considered†
Follow-up	Not required	Advisable
High risk incident and high risk exposure		
Post-exposure prophylaxis	Not recommended	Recommended
Follow-up	Not required	Required

*Where it is not possible to identify the source patient, a risk assessment should be conducted, including circumstances of exposure and epidemiological likelihood of HIV being present. Use of post-exposure prophylaxis is unlikely to be justified in most such exposures.
†Could be offered after a thorough discussion of risk.

BOX 4 RISK ASSESSMENT OF SOURCE PATIENT (BASED ON UK GUIDELINES[7] AND CASE-CONTROL STUDIES[10 11])

High risk source
- Known to be infected with one or more blood borne viruses (viral load and treatment status unknown)
- Known to have a detectable viral load for one or more blood borne viruses
- Unknown viral load but known to have advanced or untreated blood borne virus infection
- Blood borne virus status unknown but had known risk factors*

Low risk source
- Ongoing risk factors for blood borne viruses and recent blood test results were negative for all three blood borne viruses
- Infected with a blood borne virus but known to have a fully suppressed viral load
- Unknown viral load but receiving long term antiviral treatment for blood borne virus with good adherence and known to be stable
- Blood borne virus status unknown but had no known risk factors for such viruses

Source with no or minimal risk
- A recent blood test† result was negative for all three blood borne viruses

*Examples of risk factors: intravenous drug use, men who have sex with men, commercial sex workers, origin from high prevalence areas for HIV, hepatitis B virus, or hepatitis C virus.
†Can be arranged from source patient after consent if no recent results for blood borne viruses are available. However, management should not be delayed while waiting for results.

BOX 5 RECOMMENDED INVESTIGATIONS IN SOURCE PATIENT AFTER CONSENT (BASED ON EXPERT OPINION)

- Combined HIV antigen and antibody (fourth generation HIV immunoassay)
- Hepatitis B surface antigen
- Hepatitis C antibody*
- Other additional investigations could be added if a specific transmissible infectious condition is suspected—for example, malaria, human T cell leukaemia virus

*Testing for hepatitis C virus RNA or antigen should also be considered if source patient is at high risk for hepatitis C virus. This is because hepatitis C virus antibody may be negative during acute infection and may remain negative for more than 12 months in immunocompromised patients.[14]

---

discussion with the recipient about the balance between the risk of transmission and the side effects of post-exposure prophylaxis is recommended. Post-exposure prophylaxis is generally not recommended if the viral load is less than 200 copies/mL but could be offered if the recipient is anxious about the risk.[19] Thus the final decision on whether or not post-exposure prophylaxis should be used should be made with full engagement of the recipient.

The antiretroviral agents recommended for post-exposure prophylaxis differ between the guidelines from different countries. Table 2 summarises the recommended agents and their possible side effects. The current agents recommended in the UK are well tolerated, with few side effects, can be taken at any time of the day, and can be stored at room temperature. Pregnancy is not a contraindication, although the possible risk and benefits to the fetus should be discussed with the recipient. Advice from a specialist experienced in the management of HIV in pregnancy should be sought.

UK guidelines recommend starting post-exposure prophylaxis as soon as possible and no later than 72 hours after exposure, and to continue for 28 days.[7] If the source patient's HIV test result is negative, post-exposure prophylaxis can be discontinued. Before starting post-exposure prophylaxis a full drug history should be obtained from the recipient because of potential interactions between antiretroviral agents and other drugs. An excellent resource for checking drug interactions is available online.[22] Post-exposure prophylaxis may need to be adjusted if the source patient is suspected of having or known to have resistance against one or more components of the standard post-exposure prophylaxis. Such problems should be discussed with local HIV experts or the HIV doctor treating the source patient, although this should not delay post-exposure prophylaxis.

How can the transmission of hepatitis B virus be prevented?
The vaccine against hepatitis B virus can be given shortly after exposure either as the first dose of a primary course or as a booster. Table 3 shows the strategy for offering vaccination against hepatitis B virus after a sharps injury based on vaccination history, previous response to vaccination, type of exposure, and the hepatitis B virus status of the source patient. The additional use of hepatitis B immunoglobulin aims to provide passive immunity if the source patient is known to be at high risk of hepatitis B virus infection and the recipient has not been previously adequately immunised or is a known non-responder to the vaccine—that is, those with a documented absence of hepatitis B surface antibodies after a full course of hepatitis B vaccination.[12] The ideal time frame for use of post-exposure hepatitis B immunoglobulin is within 48 hours of exposure, although it can be considered up to one week.[12]

What can be done about exposure to hepatitis C virus?
A case-control study found that the risk of hepatitis C virus transmission after percutaneous exposure increased with deep injuries and procedures involving hollow bore needles placed in a source patient's blood vessel.[11] Hepatitis C virus has also been found to have prolonged survival in syringes with a high residual void volume.[23] The risk of hepatitis C virus transmission increases significantly if the source has a high viral load,[11] whereas those with an undetectable viral load are unlikely to be infectious.[24]

risk of transmission is if the viral load is undetectable. In such cases the risk is thought to be low although not zero.[17] Guidelines from the United States recommend that post-exposure prophylaxis should be offered even when source patients have undetectable viral loads.[18] In the UK a

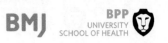

Table 2 Recommended antiretroviral agents for HIV post-exposure prophylaxis after sharps injuries (based on US,[18] UK,[20] and WHO[21] guidelines)

Source of guidelines and recommendations	Potential side effects
UK and USA	
Truvada (245 mg tenofovir disoproxil fumarate and 200 mg emtricitabine) one tablet daily	Rare, but important side effects include acute renal failure and proximal renal tubolopathy (Fanconi's syndrome)
Raltegravir 400 mg twice daily	Rare, but include insomnia, diarrhoea, and nausea and vomiting
World Health Organization	
2 nucleoside reverse transcriptase inhibitors: tenofovir+lamivudine or emtricitabine	Rare, but important side effects of tenofovir include acute renal failure and proximal renal tubolopathy (Fanconi's syndrome)
Kaletra (200 mg lopinavir and 50 mg ritonavir) or other ritonavir boosted protease inhibitor	Rare, but include rash, diarrhoea, nausea and vomiting, and abnormal liver function test results

Table 3 Hepatitis B management algorithm based on vaccination history of recipient (based on UK immunisation guidelines[12])

Hepatitis B vaccination history of recipient	≤1 dose of vaccine or uncertain vaccination history	≥2 doses of vaccine		
Hepatitis B immunity status	Unknown	Unknown	Known vaccine responder	Known vaccine non-responder
High risk exposure, source patient positive for hepatitis B surface antigen	Accelerated vaccine* course+1 dose of hepatitis B immunoglobulin†	2 doses of vaccine at 0 and 1 month	Consider booster vaccine dose	2 doses of hepatitis B immunoglobulin† at 0 and 1 month; consider booster vaccine dose
High risk exposure, hepatitis B surface antigen status of source patient unknown	Accelerated vaccine* course	1 dose of vaccine	Consider booster vaccine dose	2 doses of hepatitis B immunoglobulin† at 0 and 1 month; consider booster vaccine dose
Source patient negative for hepatitis B surface antigen or low risk exposure (regardless of hepatitis B surface antigen status)	Initiate vaccine course	Complete vaccine course	Consider booster vaccine dose	No hepatitis B immunoglobulin; consider booster vaccine dose

*Doses spaced at 0, 1, and 2 months with booster dose at 12 months.
†Hepatitis B immunoglobulin 500 units intramuscularly per dose.

Table 4 Suggested follow-up schedules after high risk sharps injuries (based on UK guidelines[7] for HIV and expert opinions for hepatitis B virus and hepatitis C virus)

Blood borne virus risk in source patient	Within first 12 weeks	Week 12*	Week 24
HIV	If post-exposure prophylaxis is started, review within seven days to monitor any side effects. Carry out tests for full blood count, urea and electrolytes, liver function, and bone profile, and carry out urine analysis	Test for combined HIV antigen and antibody (fourth generation HIV immunoassay)	Not routinely recommended
Hepatitis B virus	Attendance for hepatitis B vaccination with or without second dose of hepatitis B immunoglobulin according to recommended schedule	Test for hepatitis B surface antigen and hepatitis B surface antibody	Not routinely recommended unless hepatitis B immunoglobulin was given
Hepatitis C virus	Test for hepatitis C virus RNA at week 6	Test for hepatitis C virus antibody and hepatitis C virus RNA	Not routinely recommended unless risk of hepatitis C virus transmission is high

*If HIV post-exposure prophylaxis has been started, week 12 is calculated from end of post-exposure prophylaxis.

Currently no vaccine or post-exposure prophylaxis is effective in the prevention of hepatitis C virus transmission. However, treatment of acute hepatitis C infection is known to be highly effective.[25] Early detection of hepatitis C virus transmission and referral to an appropriate specialist for assessment and treatment is therefore essential.

How is care accessed in different healthcare settings?

Local policy should clearly identify which department to contact during and out of normal working hours. The emergency department is usually the location for immediate access to advice, medicines, and vaccines, although in some hospitals additional post-exposure prophylaxis packs are stored in strategic locations such as operating theatres or delivery suites.

In the community setting or in dental practices, the initial management of the injury has to be started on-site, immediately after the incident. A system to enable injured healthcare workers to access urgent expert advice should

be locally agreed. As this occurs in an outpatient setting, it is important that source patients should be assessed before discharge and consent obtained for any potential blood tests. Hepatitis B virus vaccines are widely available in general practice, but access to HIV post-exposure prophylaxis would require a visit to the local emergency department. Because of the need to start these drugs early, attendance at an emergency department should not be delayed if this is deemed necessary after risk assessment.

How should injured healthcare workers be followed up?

After important exposure to body fluid, recipients should be followed up for at least 12 weeks. Table 4 summarises the testing required and timing of follow-up. Healthcare workers who have sustained a high risk injury and receive post-exposure prophylaxis should not be considered infectious and should be reassured that it is safe for them to return to clinical work, including performing procedures that are prone to exposure.[26] They should, however, be advised

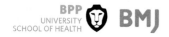

to use barrier contraception and to avoid blood or tissue donations, pregnancy, and breast feeding, especially during the first six to 12 weeks after exposure.[18]

SOURCES AND SELECTION CRITERIA

We searched PubMed and the Cochrane Library for articles published over the past 20 years using the terms "sharps injury", "needle stick injury", and "body fluid exposure" and hand selected the most relevant and appropriate articles. To search for relevant UK national guidelines we also accessed the UK Department of Health and Public Health England (formerly Health Protection Agency) websites. We consulted guidelines from the World Health Organization, Centers for Disease Control and Prevention, British HIV Association, and British Society for Sexual Health and HIV.

ADDITIONAL EDUCATIONAL RESOURCES

Resources for healthcare professionals

- Health and Safety Executive. Sharps injuries—what you need to do (www.hse.gov.uk/healthservices/needlesticks/actions. htm)—provides a perspective from the regulatory aspect of sharps injury

- NHS Choices. What should I do if I injure myself with a used needle? (www.nhs.uk/chq/Pages/2557.aspx?CategoryID=72)—provides a concise and practical approach to needlestick injury; also useful for non-healthcare workers

- Royal College of Nursing. Needlestick and sharps injuries (www.rcn.org.uk/support/the_working_environment/health_ and_safety/needlestick_and_sharps_injuries)—has a link to the Royal College of Nursing guidance on sharps safety

- Patient.co.uk. Needlestick injury (www.patient.co.uk/doctor/ needlestick-injury)—provides good tips on how to prevent sharps injury

- Health Education England. e-learning for Healthcare (http://www.e-lfh.org.uk/)—several e-learning modules under Pathology (PATH)/e-Path 07-Virology provide useful information on prevention and management of sharps injury: 07_052 Sharps Injuries; 07_060 HBV; 07_104 HIV prevention

- Medscape (http://emedicine.medscape.com/article/782611-overview)—a comprehensive overview of the American approach to management of exposure to body fluids

- HIV-drug interaction.org (www.hiv-druginteractions.org)—maintained by the University of Liverpool, which provides a clinically useful, up to date and evidence based drug-drug interaction resource, freely available to healthcare workers, patients, and researchers

---

This article was critically reviewed by several healthcare workers: Ali Hashtroudi, Ceris Evans, Eilidh Stewart, James Donaldson, Jan Kunkel, Jayshree Dave, Neil Slabbert, and Ranjababu Kulasegaram.

Contributors: CYWT conceived this review. He is the guarantor. All authors contributed equally to the writing and editing of this article and all approved its content.

Competing interests: We have read and understood the BMJ policy on declaration of interests and declare the following: none.

Provenance and peer review: Not commissioned; externally peer reviewed.

1   Woode Owusu M, Wellington E, Rice B, Gill ON, Ncube F & contributors. Eye of the needle. United Kingdom surveillance of significant occupational exposure to bloodborne viruses in healthcare workers. 2014. Public Health England. www.gov.uk/government/ uploads/system/uploads/attachment_data/file/385300/EoN_2014_-_ FINAL_CT_3_sig_occ.pdf.

2   Diprose P, Deakin CD, Smedley J. Ignorance of post-exposure prophylaxis guidelines following HIV needlestick injury may increase the risk of seroconversion. Br J Anaesth2000;84:767-70.

3   Tarantola A, Rachline A, Konto C, Houzé S, Sabah-Mondan C, Vrillon H, et al. Occupational Plasmodium falciparum malaria

4   Menna-Barreto M. HTLV-II transmission to a health care worker. Am J Infect Control2006;34:158-60.

5   Günther S, Feldmann H, Geisbert TW, et al. Management of accidental exposure to Ebola virus in the biosafety level 4 laboratory, Hamburg, Germany. J Infect Dis2011;204:S785-90.

6   Expert Advisory Group on AIDS and the Advisory Group on Hepatitis. Guidance for clinical healthcare workers: protection against infection with bloodborne viruses. UK Health Departments. 1998. http:// webarchive.nationalarchives.gov.uk/20130107105354/http://www. dh.gov.uk/prod_consum_dh/groups/dh_digitalassets/@dh/@en/ documents/digitalasset/dh_4014474.pdf.

7   Department of Health. HIV post-exposure prophylaxis: guidance from the UK Chief Medical Officer's Expert Advisory Group on AIDS. Department of Health. 2008. www.gov.uk/government/uploads/ system/uploads/attachment_data/file/203139/HIV_post-exposure_ prophylaxis.pdf.

8   Hawkins DA, Asboe D, Barlow K, Evans B. Seroconversion to HIV-1 following a needlestick injury despite combination post-exposure prophylaxis. J Infect2001;43:12-5.

9   Naghavi SH, Shabestari O, Alcolado J. Post-traumatic stress disorder in trainee doctors with previous needlestick injuries. Occup Med (Lond)2013;63:260-5.

10   Cardo DM, Culver KH, Ciesielski C, et al. A case-control study of HIV seroconversion in health-care workers after percutaneous exposure. N Engl J Med1997;337:1485-90.

11   Yazdanpanah Y, De Carli G, Migueres B, et al. Risk factors for hepatitis C virus transmission to health care workers after occupational exposure: a European case-control study. Clin Infect Dis2005;41:1423-30.

12   Public Health England. Immunisation against infectious disease: the Green Book. Public Health England; 2013:161-85. www.gov.uk/ government/uploads/system/uploads/attachment_data/file/263311/ Green_Book_Chapter_18_v2_0.pdf.

13   General Medical Council. Consent: patients and doctors making decisions together. General Medical Council. June 2008. www.gmc-uk. org/static/documents/content/Consent_-_English_0914.pdf.

14   Thomson EC, Nastouli E, Main J, et al. Delayed anti-HCV antibody response in HIV-positive men acutely infected with HCV. AIDS2009;23:89-93.

15   Young TN, Arens FJ, Kennedy GE, Laurie JW, Rutherford GW. Antiretroviral post-exposure prophylaxis (PEP) for occupational HIV exposure. Cochrane Database Syst Rev2007;1:CD002835.

16   Tsai CC, Emau P, Follis KE, et al. Effectiveness of postinoculation (R)-9-(2-phosphonylmethoxypropyl) adenine treatment for prevention of persistent simian immunodeficiency virus SIVmne infection depends critically on timing of initiation and duration of treatment. J Virol1998;72:4265-73.

17   Webster D. Is HIV post-exposure prophylaxis required following occupational exposure to a source patient who is virologically suppressed on antiretroviral therapy? HIV Med2015;16:73-5.

18   Kuhar DT, Henderson DK, Struble KA, et al. Updated US Public Health Service guidelines for the management of occupational exposures to human immunodeficiency virus and recommendations for postexposure prophylaxis. Infect Control Hosp Epidemiol2013;34:875-92.

19   Expert Advisory Group on AIDS. Updated recommendation for HIV post-exposure prophylaxis (PEP) following occupational exposure to a source with undetectable HIV viral load. Department of Health. 2013. www.gov.uk/government/uploads/system/uploads/attachment_data/ file/275060/EAGA_advice_on_PEP_after_exposure_to_UD_source_Dec13. pdf.

20   Expert Advisory Group on AIDS. Changes to recommended regimen for post-exposure prophylaxis. Department of Health. 2014. www.gov.uk/ government/uploads/system/uploads/attachment_data/file/351633/ Change_to_recommended_regimen_for_PEP_starter_pack_final.pdf.

21   Ford N, Shubber Z, Calmy A, et al. Choice of antiretroviral drugs for postexposure prophylaxis for adults and adolescents: a systematic review. Clin Infect Dis2015;60(Suppl 3):S170-6.

22   University of Liverpool. Drug interaction charts. www.hiv-druginteractions.org. 29 June 2015. www.hiv-druginteractions.org/ InteractionCharts.aspx.

23   Paintsil E, He H, Peters C, Lindenbach BD, Heimer R. Survival of hepatitis C virus in syringes: implication for transmission among injection drug users. J Infect Dis2010;202:984-90.

24   English National Blood Service HCV Lookback Collation Collaborators. Transfusion transmission of HCV infection before anti-HCV testing of blood donations in England: results of the national HCV lookback program. Transfusion2002;42:1146-53.

25   Tomkins SE, Rice BD, Roy K, Cullen B, Ncube FM. Universal treatment success among healthcare workers diagnosed with occupationally acquired acute hepatitis C. J Hosp Infect2015;89:69-71.

26   Department of Health. Annex A: examples of UKAP advice on exposure prone procedures. Department of Health. 2010. http:// webarchive.nationalarchives.gov.uk/+/www.dh.gov.uk/en/ Publicationsandstatistics/Publications/PublicationsPolicyAndGuidance/ Browsable/DH_5368137.

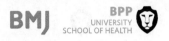

The risks of radiation exposure related to diagnostic imaging and how to minimise them

H E Davies, consultant respiratory physician[1], C G Wathen, consultant respiratory physician[2], F V Gleeson, consultant radiologist[3 4]

[1]Department of Respiratory Medicine, University Hospital of Wales, Vale of Glamorgan CF64 2XX, UK

[2]Wycombe Hospital, Buckinghamshire Hospitals NHS Trust, High Wycombe, UK.

[3]Department of Radiology, Churchill Hospital, Oxford Radcliffe Hospital, Oxford, UK

[4]Oxford NIHR Biomedical Research Centre, Oxford, UK

Correspondence to: HE Davies
hedavies@doctors.net.uk

Cite this as: BMJ 2011;342:d947

DOI: 10.1136/bmj.d947

http://www.bmj.com/content/342/bmj.d947

Since the 1970s, when computed tomography was introduced into clinical practice, the array of imaging tests that expose patients to radiation has vastly increased. This is a result of improved computed tomography techniques, advances in other techniques such as digital subtraction angiography, and the development of modalities such as positron emission tomography coregistered with computed tomography and single photon emission tomography coregistered with computed tomography. Improvements in non-ionising radiation imaging techniques, such as magnetic resonance imaging with increased field strength (3T) and multichannel technology, and Doppler and colour flow applications in ultrasound, have also occurred.

The demand for imaging has grown for several reasons. The development of picture archiving computer systems, which enable the referring doctor to view images easily, may have led to an increase in requests for diagnostic imaging. The public has become more aware of imaging tests and their potential benefit, especially in screening for cancer and cardiac disease, and faster scanners have allowed for imaging in previously unsuitable patients. Enhanced spatial resolution of images has resulted in the detection of previously unseen abnormalities of unknown relevance that often require further investigation and follow-up scanning. The treatment effects for many common diseases are now monitored using repeated imaging. Simultaneously, computed tomography has become more readily available, particularly in acute clinical areas.

Although the risks of cancer from computed tomography scans have been estimated recently,[1 2 3 4] such risks may be poorly understood by doctors and poorly communicated, especially in the case of young patients and those with benign disease. In one survey of health providers in the United States, only 9% of emergency department doctors and 47% of radiologists were aware of the increased cancer risk associated with computed tomography.[w1]

Here, we examine the risks of exposure to radiation associated with some routine diagnostic imaging investigations and discuss practical ways to minimise such risks. This review is based on evidence from retrospective cross sectional studies, special reports, prospective cohort studies, surveys, observational studies, and current international guidelines.

Why is exposure to radiation from medical imaging increasing?

In the developed world, medical "technology creep" has promoted the use of modern technology while ignoring more conventional imaging tests. For example, two recent reviews of imaging in pulmonary embolic disease in leading medical journals did not mention chest radiography but suggested using computed tomography pulmonary angiography as the initial test.[5 6 7]

The past 30 years has seen more than a 20-fold increase in the number of computed tomography scans obtained annually in the US.[8] In the United Kingdom, use of computed tomography has doubled in the past decade.[w2] We predict that computed tomography based screening programmes for the prevention of primary and secondary disease will escalate markedly and further contribute to iatrogenic radiation exposure. As an example, a recent press release in the US stated the benefit of lung cancer screening using computed tomography.[w3]

New approaches to treatment often now require imaging at diagnosis and at intervals during treatment to assess the response. As examples, guidelines from the Fleischner Society advise that a 5 mm pulmonary nodule should be followed up with regular scans for two years,[w4] and the reclassification of gastrointestinal stromal tumours and their treatment with imatinib mean that computed tomography and positron emission tomography with computed tomography are now used in patient groups previously not scanned.[w5 w6]

What levels of radiation accompany routinely performed procedures?

Table 1 shows representative mean effective doses of radiation associated with various procedures.

The term "effective dose" is used in radiation protection and indicates the radiation effect of a specific imaging modality in terms of an estimated equivalent whole body radiation dose. This allows the level of exposure associated with different techniques to be compared. This biological effect is measured in millisieverts (mSv), which are the product of the "absorbed dose" (in grays; Gy) and a dimensionless weighting factor (often known as the quality factor or Q); Q varies according to the body part irradiated, the radiation type, and the regimen delivered.

The "organ specific dose" reflects the calculated radiation delivered to any selected organ (table 2) and is the preferred measure for estimating radiation risk.[2]

How much radiation exposure is usual?

Natural background radiation emanates from two primary sources—cosmic radiation and terrestrial or environmental radionuclides, which vary according to the latitude and altitude of the location. Little can be done to influence natural radiation levels. Radon gas is one of the main contributors; it emits α radiation, which can build up within

SUMMARY POINTS

- The demand for imaging, especially computed tomography, has increased vastly over the past 20 years
- An estimated 30% of computed tomography tests may be unnecessary
- Ionising radiation may be associated with cancer and other non-neoplastic sequelae
- The risks of iatrogenic radiation exposure are often overlooked and patients are seldom made aware of these risks
- The requesting doctor must balance the risks and benefits of any high radiation dose imaging test, adhering to guideline recommendations if possible
- Difficult cases should be discussed with a radiologist, ideally at a clinicoradiological or multidisciplinary team meeting

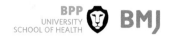

Table 1 Average* effective doses of radiation for various diagnostic radiology procedures[9-11]

Procedure†	Average effective dose of radiation (mSv)	Equivalent number of radiographs	Equivalent period of average natural background radiation (days)
Posteroanterior chest radiography	0.02	1	3
Skull radiography	0.1	5	15
Mammography	0.4	20	61
Pelvic radiography	0.6	30	91
Abdominal radiography	0.7	35	106
Lung perfusion scintigraphy (99mTc-MMA)	2.0	100	304
CT brain	2.0	100	304
Intravenous urography	3.0	150	456
Bone isotope scintigraphy (99mTc-MDP)	6.3	315	958
CT chest	7.0	350	1065
CT abdomen	8.0	400	1217
Barium enema	8.0	400	1217
CT pulmonary angiography	15.0	750	2281
CT coronary angiography	16.0	800	2433

*Exact doses vary according to the imaging technique used. As an example, for CT of the chest, whether volumetric 0.675 mm or 2.5 mm settings are used and whether overlapping or contiguous image acquisition is used.
CT=computed tomography; 99mTc-MMA=technetium-99m-methyl methacrylate; 99mTc-MDP=technetium-99m-methylene diphosphonate.

Table 2 Typical organ specific radiation doses for various radiology procedures[2 4]

Procedure	Organ	Organ specific radiation dose (mSv)
Posteroanterior chest radiography	Lung	0.01
Mammography	Breast	3.5
CT chest	Breast	21.4
CT coronary angiography	Breast	51.0
Abdominal radiography	Stomach	0.25
CT abdomen	Stomach	10.0
	Colon	4.0
Barium enema	Colon	15.0

CT=computed tomography.

Table 3 Potential risks associated with commonly performed clinical procedures[4 14 w16-w20]

Procedure	Complication	Approximate risk
Paediatric CT	Risk of fatal cancer	1/1000
CT coronary angiography	Lifetime cancer risk	1/270 (aged 40)
Lumbar puncture	Postdural puncture headache	0-70/100
Spinal or epidural surgery	Paraplegia	7/1 720 000
Cataract extraction	Infective endophthalmitis	1.28/1000
Bronchoscopy	Death	1-4/10 000

CT=computed tomography.

the home (particularly if well insulated). The average person receives an effective dose of about 2.4 mSv each year,[11] but this varies between populations. About 10% of people worldwide are exposed to annual effective doses greater than 3 mSv.[w7]

Global radiation doses to the public have increased by 20% since the start of the 20th century, mainly because of the expansion of diagnostic imaging techniques. Indeed medical radiation accounts for around 15% of the total exposure in the UK's population.[12]

What are the known consequences of radiation exposure?

Most information about the adverse effects of radiation has been extrapolated from data collected from atomic bomb survivors at Hiroshima and Nagasaki, populations living near nuclear disasters such as Chernobyl, or people with medical or occupational exposures. Whether such projections accurately assess the effects on people exposed to lower clinical radiation doses is unknown, but biological experiments suggest that all radiation exposure may cause harm.[13]

Cancer

Epidemiological data have shown that ionising radiation causes cancer in humans.[14 15 16] The risk of adverse sequelae increases with higher doses of radiation and for tissues with a high sensitivity to ionising radiation, such as the breast and thyroid. In 2004, x ray related radiation was estimated to be responsible for 0.6% of all cancers diagnosed in the UK,[17] and recent estimates indicate that one in 270 women aged 40 years who undergo computed tomographic coronary angiography will develop cancer as a result.[4] These figures may seem alarming, but they must be viewed in the context of the absolute excess risk associated with medical radiation compared with the lifetime risk of disease.

Non-neoplastic effects

Radiation can cause genetic mutations, intellectual or developmental disabilities in the children of mothers exposed to radiation during pregnancy, and an increased incidence of cardiovascular disease.[w8 w9] Direct effects include skin injury, the development of cataracts, and hair loss; these most commonly occur after radiotherapy, although diagnostic computed tomographic perfusion examinations have been implicated as the cause of hair loss in patients in the US, with litigation ensuing.[18]

Understanding the size of increased risks

The recent Biologic Effects of Ionizing Radiation (BEIR) VII report on the effects of ionising radiation predicted a lifetime attributable risk from a 10 mSv effective dose of one radiation induced cancer per 1000 patients.[13] This lifetime risk model estimates that a single 100 mSv exposure would cause one in 100 people to develop a solid cancer or leukaemia, compared with a lifetime risk of about 42 in 100 from unrelated causes.[13] This suggests that the excess number of cases (inclusive of non-fatal cases) of solid tumours in the UK population is 800 a year (95% confidence interval 400 to 1600) in men and 1300 a year (690 to 2500) in women; excess deaths in the UK a year from exposure to 100 mSv would be 410 (200 to 830) and 610 (300 to 1200) for men and women, respectively.[13 w10]

Although these numbers seem small compared with the estimated one in three absolute lifetime risk per person of developing cancer in the UK,[w11] they are worrying for the following reasons. The risk arises from an iatrogenic cause; large numbers of people are exposed; children may be exposed; and risks may be underestimated, particularly in those who have repeated tests, such as young patients with suspected renal colic who have repeated abdominal computed tomograms.

Who is most at risk?

Pregnant women

The use of diagnostic imaging in pregnant women should be carefully considered because of potential teratogenic and oncogenic effects of radiation on the fetus. The minimum dose at which adverse sequelae may occur has not been firmly established. However, the International Commission on Radiological Protection (ICRP) regards radiation doses greater than 100 mGy as potentially teratogenic, with a risk of fetal growth retardation, cognitive impairment, and damage to the central nervous system.[19 20]

The absolute risk of future malignancy remains low. For example, if chest radiography, ventilation-perfusion scanning, and computed tomographic pulmonary angiography are performed in a pregnant patient with suspected pulmonary emboli, the fetus is exposed to a total radiation dose of about 4 mGy. The ICRP states that fetal exposure to 10 mGy increases the probability of cancer before 20 years of age from 0.03% to 0.04% and suggests that this is not a clinically important increase in risk.[21]

However, risks to the mother must also be considered. There is a concerning lack of evidence about the safety of computed tomographic pulmonary angiography during pregnancy, because pregnant patients have been excluded from the large prospective trials performed to date.[22] Although this test exposes the fetus to less radiation than when ventilation perfusion scintigraphy is used,[23] it exposes the maternal breast to about 150 times more radiation than does ventilation perfusion scintigraphy.[6] During pregnancy, breast tissue is more susceptible than normal to radiation damage. Protective shields may reduce radiation exposure by more than 50%,[w12 w13] but these are not always used in UK radiology departments. Alternative imaging modalities, such as half dose perfusion scans, should be performed wherever possible in pregnant women.

Children
Computed tomography is now performed more often than previously in children because technological advances have eliminated the need for anaesthesia to prevent movement artefacts in all except the very young. National surveys have estimated that in the US 6-11% of all computed tomography studies are currently performed in children.[24 25]

The risks from exposure to radiation are greater for children than for adults because paediatric tissues are more radiosensitive and because children have a longer life expectancy during which radiation related effects may develop.

How to reduce the risk?
National guidelines have been developed to help doctors and to optimise the use of radiology services.[26 27] However, to reduce the numbers of unnecessary scans, this advice needs to be integrated into clinical practice. Some strategies that may help to cut exposure to radiation by reducing the number of imaging tests are as follows.

Calculate before you order
Several online tools are available to enable doctors (and patients) to calculate the estimated effective radiation dose from specific investigations and the equivalent period of background exposure (www.doseinfo-radar.com/RADARDoseRiskCalc.html; www.xrayrisk.com/calculator/calculator.php). An iPhone application is available to calculate and record accumulating radiation exposure from radiological examinations (Radiation Passport, Tidal Pool Software). Calculating single and accumulated exposure to ionising radiation may lead to more considered decisions being made about the need for imaging, particularly for patients who need repeated tests.

Reduce unnecessary computed tomography examinations
Estimates from cohort studies suggest that about 30% of computed tomography scans are unnecessary.[4] Adherence to local or national radiological guidelines, such as the American College of Radiology's appropriateness criteria and the Royal College of Radiologists' publications, should reduce the number of unnecessary tests.[27 28] One example

is the use of brain computed tomography for patients admitted after an acute head injury. Recommendations from the National Institute for Health and Clinical Excellence and the Scottish Intercollegiate Guidelines Network set clear parameters on which patients require an urgent scan.[w14 w15] Recommendations for certain patients, such as those presenting 24 hours after the injury, are unclear however, and for these patients discussion with radiology colleagues is prudent. Similarly, the measurement of the clinical probability score and D-dimer in patients with suspected pulmonary emboli may reduce the number of unnecessary computed tomographic pulmonary angiography scans performed.[29]

Use other imaging techniques if possible
Magnetic resonance imaging and ultrasound procedures do not deliver radiation to the patient and should be used instead of radiological imaging wherever possible.

Standardise operating procedures for radiological examinations
Implementation of standard operating procedures for radiological tests at a local and national level could negate discrepancies in the radiation doses given for the same test at different sites.

Use technological advances to increase safety
New computed tomography scanners that can detect signal at lower radiation doses could enable the delivery of lower doses of radiation. Low dose computed tomography protocols should be used as standard to follow up pulmonary nodules and renal calculi.

What should patients be told?
Although patients are routinely told about the potential adverse events of interventional diagnostic procedures and their informed consent required, patients undergoing radiological imaging studies do not usually receive similar information and neither are they asked for consent. These tests are usually performed in the patients' best interests, but in certain circumstances an awareness of the radiation risk and knowledge of alternative options might affect the patient's decision and alter the course of their management. In our experience, some pregnant mothers choose to undergo computed tomographic pulmonary angiography when pregnant rather than a half dose perfusion scan because they wish to reduce the radiation exposure to their fetus even when reassured that the perfusion scan is safe.

We believe that the risks associated with some diagnostic radiation exposures, particularly from procedures involving much higher doses than conventional radiography, should be discussed with patients or their guardians before the examination. Table 3 outlines the risks associated with some commonly performed procedures that may be communicated to patients.

Current legislation does not give dose limits for common medical imaging exposures, although radiology departments in the UK usually adhere to an "as low as reasonably practicable" policy. The position of the doctor in recommending a screening computed tomography scan is not clear and has recently been reviewed by the Department of Health's committee on medical aspects of radiation in the environment.[30]

Patients should be provided with the information needed to understand the potential benefits and risks of the

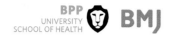

intervention and assign subjective weight to these factors, in order to make an informed choice (box). Provision of these data is often overlooked.

It is important to ensure meticulous documentation to outline the indication for the test, and to discuss the choice of test with the patient or their representative and with colleagues. Wherever possible, to promote good practice, such decisions should be discussed in clinicoradiological or multidisciplinary meetings.

Conclusion

Over recent years increasing numbers of imaging studies have been performed, and this trend looks set to continue on a global scale. As technological progress creates more sensitive faster scanners, and worldwide access improves, greater numbers of patients will be exposed to radiation and contribute to an increasing public health problem.

Communication between the doctor and radiologist is crucial in deciding whether computed tomography is appropriate. To ensure that only justifiable tests are performed, imaging requests should either be discussed with a radiologist or agreed protocols should be adhered to. It is the responsibility of the clinician to assess the benefits and risks of any proposed test, to incorporate recommendations from existing guidelines, and to provide patients with the information needed to ensure an informed decision is made before high radiation dose imaging tests are performed.

SOURCES AND SELECTION CRITERIA

We searched PubMed and used our personal reference collections. We also reviewed guidelines from the British Thoracic Society, Royal College of Radiologists, and American College of Radiology. In addition, we retrieved national recommendations from the National Institute for Health and Clinical Excellence (NICE).

CONSIDERATIONS BEFORE ANY RADIOLOGICAL EXAMINATION

- Review the circumstances of each case individually
- Assess whether the patient needs the test? Why is it needed? Will the result change management?
- Consider whether a non-radiological alternative exists
- Explain to the patient, his or her family, or the carer what the test involves and the associated radiation exposure; this may be most clearly shown in terms of equivalent numbers of chest radiographs (see table 1)
- Outline the risks versus the benefits of the test (see table 2)
- Agree an alternative management plan if the patient declines the examination

---

Contributors: HED drafted the manuscript. CGW and FVG contributed to the manuscript and critically evaluated and revised the text. FVG is guarantor.

Competing interests: All authors have completed the Unified Competing Interest form at www.icmje.org/coi_disclosure.pdf (available on request from the corresponding author) and declare: no support from any organisation for the submitted work; no financial relationships with any organisations that might have an interest in the submitted work in the previous three years; no other relationships or activities that could appear to have influenced the submitted work.

Provenance and peer review: Not commissioned; externally peer reviewed.

1. Berrington DG, Mahesh M, Kim KP, Bhargavan M, Lewis R, Mettler F, et al. Projected cancer risks from computed tomographic scans performed in the United States in 2007. Arch Intern Med 2009;169:2071-7.
2. Brenner DJ, Hall EJ. Computed tomography—an increasing source of radiation exposure. N Engl J Med 2007;357:2277-84.
3. Hall EJ, Brenner DJ. Cancer risks from diagnostic radiology. Br J Radiol 2008;81:362-78.
4. Smith-Bindman R, Lipson J, Marcus R, Kim KP, Mahesh M, Gould R, et al. Radiation dose associated with common computed tomography examinations and the associated lifetime attributable risk of cancer. Arch Intern Med 2009;169:2078-86.
5. Agnelli G, Becattini C. Acute pulmonary embolism. N Engl J Med 2010;363:266-74.
6. Bourjeily G, Paidas M, Khalil H, Rosene-Montella K, Rodger M. Pulmonary embolism in pregnancy. Lancet 2010;375:500-12.
7. Patel C, Scarsbrook A, Gleeson F. Pulmonary embolism in pregnancy. Lancet 2010;375:1778-9.
8. IMV Medical Information Division. IMV 2006 CT market summary report. 2006. www.imvinfo.com/user/documents/content_documents/nws_rad/MS_CT_DSandTOC.pdf.
9. Mettler FA Jr, Huda W, Yoshizumi TT, Mahesh M. Effective doses in radiology and diagnostic nuclear medicine: a catalog. Radiology 2008;248:254-63.
10. National Radiological Protection Board (NRPB). X-rays: how safe are they? 2001. www.hpa.org.uk/Publications/Radiation/NPRBArchive/NRPBEducationalPublications/radXrayshowsafearetheyleaflet/.
11. Report of the United Nations Scientific Committee on the Effects of Atomic Radiation. General Assembly Official Records. 63rd Session. Suppl 46. 2008. www.undemocracy.com/A-63-398.pdf.
12. Hughes JS, Watson SJ, Jones AL, Oatway WB. Review of the radiation exposure of the UK population. J Radiol Prot 2005;25:493-6.
13. National Research Council BEIR VII Committee. BEIR VII: health risks from exposure to low levels of ionizing radiation. 2005. http://dels-old.nas.edu/dels/rpt_briefs/beir_vii_final.pdf.
14. Brenner DJ, Elliston CD, Hall EJ, Berdon WE. Estimates of the cancer risks from pediatric CT radiation are not merely theoretical: comment on "point/counterpoint: in x-ray computed tomography, technique factors should be selected appropriate to patient size. Against the proposition." Med Phys 2001;28:2387-8.
15. Cardis E, Vrijheid M, Blettner M, Gilbert E, Hakama M, Hill C, et al. The 15-Country Collaborative Study of Cancer Risk among Radiation Workers in the Nuclear Industry: estimates of radiation-related cancer risks. Radiat Res 2007;167:396-416.
16. Pierce DA, Vaeth M, Shimizu Y. Selection bias in cancer risk estimation from A-bomb survivors. Radiat Res 2007;167:735-41.
17. Berrington dG, Darby S. Risk of cancer from diagnostic X-rays: estimates for the UK and 14 other countries. Lancet 2004;363:345-51.
18. Smith-Bindman R. Is computed tomography safe? N Engl J Med 2010;363:1-4.
19. Brent RL. Saving lives and changing family histories: appropriate counseling of pregnant women and men and women of reproductive age, concerning the risk of diagnostic radiation exposures during and before pregnancy. Am J Obstet Gynecol 2009;200:4-24.
20. International Commission on Radiological Protection. Pregnancy and medical radiation. ICRP Publication 84. Ann ICRP 2000;3-41.
21. Streffer C, Shore R, Konermann G, Meadows A, Uma DP, Preston WJ, et al. Biological effects after prenatal irradiation (embryo and fetus). A report of the International Commission on Radiological Protection. Ann ICRP 2003;33:5-206.
22. Stein PD, Fowler SE, Goodman LR, Gottschalk A, Hales CA, Hull RD, et al. Multidetector computed tomography for acute pulmonary embolism. N Engl J Med 2006;354:2317-27.
23. Winer-Muram HT, Boone JM, Brown HL, Jennings SG, Mabie WC, Lombardo GT. Pulmonary embolism in pregnant patients: fetal radiation dose with helical CT. Radiology 2002;224:487-92.
24. Conference of Radiation Control Program Directors IC. Nationwide evaluation of x-ray trends (NEXT): 2000 computed tomography. 2006. www.crcpd.org/next.aspx.
25. Mettler FA Jr, Wiest PW, Locken JA, Kelsey CA. CT scanning: patterns of use and dose. J Radiol Prot 2000;20:353-9.
26. Amis ES Jr, Butler PF, Applegate KE, Birnbaum SB, Brateman LF, Hevezi JM, et al. American College of Radiology white paper on radiation dose in medicine. J Am Coll Radiol 2007;4:272-84.
27. Royal College of Radiologists. Making best use of clinical radiology services (MBUR). 6th ed. 2007. www.rcr.ac.uk/content.aspx?pageID=995.
28. American College of Radiology. ACR appropriateness criteria. 1993. www.acr.org/secondarymainmenucategories/quality_safety/app_criteria.aspx.
29. British Thoracic Society guidelines for the management of suspected acute pulmonary embolism. Thorax 2003;58:470-83.
30. Health Protection Agency. Committee on Medical Aspects of Radiation in the Environment (COMARE). 12th report. 2007. www.comare.org.uk/comare_docs.htm#statements.

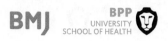

Facemasks for the prevention of infection in healthcare and community settings

C Raina MacIntyre, professor of infectious diseases epidemiology and head of school, Abrar Ahmad Chughtai, research assistant

School of Public Health and Community Medicine, Faculty of Medicine, University of New South Wales, Sydney, 2052, NSW, Australia

Correspondence to: C R MacIntyre
r.macintyre@unsw.edu.au

Cite this as: *BMJ* 2015;350:h694

DOI: 10.1136/bmj.h694

http://www.bmj.com/content/350/bmj.h694

ABSTRACT

Facemasks are recommended for diseases transmitted through droplets and respirators for respiratory aerosols, yet recommendations and terminology vary between guidelines. The concepts of droplet and airborne transmission that are entrenched in clinical practice have recently been shown to be more complex than previously thought. Several randomised clinical trials of facemasks have been conducted in community and healthcare settings, using widely varying interventions, including mixed interventions (such as masks and handwashing), and diverse outcomes. Of the nine trials of facemasks identified in community settings, in all but one, facemasks were used for respiratory protection of well people. They found that facemasks and facemasks plus hand hygiene may prevent infection in community settings, subject to early use and compliance. Two trials in healthcare workers favoured respirators for clinical respiratory illness. The use of reusable cloth masks is widespread globally, particularly in Asia, which is an important region for emerging infections, but there is no clinical research to inform their use and most policies offer no guidance on them. Health economic analyses of facemasks are scarce and the few published cost effectiveness models do not use clinical efficacy data. The lack of research on facemasks and respirators is reflected in varied and sometimes conflicting policies and guidelines. Further research should focus on examining the efficacy of facemasks against specific infectious threats such as influenza and tuberculosis, assessing the efficacy of cloth masks, investigating common practices such as reuse of masks, assessing compliance, filling in policy gaps, and obtaining cost effectiveness data using clinical efficacy estimates.

Introduction

Most efforts on the prevention of respiratory infections have focused on drug based interventions. In an emerging outbreak of infectious disease, non-pharmaceutical measures including facemasks and respirators may be the only available protection.

Various devices are used in healthcare and community settings worldwide, ranging from cloth, cotton, or gauze masks (cloth masks); medical, surgical, or procedure mask (medical masks); and N95, N99, N100, P2, P3, FFP2, and FFP3 respirators (respirators) (see fig 1). The difference between the products arises from their design and intended use. Medical masks and cloth masks (hereafter "facemasks") were designed to prevent the spread of infection from wearers to others, but are commonly used to protect the wearer from splashes or sprays of blood or body fluids. Facemasks are not subject to regulation, do not provide a seal around the face, and vary widely in type and quality.[1] [2] A respirator is a fitted device designed to protect the wearer from respiratory infections, which provides a seal around the face and is defined and regulated by its filtration capacity.[1] [2]

No consensus exists around the choice between facemasks and respirators for respiratory protection, as is starkly illustrated by the widely discrepant guidelines for protection against the Ebola virus in the midst of the worst epidemic in history.[3] Although the efficacy of hand washing against respiratory and gastrointestinal infection has long been established in randomised clinical trials (RCTs),[4] [5] [6] evidence for facemasks has lagged behind. The threat of pandemic A/H5N1 influenza and resultant pandemic planning drove the first RCTs of facemasks in various settings.[7] [8] [9] [10] [11] [12] [13] [14] [15] [16] [17] [18] [19] The aim of this review is to inform policy makers and stakeholders by examining and summarising the available evidence related to the efficacy of facemasks and respirators, current practice, and guidelines, as well as highlighting the gaps in evidence.

Sources and selection criteria

We used the following keywords: "facemask", "mask", "surgical mask", "medical mask", "cotton/cloth mask", "respirator", "N95/N97, N99 respirator", "FFP2/FFP3 respirator", "P2/P3 respirator" "respiratory protection", "respiratory protective device", "infection control", "respiratory infections and facemasks/mask/respirator", "influenza and facemasks/mask/respirator", "flu and facemasks/mask/respirator", "pandemic influenza and facemasks/mask/respirator", "SARS and facemasks/mask/respirator" "tuberculosis and facemasks/mask/respirator", "TB and facemasks/mask/respirator" and emerging infections and facemasks/mask/respirator". The GRADE (grading of recommendations assessment, development and evaluation) approach was used to examine the type of evidence.[20] RCTs were considered as level 1 (high) evidence, observational studies (cohort, case control, before after, time series, case series, and case reports) as level 2 (low) evidence, and any other evidence as level 3 (very low) evidence.[20] Only high level evidence (from RCTs) is summarised in the tables and figures. Because this article is not a systematic review, we did not further grade individual RCTs into high, moderate, low, and very low quality evidence but summarised each RCT's specific limitations. AAC reviewed the titles of the search articles and prepared an initial list of articles to be included in the study. Both authors then independently reviewed the abstracts included in the list and selected studies to be included in the figures.

We examined infection control policies and guidelines from the World Health Organization, US Centres for Disease Prevention and Control (CDC), European Centre for Disease Prevention and Control (ECDC), and other health organisations for recommendations on the use of facemasks and respirators. We also did a Google search and searched the websites of other health related organisations. Policies and guidelines on the use of facemasks were also searched

Study, year of publication	Design, methods	Mask type, intervention	Outcome	Results	Comments, limitations, biases
Jacobs[7] 2009	• Block RCT • Tertiary care hospitals in Tokyo Japan, 2007 • 32 HCWs (2464 subject days)	• Medical masks • Control group	• Self reported cold symptoms	• No difference in outcome (cold symptoms) in intervention v control arm (P=0.81)	• Self reported compliance 84.3% • Small study • Underpowered • Symptoms self reported—not laboratory confirmed
Loeb et al[8] 2009	• Non-inferiority randomised clinical trial, no controls • 8 tertiary care hospitals in Ontario, Canada 2008-09 • 446 nurses	• Targeted use of medical masks • Fit tested N95 respirators	• Laboratory confirmed influenza infection assessed by PCR or seroconversion during 2008-09	• No difference in the outcome • Rate of mostly serologically defined influenza in the medical mask group 23.6% v 22.9% in the respirator group (absolute risk difference −0.73%, 95% CI −8.8% to −7.3%)	• No data on compliance • No control arm, no information on training or fit testing • Despite statement to the contrary, reported numerator and denominator data show that seropositive vaccinated subjects included in definition of "influenza" • Study was stopped early owing to influenza A/H1N1-pdm09, as respirator use became mandatory • Stated as "non-inferiority" but superiority of any tested intervention not previously proved in any RCT
MacIntyre[9] 2011	• Cluster RCT • 15 hospitals in Beijing China, 2008-09 • 1441 HCWs, 481 convenience controls	• Medical masks • N95 respirators (fit tested) • N95 respirators (not fit tested) • Convenience control group	• Self reported CRI • Self reported ILI • Laboratory confirmed viral infection and influenza by PCR	• Compared with medical masks, all outcomes were consistently lower for the N95 group • CRI (OR 0.38, 0.17 to 0.86) and laboratory confirmed viral infection (0.19, 0.05 to 0.67) significantly lower in N95 group	• Self reported compliance 68-86% • Use of convenience control group • N95 protective compared with medical masks (excluding controls) • Lack of power for PCR confirmed influenza
MacIntyre[10] 2013	• Cluster RCT, no controls • Beijing China 2010-11 • 1669 HCWs in 68 wards (19 hospitals)	• Continuous use of N95 respirators • Targeted use of N95 respirators for high risk situations • Continuous use of medical masks	• Self reported CRI • Self reported ILI • Laboratory confirmed viral infection and influenza by PCR	• Rates of CRI (HR 0.39, 0.21 to 0.71) and bacterial colonisation (0.40, 0.21 to 0.73) significantly lower in the continuous N95 respirator use arm	• Self reported compliance 57-82% • Lack of power for PCR confirmed influenza
MacIntyre[45] 2014*	• Cluster RCT • 15 hospitals in Beijing China, 2008-09 • 1441 HCWs	• Medical masks • N95 respirators (fit tested and not fit tested) • Convenience control group	• Laboratory confirmed bacterial colonisation	• Bacterial colonisation was significantly lower among HCWs who used N95 respirators (RR 0.34, 0.21 to 0.56) • Dual infections significantly lower in N95 arm	• Analysis of bacterial outcomes from previous RCT • Bacterial testing was done on symptomatic subjects only, so cannot determine if bacterial colonisation higher in symptomatic versus asymptomatic subjects

*Same as the RCT by MacIntyre,[9] but reports the outcome of bacterial infection.
CI=confidence interval; CRI=clinical respiratory infection; HCW=healthcare worker; HR=hazard ratio; ILI=influenza-like illness; OR=odds ratio; PCR=polymerase chain reaction; RCT=randomised controlled trial; RR=relative risk

Fig 1 Summary of high level evidence (GRADE guidelines) on facemasks and respirators in the healthcare setting

using the following keywords: "infection control guideline/ policy/plan", "pandemic influenza guideline/policy/plan", "personal protective equipment use/guideline", "personal protective equipment use/guideline for infection control", "masks use/guideline for infection control", "respirator use/guideline for infection control". Only English language articles were reviewed.

Use of facemasks and respirators in healthcare settings

Studies in the late 19th century first examined cloth masks for the prevention of the spread of infection from surgeons to patients in the operating theatre.[21] [22] Cloth masks have been used for respiratory protection since the early 20th century.[23] The first study of the use of facemasks by healthcare workers in 1918 found low rates of infection in those who used a cloth mask.[24] Masks were also used to protect healthcare workers from scarlet fever, measles,[25] influenza,[26] [27] plague,[28] and tuberculosis.[29]

The use of disposable medical masks became common in the mid-20th century,[30] [31] with very little research on cloth masks since, despite their continued widespread use in developing countries.[23] Respirators were later specifically designed for respiratory protection. We identified 13 RCTs on face masks and respirators, which studied a diverse range of interventions and outcomes. Of these, four were conducted in the healthcare setting and nine in various community and household settings.[7] [8] [9] [10] [11] [12] [13] [14] [15] [16] [17] [18] [19] Three unpublished RCTs were identified from clinical trial registries, two of which were carried out in healthcare settings and one in the Hajj.[32] [33] [34] We also found systematic reviews of some RCTs, and several observational studies.[35] [36] [37] [38] [39] [40] [41] [42] [43]

Efficacy of facemasks and respirators in healthcare settings

Randomised controlled trials

In line with GRADE, we considered RCTs as the best available evidence. We identified only four RCTs of the clinical efficacy of facemasks or respirators in healthcare workers, which studied a diverse range of interventions and outcomes (fig 2).[7] [8] [9] [10] The updated 2014 WHO guidelines on personal protective equipment (PPE) cite two of these four trials,[44] but exclude the larger two.[9] [10]

The first trial, which was carried out in healthcare workers in Japan, randomised 32 workers to a medical mask group or a control arm. It found no significant difference in respiratory illnesses (P=0.81) but was underpowered to examine efficacy.[7] The second trial compared targeted use of medical masks and N95 respirators in 446 nurses in Canada and reported equal efficacy in preventing influenza (23.6% with medical masks v 22.9% with respirators; absolute risk difference, −0.73%, 95% confidence interval −8.8% to 7.3%).[8] However, because the study did not have a control group it technically cannot determine efficacy—both arms may have been equally ineffective, as suggested by the high rate of influenza in both groups. Similar rates of influenza of 23% have been described in unprotected healthcare workers during hospital influenza outbreaks.[46] Studies of nosocomial influenza generally describe lower attack rates than this second study, which suggests that targeted masks and respirators are equally inefficacious (rather than equally efficacious).[47]

The third trial, which investigated 1922 healthcare workers in China, compared continuous use of medical

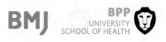

masks, N95 respirators (fit tested and not fit tested), and a control group.[9] N95 respirators protected against clinical respiratory infection (odds ratio 0.38, 0.17 to 0.86 but not against polymerase chain reaction (PCR) confirmed influenza.[9] Trends for all outcomes, including influenza, showed the highest infection rates in the control arm and the lowest in the N95 arm.

The fourth RCT, which looked at 1669 healthcare workers in China, compared continuous use of N95 respirators, targeted use of N95 respirators while doing high risk procedures, and continuous use of medical masks. The study showed efficacy of continuous N95 use against clinical respiratory infection (hazard ratio 0.39, 0.21 to 0.71) and bacterial colonisation (0.40, 0.21 to 0.73). No difference was seen between targeted N95 use and medical mask use, which suggests that a N95 respirator needs to be worn throughout the shift to be protective.[10] None of the four RCTs showed that medical masks were efficacious, although efficacy might have been at a lower level than the trials were able to detect.[9] [10]

Bacterial colonisation

An analysis published in 2014 showed that laboratory confirmed bacterial colonisation (mainly *Streptococcus pneumoniae* and *Haemophilus influenzae*) is common in healthcare workers with symptoms of respiratory illness.[45] Importantly, N95 respirators significantly reduced the risk of bacterial colonisation by 62% compared with no mask and by 46% compared with medical masks, which were not efficacious. These findings may have important implications for policy and practice, but the role of respirators to help combat antibiotic resistant bacteria has not been tested in an RCT. The analysis also found that simultaneous infection of healthcare workers with two bacteria and a virus, or a bacterium and two viruses was common,[45] and that an N95 respirator significantly protected against dual infections.

Non-randomised studies

Lower levels of evidence are available from cohort,[48] case-control,[49 50 51 52 53 54 55] cross sectional,[56 57 58 59 60 61] laboratory experimental,[62 63 64 65 66 67 68] and observational (including time series and case series) studies.[69 70 71 72 73 74 75 76 77 78] Most were conducted during the severe acute respiratory syndrome (SARS) outbreak,[50 51 52 53 54 55 59 60 61 69 72 73 74 75 79] but others examined tuberculosis,[77 80 81] respiratory syncytial virus (RSV),[48] and pertussis.[58]

With a few exceptions,[53 60 74] evidence from SARS favoured the use of facemasks or respirators (or both) in healthcare workers. Respirators are generally recommended for tuberculosis, although most of these studies examined a combination of simultaneous infection control practices (environmental and source control measures).[77 80 81] No study has measured the efficacy of facemasks or respirators in preventing tuberculosis (either asymptomatic infection or disease) in healthcare workers. A small study found no significant difference in the rate of RSV between hand hygiene versus mask wearing or hand hygiene versus gown wearing.[48] An observational study showed that medical masks protected against nosocomial transmission of pertussis in staff and patients.[58]

In vivo studies report varying levels of filtration performance and protection for different types of barrier, with the degree of protection increasing from cloth masks, to medical masks, and finally to respirators.[37 64 68] Conflicting advice is given by different agencies for other infections

such as Middle East respiratory syndrome coronavirus (MERS-CoV) and Ebola virus disease.[3 82]

Role of cloth masks

Cloth masks are commonly used in developing countries and many non-standard practices around cleaning and reuse have evolved. However, no RCTs of cloth masks have been published. Most studies were conducted before the development of disposable masks.[23] Data on the use of cloth masks for the prevention of diphtheria, measles, and tuberculosis are limited and outdated.[24 25 29] The penetration through cloth is reported to be high—40-90% of particles penetrated in one study.[63] Without an RCT it is unclear whether cloth masks provide clinical protection. Given their widespread use in developing countries, including Asia, where the risk of emerging infectious diseases is high, research on the clinical efficacy of cloth masks is needed. Healthcare workers in the west African Ebola outbreak use cloth masks when other supplies are not available (personal communication, W Beckley, 2014). Guidelines make cautious recommendations about the use of such masks when medical masks and respirators are in high demand and supplies are exhausted.[83 84]

Facemasks as source control

Facemasks were first used in operating theatres to maintain a sterile operating field and to prevent transmission of infection from surgeons to patients. However, studies fail to show any efficacy for this indication.[85 86 87] Only one randomly controlled clinical trial reported high infection rates after gynaecological and abdominal surgery—three of five women developed infection in the "no mask" group compared with no infections in the four women operated on by a masked surgeon.[88] Guidelines have recommended medical masks for use in operating theatres to protect staff from the splash and spray of blood and body fluids.[89] A visor or protective face shield may be used, subject to adequate air circulation and ventilation,[90] but no studies have directly compared these options. Although the use of facemasks for source control has not been proved in the operating theatre setting, their use is standard across most healthcare sites.

As source control, facemasks are also used by sick people to prevent the spread of infection to others. An experimental study showed that the spread of influenza virus from a sick patient may be reduced by the patient wearing a facemask or a respirator.[91] A study on volunteers with influenza-like illnesses symptoms reported a more than threefold reduction of viral particles in exhaled samples with use of medical masks.[92] During the SARS outbreak, medical and cloth masks were used as source control and were reported to be effective.[61] Evidence shows that the use of facemasks by infective patients with tuberculosis reduces the risk of tuberculosis transmission.[93] Despite the lack of data from human clinical trials, medical masks are highly recommended by WHO, the CDC, and the ECDC for source control in tuberculosis.[44 94 95]

The use of facemasks in the community setting

Facemasks are used in the community in Asian countries, not only to protect people from acquiring respiratory infections but also to minimise spread of infection from the wearer. Such use often increases during outbreaks and pandemics. Cloth masks were reportedly used by the general public during the 1918 influenza pandemic.[26 27] During the SARS outbreaks, masks were widely used in diverse community settings.[96 97]

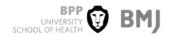
Study, year of publication	Design, participants	Mask type, intervention	Outcome	Results	Comments, limitations, biases
Cowling[11] 2008	• Cluster RCT • 198 index cases and household contacts • Hong Kong	• Medical masks • Hand hygiene • Control	• Self reported influenza symptoms • Laboratory confirmed influenza (by culture or RT-PCR) in household	• No significant difference in rates of laboratory confirmed influenza (OR 1.16, 95% CI 0.31 to 4.34) and ILI (0.88, 0.34 to 2.27) in the medical masks arm versus control arm	• Both index cases and household contacts used medical masks • This pilot study was small and underpowered • Compliance 45% in index cases and 21% in household contacts • Compliance data showed that some index cases in the control and hand hygiene arms used medical masks
Cowling[12] 2009	• Cluster RCT • 407 index cases and 794 household contacts • Hong Kong	• Hand hygiene • Masks + hand hygiene • Control (education)	• Self reported influenza symptoms • Laboratory confirmed influenza (by RT-PCR) in household	• No significant difference in rate of laboratory confirmed influenza in three arms • Significant difference if masks + hand hygiene together applied within 36 hours of illness (OR 0.33, 0.13 to 0.87) • Hand hygiene alone was not significant	• No separate medical mask arm, making it difficult to evaluate the efficacy of masks • Both index cases and household contacts used masks • Compliance 49% in index cases and 26% in household contacts using masks • Compliance data showed that some index cases in the control and hand hygiene arms used medical masks
MacIntyre[13] 2009	• Cluster RCT • 145 child index cases and well adult household contacts • Australia	• Medical masks for contacts • P2 respirators (equivalent to N95) for contacts • Control	• Self reported ILI • Laboratory confirmed respiratory infection	• No significant difference in ILI and laboratory confirmed respiratory infections in all three arms • Adherent use of P2 or medical masks significantly reduced the risk of ILI (HR 0.26, 0.09 to 0.77)	• Only household contacts used medical masks • Low compliance: 21% of household contacts wore masks often/always
Aiello[14] 2010	• Cluster RCT • 1437 well university residents • Michigan, USA	• Medical masks • Medical masks + hand hygiene • Control	• Self reported ILI • Laboratory confirmed influenza (by culture or RT-PCR)	• No significant difference in ILI in three arms • Significant reduction in ILI in the medical masks + hand hygiene arm over 4-6 weeks (P<0.05)	• Self reported ILI • Not all ILI cases (n=368) were laboratory tested (n=94) • No data on compliance
Larson[15] 2010	• Block RCT • 617 households • Manhattan, USA	• HE • HE + hand sanitiser • HE + hand sanitiser + medical masks	• Self reported ILI • Self reported URI • Laboratory confirmed influenza through culture or PCR	• No significant difference in rates of URI, ILI, or laboratory confirmed influenza between the three arms • Significantly lower secondary attack rates of URI/ILI/influenza in the HE + hand sanitiser + medical mask arm (OR 0.82, 0.70 to 0.97).	• No separate medical masks group • Household contacts used medical masks • Low compliance and around half of household in the masks arm used masks within 48 hours • There was no index case at home
Canini[16] 2010	• Cluster RCT • 105 index cases and 306 households • France	• Medical mask (as source control to be used by index case) • Control	• Self reported ILI in household	• No significant difference in the rates of ILI between the two arms (OR 0.95, 0.44 to 2.05)	• Trial stopped early owing to low recruitment and influenza A/H1N1-pdm09 in subsequent year
Simmerman[17] 2011	• Cluster RCT • 465 index patients and their families • Thailand	• Hand hygiene • Hand hygiene + medical masks • Control	• Self reported ILI • Laboratory confirmed influenza by PCR and serology in family members	• No significant difference in secondary influenza infection rates between hand hygiene arm (OR 1.20, 0.76 to 1.88) and hand hygiene plus medial masks arm (1.16, 0.74 to 1.82)	• No separate medical mask group • Owing to H1N1 pandemic, hand and respiratory hygiene campaigns and mask use substantially increased among the index cases (from 4% to 52%) and families (from 17.6% to 67.7%) in control arm
Aiello[18] 2012	• Cluster RCT • 1178 university residents • Michigan, USA	• Medical masks • Medical masks + hand hygiene • Control	• Clinically diagnosed and laboratory confirmed influenza (by RT-PCR)	• No overall difference in ILI and laboratory confirmed influenza in three arms • Significant reduction in ILI in the medical masks + hand hygiene arm over 3-6 weeks (P<0.05)	• Good compliance: medical mask + hand hygiene group used masks for 5.08 h/day (SD 2.23) and medical mask group used masks for 5.04 h/day (SD 2.20) • Self reported ILI • Effect may have been due to hand hygiene because medical masks alone not significant
Suess[19] 2012	• Cluster RCT • 84 index cases and 218 household contacts • Berlin, Germany	• Masks • Masks + hand hygiene • Control	• Laboratory confirmed influenza infection and ILI	• No significant difference in rates of laboratory confirmed influenza and ILI in all arms by intention to treat analysis • The risk of influenza was significantly lower if data from two intervention arms (masks and masks + hand hygiene) were pooled and intervention was applied within 36 hours of the onset of symptoms (OR 0.16, 0.03 to 0.92)	• Around 50% participants wore masks "mostly" or "always" • Participants paid to provide respiratory samples

CI=confidence interval; CRI=clinical respiratory infection; HCW=healthcare worker; HE=health education; HR=hazard ratio; ILI=influenza-like illness; OR=odds ratio; PCR=polymerase chain reaction; RCT=randomised controlled trial; RR=relative risk. RT=reverse transcriptase; SD=standard deviation; URI=upper respiratory tract infection.

Fig 2 Summary of high level evidence (GRADE guidelines) on facemasks in the household setting

Efficacy of facemasks in the community

We identified nine RCTs of facemasks in various household and community settings,[11 12 13 14 15 16 17 18 19] and in all but one they were used for respiratory protection. In one household trial the use of facemasks was tested as source control to prevent the spread of infections from the wearer.[16] These RCTs had diverse settings, designs, and interventions—many of which were mixed, such as hand washing and facemasks (fig 3).

An RCT in Hong Kong randomised index cases (198 laboratory confirmed influenza cases) and their households into medical masks, hand hygiene, or a control arm. Rates of laboratory confirmed influenza and influenza-like illness were not significantly different in the medical mask arm versus the control arm (influenza: odds ratio 1.16, 0.31 to 4.34; influenza-like illness: 0.88, 0.34 to 2.27).[11] In a second trial by the same group, medical masks plus hand hygiene and hand hygiene alone groups were compared with a control group (total 407 index cases). There was no significant difference across the three arms, although medical masks plus hand hygiene were protective when

the intervention was implemented early (within 36 hours of onset of symptoms in the index case, adjusted odds ratio 0.33, 0.13 to 0.87).[12]

An Australian study randomised 145 index cases and their household members to one of three arms—medical masks, P2 respirators (equivalent to N95), or control.[13] In contrast to the second trial above, where both index cases and household members used a mask,[12] only household contacts used a medical mask in this study. No significant difference in the risk of influenza-like illness was seen between the three arms in the per protocol analysis, but risk was significantly lower with the adherent use of P2 or medical masks (hazard ratio 0.26, 0.09 to 0.77).[13]

Two RCTs in university residence halls in the United States over two influenza seasons randomised well students into medical masks plus hand hygiene, medical masks alone, or control.[14 18] Influenza-like illness and laboratory confirmed influenza were not significantly reduced after either intervention, although during the first four to six weeks, influenza-like illness was significantly lower in the medical masks plus hand hygiene arm in both trials (P<0.05).[14 18]

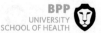

Table 1 Summary indications for use of masks and respirators for selected infectious diseases

Disease	Healthcare setting*		Community setting†	
	Low risk	High risk	Low risk	High risk
Seasonal influenza	First choice: medical mask‡§; Second choice: cloth mask**	First choice: respirator‡§; Second choice: medical mask**; Third choice: cloth mask**	Not recommended‡§	Not recommended‡§
Pandemic influenza	First choice: respirator‡ or medical mask§; Second choice: cloth mask**	First choice: respirator‡§; Second choice: medical mask**; Third choice: cloth mask**	Not recommended‡§	First choice: medical mask‡§; Second choice: cloth masks**
MERS-CoV	First choice: respirator‡ or medical mask§	First choice: respirator‡§	Not recommended	Not recommended
Tuberculosis	First choice: respirator‡§	First choice: respirator‡§	Not recommended‡§	Not recommended*†
Ebola virus	First choice: respirator‡ or medical mask§; Second choice: cloth mask**	First choice: respirator‡§; Second choice: medical mask**; Third choice: cloth mask**	Not recommended§	First choice: medical mask§; Second choice: cloth masks**

*Low risk: routine patient care, not within 1-2 m of infective patient; High risk: high risk procedures such as aerosol generating procedures, new or drug resistance organism.

†Low risk: home, non-crowded settings; high risk: crowded settings (such as public transport), pre-existing illness, pregnancy, older age (pandemic influenza), contact with human remains or infected animals (Ebola virus).

‡Centres for Disease Control and Prevention (CDC).

§World Health Organization.

**Not stated explicitly—inference drawn from Institute of Medicine (IOM) guidelines and other policy documents prepared for low recourse settings (As efficacy data is not available, cloth masks should be used only when no other option is available).

MERS-CoV=Middle East respiratory syndrome coronavirus.

This suggests that hand hygiene might have been the major contributor to protection.

An RCT in the US randomised 617 households to education, hand sanitiser alone, or hand sanitiser plus medical masks. Although the rates of upper respiratory tract infections, influenza-like illness, and laboratory confirmed influenza were low in the hand sanitiser and hand sanitiser plus medical masks groups, the difference was not significant after adjusting for other factors. However, the hand sanitiser plus medical masks group had significantly lower secondary attack rates for influenza, influenza-like illness, and upper respiratory tract infections (odds ratio 0.82, 0.70 to 0.97) compared with the education group. Results for the hand sanitiser only group were not significant (1.01, 0.85 to 1.21).[15]

An RCT in Thailand randomised 465 index patients and their families to hand hygiene, hand hygiene plus medical masks, and a control arm. No significant difference between secondary influenza rate was seen.[17]

In a cluster randomised controlled trial in Germany, 84 index cases and 218 household contacts were randomised into a mask arm, masks plus hand hygiene arm, and a control arm. There was no significant difference in rates of laboratory confirmed influenza and influenza-like illness in all arms by intention to treat analysis. However, the risk of influenza was significantly lower if the data from two intervention arms were pooled and the intervention was applied within 36 hours of the onset of symptoms (odds ratio 0.16, 0.03 to 0.92).[19]

A household trial in France examined the role of medical masks as source control—index patients were randomised into medical mask (52 household and 148 contacts) and control groups (53 household and 158 contacts). There was no difference between the groups (0.95, 0.44 to 2.05), and the trial was finished early owing to low recruitment and subsequent H1N1-pdm09 infection.[16]

Community use of facemasks during outbreaks and pandemics

The routine use of facemasks is not recommended by WHO, the CDC, or the ECDC in the community setting.[98 99 100] However, the use of facemasks is recommended in crowded settings (such as public transport) and for those at high risk (older people, pregnant women, and those with a medical condition) during an outbreak or pandemic.[98 99]

A modelling study suggests that the use of facemasks in the community may help delay and contain a pandemic, although efficacy estimates were not based on RCT data.[101] Community masks were protective during the SARS outbreaks, and about 76% of the population used a facemask in Hong Kong.[102] There is evidence that masks have efficacy in the community setting, subject to compliance[13] and early use.[12 18 19] It has been shown that compliance in the household setting decreases with each day of mask use, however, which makes long term use over weeks or months a challenge.[13]

The statistical power of each individual RCT may have been too low to determine efficacy by intention to treat, and larger trials may be needed. A meta-analysis of the existing community trials would be difficult because of the diverse settings, interventions, outcomes, and measurements. The study designs of all but one of the RCTs used mixed interventions, where one intervention was present in both intervention arms (such as hand hygiene alone compared with masks plus hand hygiene; fig 3), which makes it more difficult to determine the efficacy of masks alone.

Choice of facemask versus respirator

In communities where facemasks are commonly used, such as in Asia, the choice is between medical masks and cloth masks. In the healthcare setting, the choice is between respirators or medical masks in developed countries, and between respirators, medical masks, or cloth masks in developing countries (table 1). In the healthcare sector the purpose of PPE is the occupational health and safety of healthcare workers, and the choice should be made using a risk analysis framework.[3] The framework should be based on expected mode of transmission, level of exposure or risk, severity of the disease in question, availability of other preventive or therapeutic agents, and uncertainty about transmission. Cost considerations, organisational factors, and individual factors (such as compliance) may affect implementation but should not drive best practice guidelines. In developing countries, the cost of N95

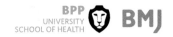

Table 2 Primary modes of transmission of respiratory infections

Presumed main mode of transmission	Examples of virus	Examples of bacteria
Droplet	Influenza virus A and B*, coronavirus*	*Streptococcus pneumoniae*, *Haemophilus influenzae*
Airborne	Rhinovirus A and B	Tuberculosis, *Bordetella pertussis**
Contact	Adenovirus, parainfluenza virus, respiratory syncytial virus, Middle East respiratory syndrome coronavirus*	

*Primary mode is by droplet transmission, but airborne transmission may occur in high risk situations.

respirators may limit their use, and cloth masks are popular because they can be cleaned and reused.

Transmission modes

Infectious diseases can spread though droplets, respiratory aerosols, or direct and indirect contact with contaminated surfaces (table 2). Droplets are large particles (>5 μm), generally emitted while coughing or sneezing, which do not remain suspended in the air, whereas aerosols are small particles (<5 μm), which can remain suspended in the air for several hours and transmit infection over long distances.[2] [103]

A medical mask is theoretically sufficient to prevent droplet infection, whereas a respirator is needed to prevent airborne infection. In terms of facemask use, the physical barrier may also prevent contact transmission such as hand to face, mouth, or nose. A facemask or a respirator may provide protection against multiple modes of transmission, including droplet, airborne, and hand to mouth (or nose) transmission.

The relative contribution of each mode is difficult to quantify and is controversial,[104] [105] but the debate about mode of transmission is academic if an intervention is shown to prevent infection in a clinical trial. Clinical efficacy data should take precedence over theoretical debates about modes of transmission, which have long dominated the discourse on PPE.

The current paradigm of droplet and airborne transmission is based on outmoded experiments from the 1950s, done using outdated equipment, and it oversimplifies the complexity of pathogen transmission.[106] Enough evidence exists for us to know that pathogens are not transmitted by three mutually exclusive routes, and that the term "aerosol transmissible" is preferable to droplet or airborne.[106] For example, evidence exists that influenza, which has been thought of as predominantly droplet spread,[104] can also be spread by the airborne route.[103] [105] [107] Pathogens that are spread predominantly through droplets do not need to travel long distances in air currents (as in the current definition of airborne) to be inhaled and cause infection. They can be transmitted in short range aerosols, for which a facemask does not offer sufficient protection.[106]

It is further argued that aerosol transmission and airborne transmission are not the same. Airborne transmission can occur through inhalation of small infectious particles at long or short distances from the infectious person, even in the absence of aerosols or aerosol generating procedures owing to evaporation of larger droplets.[106] Diseases transmitted mainly through the airborne route, such as tuberculosis, require a properly fitted N95 or higher respirator. Aerosol transmission may also occur during high risk procedures with organisms that are normally transmitted by other routes. Similarly, evidence suggests that infective aerosols may be generated from vomitus and faecal matter in people infected with norovirus and SARS.[108] [109] [110] [111] Respirators have also been shown to be more effective against aerosol transmission.[112]

When the transmission dynamics of a newly emergent infection are unknown, a respirator should be used as a precaution.[44] For example, respirators were initially recommended for SARS and H1N1-pdm09,[99] [113] but recommendations were later changed in favour of masks.[44] [114] It is unclear what evidence underpinned this change.

High risk situations

Healthcare workers who undertake high risk aerosol generating procedures have a threefold higher risk of acquiring nosocomial respiratory infections than those who do not.[112] WHO and the CDC recommend medical masks to protect from seasonal influenza; however, a respirator is recommended when high risk procedures are performed.[44] [115] Recent debate about "surgical smoke" (aerosols generated during surgery that uses lasers or diathermy) indicates that superior respiratory protection is needed for operating theatre staff.[116]

During the SARS epidemic, high risk procedures put healthcare workers at high risk of acquiring infection.[117] In a study in Hong Kong, none of the staff who wore medical masks or respirators became infected. However, the study excluded one hospital in which cases occurred as a result of a high risk procedure (drug nebulisation), and the authors concluded that medical masks are sufficient to protect against SARS if there is no risk of aerosol transmission.[50] Inconsistent use of N95 respirators was not associated with the acquisition of infection during the SARS outbreak in the US, and this was attributed to low rates of aerosol generating procedures.[60] In the Ebola virus outbreak of 2014, the CDC and other agencies changed their guidelines from surgical masks to respirators after nurses became infected.[118]

Organisational and individual factors

Organisational and individual factors play a role in use of respiratory protection. Healthcare workers may be limited by what is available in the workplace. Availability, cost, and the ability to conduct annual fit testing are important.

Few options are available in most low resource settings, and healthcare workers may have to buy their own masks.[119] During the H1N1-pdm09 pandemic, the supply of respirators was exhausted in many hospitals, and healthcare workers had to reuse respirators or rely on other types of facemask.[120] [121]

Current stockpiling guidelines are based on assumptions about the size and duration of a pandemic, hospital stay, number of healthcare workers, and length of shifts,[122] but these may be inaccurate.[123] [124] It has been documented that non-standard practices occur during outbreaks, especially when there is a shortage of supplies.[119] There is very little research on such practices, which include reuse, cleaning of facemasks, and double masking.[125]

The balance between risk perception and discomfort affects individual decisions to use facemasks and respirators. When the risk of infection is thought to be high, acceptance and compliance with interventions to prevent infection are generally higher.[126] Compliance was reported to be high during the initial phase of the H1N1-pdm09 pandemic, when risk perception was high, but it later decreased when healthcare workers thought that the pandemic was less severe than initially estimated.[121]

In countries that have experienced epidemics such as SARS, mask wearing is more acceptable, but it is not commonplace in countries such as the UK, US, and Australia.[127] Compliance with the wearing of facemasks

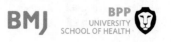

is lower than for other PPE,[128] [129] and it decreases with increased duration of use.[9] Compared with medical masks, respirators are associated with more adverse effects, such as discomfort, headache, skin irritation, and pressure on the nose.[9] [10] However, in China, despite healthcare workers reporting the same level of discomfort with respirators as in Western countries, compliance remains high.[9] [10] [127] Discomfort is therefore not the sole determinant of compliance, which is also influenced by cultural factors, risk perception, and experience of serious outbreaks such as SARS.

Healthcare workers are known to be poorly compliant with other infection control interventions, such as hand hygiene and vaccination, which points to a particularly challenging organisational culture.[130] [131] A supportive organisational environment, promotion of a safety culture, regular communication, availability of respiratory protective equipment, and training programmes improve compliance.[56] [132] [133] [134] Legislation may also work—New York State recently passed legislation that compels all frontline healthcare workers to either receive influenza vaccination or use a facemask.[135]

Regulations, training, and fit testing of respirators

The optimal use of respirators requires selection of certified respirators, training and fit testing, and inspection, as well as suitable maintenance and storage of the equipment.[136] Certified respirators should be used in the healthcare setting, and the certification process should be managed by a regulatory body, such as the US National Institute for Occupational Safety and Health (NIOSH).[137] In Europe, European Norm (EN) standards and in Australia, AS/NZS 1716 standards regulate the use of respirators.[138] [139]

Low resource countries may lack the resources to manage the regulation and certification process. A recent survey of 89 hospital in low to middle income countries showed that very few hospitals used certified respirators, and where used the various types of respirators were of unknown quality (unpublished data).

Training, fit checking (previously known as user seal checking), and fit testing are vital components of any respiratory protection programme, which must ensure a seal between the respirator and the face so that air does not leak out. Healthcare workers should be trained in donning (order and methods of putting on facemasks and respirators) and doffing (order and methods of removing facemasks and respirators) techniques so that they do not contaminate themselves. Fit checking is a qualitative process and not a substitute for fit testing; it should be done every time a respirator is donned to ensure that it is sealed to the face, with no gap between the face and the respirator.[140]

Fit testing ensures that the specific type (for example, model and size) of respirator is suitable for the wearer. Fit testing can be quantitative or qualitative, with the second option being cheaper for most workplaces.[141] Qualitative fit test is performed by releasing a bitter or sweet agent into an exposure chamber to test whether the wearer can taste the agent.[141] This test is easy to perform but indicates lack of fit only and does not measure leakage around the respirator.

In the quantitative test, air sampling is performed from inside the respirator through a fit testing instrument and the amount of leakage is calculated.[141] No clinical data are available to support the use of fit testing—the recommendation to fit test is based on laboratory evidence. The efficacy of a respirator is thought to improve with fit testing,[142] but the only trial to compare fit tested and non-fit tested respirators showed no difference in efficacy with fit testing.[9] These results are specific to the respirator used in that trial and cannot be generalised to other respirators because respirators are regulated for filtration only and not for fit, which varies widely between products.

In vivo studies showed that properly fitted respirators decrease the risk of infection transmission and block most viral particles.[142] Fit testing is recommended annually, because weight gain or changes in facial shape or size can change the adequacy of fit.

Current data suggest that rates of fit checking and fit testing are low among healthcare workers.[143] [144] Surveys of health professionals and home based healthcare workers in the US showed that respirators were supplied to most during the H1N1-pdm09 pandemic, but that less than a third were fit tested.[145] [146] Various types of respirators were fit tested in an Australian study and 28% of healthcare workers were unable to fit any available respirator owing to variations in face shape.[147]

Policies and guidelines around the use of facemasks and respirators

Different health organisations and countries have diverse policies and guidelines on the use of facemasks and respirators.[3] [148] WHO and the CDC have consistent policies for the use of facemasks and respirators to protect against seasonal influenza and tuberculosis,[44] [94] [115] [149] but policies for pandemic influenza are inconsistent.[44] [150]

For seasonal influenza, both organisations recommend medical masks in low risk situations and N95 respirators in high risk situations, such as aerosol generating procedures. For some other infections, such as Ebola virus, MERS-CoV, and during an influenza pandemic, WHO recommends the use of medical masks in low risk situations and N95 respirators in high risk situations,[44] [151] [152] whereas, the CDC now recommends respirators in both situations.[82] [118] [150] Respirators are recommended by both organisations to protect healthcare workers from tuberculosis.[94] [149]

High, middle, and low income countries also have diverse policies on the use of facemasks and adopt variations on WHO or CDC guidelines depending on resources and occupational health and safety legislation.[148] [153] For Ebola virus, which is mostly spread by contact, WHO and many countries recommend a medical mask, but this recommendation has been challenged on multiple grounds.[3] No RCTs have compared respirators with facemasks for Ebola, but several healthcare workers have contracted Ebola while using PPE.[154] Many countries look to the WHO and CDC guidelines to model their own guidelines. The CDC remains highly influential for developed countries, Australia being an example.

Different policy recommendations may reflect the paucity of evidence and varying results of the few available RCTs of facemasks in the healthcare setting. However, for end users in the hospital setting, the conflicting guidance from different sources (such as WHO and the CDC) is not ideal. A US study showed that healthcare workers used various types of facemasks and respirators during the H1N1-pdm09 pandemic as a result of the conflicting guidance from WHO and the CDC.[121]

Despite widespread use in low resource settings, most guidelines do not cover or only briefly mention cloth masks.[23] In addition, most policy documents do not discuss recommendations on the extended use and reuse of facemasks and respirators.[148]

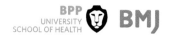

Research gaps

Limitations of existing evidence

Clinical trials of facemasks report a range of outcomes from self reported clinical syndromes to laboratory confirmed viruses,[7 8 9 10 11 12 13 15 16 17 18 19] which might not be generalisable to other specific infectious diseases. Cross sectional and observational studies of masks largely draw from the SARS outbreak, and may not be applicable to other pathogens,[36] because SARS was less infectious than many other respiratory infections and was mostly nosocomial.[155]

Laboratory based studies of masks are mostly simulated and so have limited clinical application because they cannot account for events such as compliance, coughing, talking, and other subtle actions by the wearer. Although masks and respirators are commonly used to protect the wearer against tuberculosis, no clinical trial data are available to prove their efficacy, and a trial of respirators versus a "no mask" group is unlikely to be conducted. Elastomeric respirators (reusable full face respirators with a changeable cartridge) and powered air purifying respirators are increasingly recommended in the healthcare setting but have not been tested in an RCT.[148]

Another limitation of the available facemask studies is the mixing of interventions. In four trials in the community setting facemasks were combined with hand hygiene as an intervention, which makes it difficult to ascertain the efficacy of masks alone.[12 15 17 18]

Most studies failed to control for other infection control measures (administrative and environmental controls) and the use of other types of PPE, and compliance was variably accounted for.

Many observational and cross sectional studies also examined facemasks together with other forms of PPE and hand hygiene, so the observed effect might be due to the combined effect of hand hygiene or use of other types of PPE (or both).[48 58 70 73 75] Similarly, in some community based trials both index cases and household members used a mask,[12] whereas in others only household members used a mask.[13] In the first case, it may be difficult to ascertain whether efficacy is due to mask use by the index case, by a household member, or by both.

RCTS of facemasks are difficult to design and conduct owing to the complexity of follow-up and measurement of infection outcomes, the statistical power needed to examine outcomes such as influenza, and the difficulty in identifying settings where adequate compliance can be achieved to make a trial feasible. In most clinical trials, controls followed routine practice, and trials without a control arm cannot determine efficacy if no difference is found between interventions. The use of facemasks and respirators in the non-hospital healthcare setting (for example, in home based healthcare workers, nursing homes, paramedics, and ambulatory clinics) has not been studied.

New research

For influenza, further study is needed on the role of facemasks and other types of PPE in the hierarchy of other interventions such as vaccines, antivirals, and social distancing in pandemic planning. In general, a matched pandemic vaccine will not be available for three to six months after the emergence of a new pandemic influenza strain, so masks and respirators—along with other non-pharmaceutical measures and antivirals—will be particularly important in the early phase of a pandemic. The type of product used, estimated stockpiling, and role of extended use and reuse are important factors to consider. Cloth masks may be the only option for some countries, and their role in healthcare and community settings needs also to be further explored.

Studies should also be conducted on the storage of facemasks and respirators and stockpiling for pandemics. The shelf life of respirators is around three years, whereas medical masks have no specified shelf life.[123]

Given the large cost differential between respirators and masks, health economic studies that incorporate clinical efficacy data are needed to determine cost effectiveness.

Finally, more education and research are needed on modes of transmission to supersede the blunt experiments of the 1950s, the findings of which have become entrenched in the dogma on hospital infection control.[106] Old paradigms around droplet, airborne, and contact spread need to be reviewed when formulating guidelines to take into account clinical data that prove multi-modal spread for many pathogens.[103 105 107]

Conclusion

Facemasks and respirators are important but under-studied forms of PPE, which offer protection against respiratory infections. They may be the only available protection for healthcare workers when no drugs or vaccines are available and the mode of transmission is unknown.

Community RCTs suggest that facemasks provide protection against infection in various community settings, subject to compliance and early use. For healthcare workers, the evidence suggests that respirators offer superior protection to facemasks. During pandemics and outbreaks these form part of a suite of protection offered to frontline workers to ensure occupational health and safety. Respirators are also preferable when the disease is severe, with a high case fatality rate, and no drug treatment or vaccine is available.[3]

In developed countries, the choice for healthcare workers is between disposable masks and respirators, whereas in developing countries reusable cloth masks are also widely used in hospitals. RCTs on cloth masks are lacking, and policy guidance on their use is sparse.

Compliance is a determinant of protection, and it decreases with increasing duration of continuous mask use. Policies and guidelines on mask use worldwide are inconsistent, perhaps reflecting the relatively small number of RCTs available to inform them.

Ultimately the greatest priority is to provide evidence based choices for healthcare workers, whose occupational health and safety must be protected to ensure integrity and an effective response during an epidemic.

Contributors: Both authors contributed equally to the writing of this paper. CRM devised the structure and topic areas for the review, AAC did the literature review and first draft, and both contributed equally to the final manuscript.

Competing interests: We have read and understood BMJ policy on declaration of interests and declare the following interests: CRM has received funding for investigator driven research on facemasks from 3M in the form of an Australian Research Council Industry Linkage grant (where 3M was the industry partner) and supply of masks for clinical research. She also has received funding or in-kind support from GSK, Merck, BioCSL, and Pfizer for investigator driven research on infectious diseases. 3M Australia provided support to AAC for facemask testing as part of his PhD thesis.

Provenance and peer review: Commissioned; externally peer reviewed.

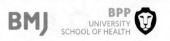

1   Institute of Medicine (IOM) National Academy of Sciences. Preventing transmission of pandemic influenza and other viral respiratory diseases: personal protective equipment for healthcare personnel update 2010. National Academies Press, 2010.

2   Siegel JD, Rhinehart E, Jackson M, Chiarello L. 2007 guideline for isolation precautions: preventing transmission of infectious agents in health care settings. Am J Infect Control2007;35(10 suppl 2):S65-164.

3   MacIntyre CR, Chughtai AA, Seale H, Richards GA, Davidson PM. Respiratory protection for healthcare workers treating Ebola virus disease (EVD): are facemasks sufficient to meet occupational health and safety obligations? Int J Nurs Stud2014;51:1421-6.

4   White C, Kolble R, Carlson R, Lipson N, Dolan M, Ali Y, et al. The effect of hand hygiene on illness rate among students in university residence halls. Am J Infect Control2003;31:364-70.

5   Luby SP, Agboatwalla M, Feikin DR, Painter J, Billhimer W, Altaf A, et al. Effect of handwashing on child health: a randomised controlled trial. Lancet 2005;366:225-33.

6   Rabie T, Curtis V. Handwashing and risk of respiratory infections: a quantitative systematic review. Trop Med Int Health 2006;11:258-67.

7   Jacobs JL, Ohde S, Takahashi O, Tokuda Y, Omata F, Fukui T. Use of surgical face masks to reduce the incidence of the common cold among health care workers in Japan: a randomized controlled trial. Am J Infect Control 2009;37:417-9.

8   Loeb M, Dafoe N, Mahony J, John M, Sarabia A, Glavin V, et al. Surgical mask vs N95 respirator for preventing influenza among health care workers: a randomized trial. JAMA 2009;302:1865-71.

9   MacIntyre CR, Wang Q, Cauchemez S, Seale H, Dwyer DE, Yang P, et al. A cluster randomized clinical trial comparing fit-tested and non-fit-tested N95 respirators to medical masks to prevent respiratory virus infection in health care workers. Influenza Other Respir Viruses2011;5:170-9.

10   MacIntyre CR, Wang Q, Seale H, Yang P, Shi W, Gao Z, et al. A randomized clinical trial of three options for N95 respirators and medical masks in health workers. Am J Respir Crit Care Med2013;187:960-6.

11   Cowling BJ, Fung RO, Cheng CK, Fang VJ, Chan KH, Seto WH, et al. Preliminary findings of a randomized trial of non-pharmaceutical interventions to prevent influenza transmission in households. PloS One2008;3:e2101.

12   Cowling BJ, Chan KH, Fang VJ, Cheng CK, Fung RO, Wai W, et al. Facemasks and hand hygiene to prevent influenza transmission in households: a cluster randomized trial. Ann Intern Med2009;151:437-46.

13   MacIntyre CR, Cauchemez S, Dwyer DE, Seale H, Cheung P, Browne G, et al. Face mask use and control of respiratory virus transmission in households. Emerg Infect Dis2009;15:233-41.

14   Aiello AE, Murray GF, Perez V, Coulborn RM, Davis BM, Uddin M, et al. Mask use, hand hygiene, and seasonal influenza-like illness among young adults: a randomized intervention trial. J Infect Dis2010;201:491-8.

15   Larson EL, Ferng YH, Wong-McLoughlin J, Wang S, Haber M, Morse SS. Impact of non-pharmaceutical interventions on URIs and influenza in crowded, urban households. Public Health Rep2010;125:178-91.

16   Canini L, Andreoletti L, Ferrari P, D'Angelo R, Blanchon T, Lemaitre M, et al. Surgical mask to prevent influenza transmission in households: a cluster randomized trial. PloS One2010;5:e13998.

17   Simmerman JM, Suntarattiwong P, Levy J, Jarman RG, Kaewchana S, Gibbons RV, et al. Findings from a household randomized controlled trial of hand washing and face masks to reduce influenza transmission in Bangkok, Thailand. Influenza Other Respir Viruses2011;5:256-67.

18   Aiello AE, Perez V, Coulborn RM, Davis BM, Uddin M, Monto AS. Facemasks, hand hygiene, and influenza among young adults: a randomized intervention trial. PloS One2012;7:e29744.

19   Suess T, Remschmidt C, Schink SB, Schweiger B, Nitsche A, Schroeder K, et al. The role of facemasks and hand hygiene in the prevention of influenza transmission in households: results from a cluster randomised trial; Berlin, Germany, 2009-2011. BMC Infect Dis2012;12:26.

20   Atkins D, Best D, Briss PA, Eccles M, Falck-Ytter Y, Flottorp S, et al. Grading quality of evidence and strength of recommendations. BMJ 2004;328:1490.

21   Weaver GH. Droplet infection and its prevention by the face mask. J Infect Dis1919;24:218-30.

22   Belkin NL. The evolution of the surgical mask: filtering efficiency versus effectiveness. Infect Control Hosp Epidemiol 1997;18:49-57.

23   Chughtai AA, Seale H, MacIntyre CR. Use of cloth masks in the practice of infection control—evidence and policy gaps. Int J Infect Control2013;9:1-12.

24   Weaver GH. The value of the face mask and other measures in prevention of diphtheria, meningitis, pneumonia, etc. JAMA 1918;70:76-8.

25   Capps JA. Measures for the prevention and control of respiratory infections in military camps. JAMA 1918;71:448-51.

26   New South Wales Department of Public Health. Report on the influenza epidemic in New South Wales in 1919. Part 1: epidemiology and administration. http://pandora.nla.gov.au/tep/83132.

27   Whitelaw TH. The practical aspects of quarantine for influenza. CMAJ1919;9:1070-4.

28   Wu L. A treatise on pneumonic plague. League of Nations, Health Organisation, 1926.

29   McNett EH. The face mask in tuberculosis. How the cheese-cloth face mask has been developed as a protective agent in tuberculosis. Am J Nurs1949;49:32-6.

30   Kiser JC, Hitchcock CR. Comparative studies with a new plastic surgical mask. Surgery1958;44:936-9.

31   Madsen PO, Madsen RE. A study of disposable surgical masks. Am J Surg1967;114:431-5.

32   Perl TM, Radonovich L, Cummings D, Simberkoff M, Price CS, Gaydos C, et al. Incidence of respiratory illness in outpatient healthcare workers who wear respirators or medical masks while caring for patients. ClinicalTrials.gov2014. https://clinicaltrials.gov/ct2/show/NCT01249625?term=N95&rank=3.

33   MacIntyre CR. Face masks in the protection of healthcare workers to pandemic influenza and emerging infections. ANZCTR2014. www.anzctr.org.au/Trial/Registration/TrialReview.aspx?id=336078.

34   Rashid H. Cluster-randomised controlled trial to test the effectiveness of facemasks in preventing respiratory virus infection among Hajj pilgrims. ANZCTR2013. www.anzctr.org.au/Trial/Registration/TrialReview.aspx?id=364770.

35   Cowling BJ, Zhou Y, Ip DK, Leung GM, Aiello AE. Face masks to prevent transmission of influenza virus: a systematic review. Epidemiol Infect2010;138:449-56.

36   Bin-Reza F, Lopez Chavarrias V, Nicoll A, Chamberland ME. The use of masks and respirators to prevent transmission of influenza: a systematic review of the scientific evidence. Influenza Other Respir Viruses2012;6:257-67.

37   Gralton J, McLaws ML. Protecting healthcare workers from pandemic influenza: N95 or surgical masks? Crit Care Med2010;38:657-67.

38   Gamage B, Moore D, Copes R, Yassi A, Bryce E. Protecting health care workers from SARS and other respiratory pathogens: a review of the infection control literature. Am J Infect Control2005;33:114-21.

39   Jefferson T, Del Mar C, Dooley L, Ferroni E, Al-Ansary LA, Bawazeer GA, et al. Physical interventions to interrupt or reduce the spread of respiratory viruses: systematic review. BMJ 2009;339:b3675.

40   Jefferson T, Del Mar CB, Dooley L, Ferroni E, Al-Ansary LA, Bawazeer GA, et al. Physical interventions to interrupt or reduce the spread of respiratory viruses. Cochrane Database Syst Rev2011;7:CD006207.

41   Jefferson T, Foxlee R, Del Mar C, Dooley L, Ferroni E, Hewak B, et al. Physical interventions to interrupt or reduce the spread of respiratory viruses: systematic review. BMJ 2008;336:77-80.

42   Aledort JE, Lurie N, Wasserman J, Bozzette SA. Non-pharmaceutical public health interventions for pandemic influenza: an evaluation of the evidence base. BMC Public Health2007;7:208.

43   Lee KM, Shukla VK, Clark M, Mierzwinski-Urban M, Pessoa-Silva CL, Conly J. Physical interventions to interrupt or reduce the spread of respiratory viruses—resource use implications: a systematic review. CADTH, 2011 www.cadth.ca/en/products/health-technology-assessment/publication/3140.

44   WHO. Infection prevention and control of epidemic- and pandemic-prone acute respiratory infections in health care. 2014. www.who.int/csr/bioriskreduction/infection_control/publication/en/.

45   MacIntyre CR, Wang Q, Rahman B, Seale H, Ridda I, Gao Z, et al. Efficacy of face masks and respirators in preventing upper respiratory tract bacterial colonization and co-infection in hospital healthcare workers. Prevent Med2014;62:1-7.

46   Elder AG, O'Donnell B, McCruden EA, Symington IS, Carman WF. Incidence and recall of influenza in a cohort of Glasgow healthcare workers during the 1993-4 epidemic: results of serum testing and questionnaire. BMJ 1996;313:1241-2.

47   Salgado CD, Farr BM, Hall KK, Hayden FG. Influenza in the acute hospital setting. Lancet Infect Dis2002;2:145-55.

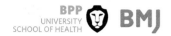

48 Murphy D, Todd JK, Chao RK, Orr I, McIntosh K. The use of gowns and masks to control respiratory illness in pediatric hospital personnel. J Pediatr1981;99:746-50.

49 Al-Asmary S, Al-Shehri AS, Abou-Zeid A, Abdel-Fattah M, Hifnawy T, El-Said T. Acute respiratory tract infections among Hajj medical mission personnel, Saudi Arabia. Int J Infect Dis2007;11:268-72.

50 Seto WH, Tsang D, Yung RW, Ching TY, Ng TK, Ho M, et al. Effectiveness of precautions against droplets and contact in prevention of nosocomial transmission of severe acute respiratory syndrome (SARS). Lancet2003;361:1519-20.

51 Yin WW, Gao LD, Lin WS, Du L, Zhang XC, Zou Q, et al. [Effectiveness of personal protective measures in prevention of nosocomial transmission of severe acute respiratory syndrome. In Chinese]. Zhonghua Liu Xing Bing Xue Za Zhi2004;25:18-22.

52 Teleman MD, Boudville IC, Heng BH, Zhu D, Leo YS. Factors associated with transmission of severe acute respiratory syndrome among health-care workers in Singapore. Epidemiol Infect2004;132:797-803.

53 Lau JT, Fung KS, Wong TW, Kim JH, Wong E, Chung S, et al. SARS transmission among hospital workers in Hong Kong. Emerg Infect Dis2004;10:280-6.

54 Nishiyama A, Wakasugi N, Kirikae T, Quy T, Ha le D, Ban VV, et al. Risk factors for SARS infection within hospitals in Hanoi, Vietnam. Jap J Infect Dis2008;61:388-90.

55 Nishiura H, Kuratsuji T, Quy T, Phi NC, Van Ban V, Ha LE, et al. Rapid awareness and transmission of severe acute respiratory syndrome in Hanoi French Hospital, Vietnam. Am J Trop Med Hyg2005;73:17-25.

56 Ng TC, Lee N, Hui SC, Lai R, Ip M. Preventing healthcare workers from acquiring influenza. Infect Control Hosp Epidemiol 2009;30:292-5.

57 Davies KJ, Herbert AM, Westmoreland D, Bagg J. Seroepidemiological study of respiratory virus infections among dental surgeons. Br Dent J1994;176:262-5.

58 Christie CD, Glover AM, Willke MJ, Marx ML, Reising SF, Hutchinson NM. Containment of pertussis in the regional pediatric hospital during the greater Cincinnati epidemic of 1993. Infect Control Hosp Epidemiol 1995;16:556-63.

59 Wilder-Smith A, Teleman MD, Heng BH, Earnest A, Ling AE, Leo YS. Asymptomatic SARS coronavirus infection among healthcare workers, Singapore. Emerg Infect Dis2005;11:1142-5.

60 Park BJ, Peck AJ, Kuehnert MJ, Newbern C, Smelser C, Comer JA, et al. Lack of SARS transmission among healthcare workers, United States. Emerg Infect Dis2004;10:244-8.

61 Chen YC, Chen PJ, Chang SC, Kao CL, Wang SH, Wang LH, et al. Infection control and SARS transmission among healthcare workers, Taiwan. Emerg Infect Dis2004;10:895-8.

62 Rengasamy S, King WP, Eimer BC, Shaffer RE. Filtration performance of NIOSH-approved N95 and P100 filtering facepiece respirators against 4 to 30 nanometer-size nanoparticles. J Occupat Environ Hyg2008;5:556-64.

63 Rengasamy S, Eimer B, Shaffer RE. Simple respiratory protection—evaluation of the filtration performance of cloth masks and common fabric materials against 20-1000 nm size particles. Ann Occupat Hyg2010;54:789-98.

64 Van der Sande M, Teunis P, Sabel R. Professional and home-made face masks reduce exposure to respiratory infections among the general population. PloS One2008;3:e2618.

65 Makison Booth C, Clayton M, Crook B, Gawn JM. Effectiveness of surgical masks against influenza bioaerosols. J Hosp Infect2013;84:22-6.

66 Balazy A, Toivola M, Adhikari A, Sivasubramani SK, Reponen T, Grinshpun SA. Do N95 respirators provide 95% protection level against airborne viruses, and how adequate are surgical masks? Am J Infect Control2006;34:51-7.

67 Quesnel LB. The efficiency of surgical masks of varying design and composition. Br J Surg1975;62:936-40.

68 Chen SK, Vesley D, Brosseau LM, Vincent JH. Evaluation of single-use masks and respirators for protection of health care workers against mycobacterial aerosols. Am J Infect Control1994;22:65-74.

69 Loeb M, McGeer A, Henry B, Ofner M, Rose D, Hlywka T, et al. SARS among critical care nurses, Toronto. Emerg Infect Dis2004;10:251-5.

70 Simon A, Khurana K, Wilkesmann A, Muller A, Engelhart S, Exner M, et al. Nosocomial respiratory syncytial virus infection: impact of prospective surveillance and targeted infection control. Int J Hyg Environ Health2006;209:317-24.

71 Hall CB, Douglas RG Jr. Nosocomial respiratory syncytial viral infections. Should gowns and masks be used? Am J Dis Child1981;135:512-5.

72 Liu JW, Lu SN, Chen SS, Yang KD, Lin MC, Wu CC, et al. Epidemiologic study and containment of a nosocomial outbreak of severe acute respiratory syndrome in a medical center in Kaohsiung, Taiwan. Infect Control Hosp Epidemiol 2006;27:466-72.

73 Chen M, Leo YS, Ang B, Heng BH, Choo P. The outbreak of SARS at Tan Tock Seng Hospital—relating epidemiology to control. Ann Acad Med Singapore2006;35:317-25.

74 Centers for Disease Control and Prevention. Cluster of severe acute respiratory syndrome cases among protected health-care workers—Toronto, Canada, April 2003. JAMA2003;289:2788-9.

75 Leung TF, Ng PC, Cheng FW, Lyon DJ, So KW, Hon EK, et al. Infection control for SARS in a tertiary paediatric centre in Hong Kong. J Hosp Infect 2004;56:215-22.

76 Fella P, Rivera P, Hale M, Squires K, Sepkowitz K. Dramatic decrease in tuberculin skin test conversion rate among employees at a hospital in New York City. Am J Infect Control1995;23:352-6.

77 Manangan LP, Collazo ER, Tokars J, Paul S, Jarvis WR. Trends in compliance with the guidelines for preventing the transmission of Mycobacterium tuberculosis among New Jersey hospitals, 1989 to 1996. Infect Control Hosp Epidemiol 1999;20:337-40.

78 Ang B, Poh BF, Win MK, Chow A. Surgical masks for protection of health care personnel against pandemic novel swine-origin influenza A (H1N1)-2009: results from an observational study. Clin Infect Dis 2010;50:1011-4.

79 Chen WQ, Ling WH, Lu CY, Hao YT, Lin ZN, Ling L, et al. Which preventive measures might protect health care workers from SARS? BMC Public Health2009;9:81.

80 Maloney SA, Pearson ML, Gordon MT, Del Castillo R, Boyle JF, Jarvis WR. Efficacy of control measures in preventing nosocomial transmission of multidrug-resistant tuberculosis to patients and health care workers. Ann Intern Med1995;122:90-5.

81 Blumberg HM, Watkins DL, Berschling JD, Antle A, Moore P, White N, et al. Preventing the nosocomial transmission of tuberculosis. Ann Intern Med1995;122:658-63.

82 Centers for Disease Control and Prevention (CDC). Interim infection prevention and control recommendations for hospitalized patients with middle east respiratory syndrome coronavirus (MERS-CoV). 2014. www.cdc.gov/coronavirus/mers/infection-prevention-control.html.

83 Institute of Medicine. Reusability of facemasks during an influenza pandemic: facing the flu. National Academy of Sciences, 2006. www.nap.edu/openbook.php?record_id=11637.

84 Association for Professionals in Infection Control and Epidemiology (APIC). APIC position paper: extending the use and/or reusing respiratory protection in healthcare settings during disasters. 2009. www.apic.org/Resource_/TinyMceFileManager/Advocacy-PDFs/APIC_Position_Ext_the_Use_and_or_Reus_Resp_Prot_in_Hlthcare_Settings1209l.pdf.

85 Orr N. Is a mask necessary in the operating theatre? Ann R Coll Surg Engl1982;64:205.

86 Mitchell NJ, Hunt S. Surgical face masks in modern operating rooms—a costly and unnecessary ritual? J Hosp Infect 1991;18:239-42.

87 Tunevall TG. Postoperative wound infections and surgical face masks: a controlled study. World J Surg1991;15:383-7; discussion 7-8.

88 Chamberlain GV, Houang E. Trial of the use of masks in the gynaecological operating theatre. Ann R Coll Surg Engl1984;66:432-3.

89 Mangram AJ, Horan TC, Pearson ML, Silver LC, Jarvis WR. Guideline for prevention of surgical site infection, 1999. Hospital Infection Control Practices Advisory Committee. Infect Control Hosp Epidemiol 1999;20:250-78; quiz 79-80.

90 Belkin NL. Surgical face masks in the operating theatre: are they still necessary? J Hosp Infect2002;50:233; author reply 4-5.

91 Johnson DF, Druce JD, Birch C, Grayson ML. A quantitative assessment of the efficacy of surgical and N95 masks to filter influenza virus in patients with acute influenza infection. Clin Infect Dis 2009;49:275-7.

92 Milton DK, Fabian MP, Cowling BJ, Grantham ML, McDevitt JJ. Influenza virus aerosols in human exhaled breath: particle size, culturability, and effect of surgical masks. PLoS Pathogens2013;9:e1003205.

93 Dharmadhikari AS, Mphahlele M, Stoltz A, Venter K, Mathebula R, Masotla T, et al. Surgical face masks worn by patients with multidrug-resistant tuberculosis: impact on infectivity of air on a hospital ward. Am J Respir Crit Care Med2012;185:1104-9.

94 Jensen PA, Lambert LA, Iademarco MF, Ridzon R. Guidelines for preventing the transmission of Mycobacterium tuberculosis in health-care settings, 2005. MMWR Rec Rep2005;54(RR-17):1-141.

95 Migliori GB, Zellweger JP, Abubakar I, Ibraim E, Caminero JA, De Vries G, et al. European union standards for tuberculosis care. Eur Respir J2012;39:807-19.

96 Lau JT, Tsui H, Lau M, Yang X. SARS transmission, risk factors, and prevention in Hong Kong. Emerg Infect Dis2004;10:587-92.

97 Wu J, Xu F, Zhou W, Feikin DR, Lin CY, He X, et al. Risk factors for SARS among persons without known contact with SARS patients, Beijing, China. Emerg Infect Dis2004;10:210-6.

98 Bell D, Nicoll A, Fukuda K, Horby P, Monto A, Hayden F, et al. Non-pharmaceutical interventions for pandemic influenza, national and community measures. Emerg Infect Dis2006;12:88-94.

99 Center for Disease Control and Prevention. Interim recommendations for facemask and respirator use to reduce 2009 influenza A (H1N1) virus transmission. 2009. www.cdc.gov/h1n1flu/masks.htm.

100 European Centre for Disease Prevention and Control. Q&A on seasonal influenza 2014. www.ecdc.europa.eu/EN/HEALTHTOPICS/SEASONAL_INFLUENZA/BASIC_FACTS/Pages/QA_seasonal_influenza.aspx.

101 Brienen NC, Timen A, Wallinga J, van Steenbergen JE, Teunis PF. The effect of mask use on the spread of influenza during a pandemic. Risk Anal2010;30:1210-8.

102 Lo JY, Tsang TH, Leung YH, Yeung EY, Wu T, Lim WW. Respiratory infections during SARS outbreak, Hong Kong, 2003. Emerg Infect Dis2005;11:1738-41.

103 Blachere FM, Lindsley WG, Pearce TA, Anderson SE, Fisher M, Khakoo R, et al. Measurement of airborne influenza virus in a hospital emergency department. Clin Infect Dis 2009;48:438-40.

104 Brankston G, Gitterman L, Lemieux C, Gardam M. Transmission of influenza A in human beings. Lancet Infect Dis2007;7:257-65.

105 Tellier R. Aerosol transmission of influenza A virus: a review of new studies. J R Soc2009;6(suppl 6):S783-90.

106 Brosseau LM, Jones R. Health workers need optimal respiratory protection for Ebola. Center for Infectious Disease Research and Policy (CIDRAP), 2014. www.cidrap.umn.edu/news-perspective/2014/09/commentary-health-workers-need-optimal-respiratory-protection-ebola.

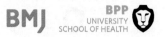

107 Lindsley WG, Blachere FM, Thewlis RE, Vishnu A, Davis KA, Cao G, et al. Measurements of airborne influenza virus in aerosol particles from human coughs. PloS One2010;5:e15100.

108 Marks P, Vipond I, Regan F, Wedgwood K, Fey R, Caul E. A school outbreak of Norwalk-like virus: evidence for airborne transmission. Epidemiol Infect2003;131:727-36.

109 McKinney KR, Gong YY, Lewis TG. Environmental transmission of SARS at Amoy Gardens. J Environ Health2006;68:26-30; quiz 51-2.

110 Yu IT, Li Y, Wong TW, Tam W, Chan AT, Lee JH, et al. Evidence of airborne transmission of the severe acute respiratory syndrome virus. N Engl J Med2004;350:1731-9.

111 Barker J, Vipond I, Bloomfield S. Effects of cleaning and disinfection in reducing the spread of Norovirus contamination via environmental surfaces. J Hosp Infect2004;58:42-9.

112 Macintyre CR, Seale H, Yang P, Zhang Y, Shi W, Almatroudi A, et al. Quantifying the risk of respiratory infection in healthcare workers performing high-risk procedures. Epidemiol Infect2014;142:1802-8.

113 WHO. Practical guidelines for infection control in health care facilities. 2003. www.wpro.who.int/publications/docs/practical_guidelines_ infection_control.pdf.

114 Society for Healthcare Epidemiology of America (SHEA). SHEA position statement: interim guidance on infection control precautions for novel swine-origin influenza A H1N1 in healthcare facilities. 2009. www.shea-online.org/Assets/files/policy/061209_H1N1_Statement.pdf.

115 Centers for Disease Control and Prevention. Prevention strategies for seasonal influenza in healthcare settings. 2014 www.cdc.gov/flu/ professionals/infectioncontrol/healthcaresettings.htm.

116 Ulmer BC. The hazards of surgical smoke. AORN J2008;87:721-34; quiz 35-8.

117 Tran K, Cimon K, Severn M, Pessoa-Silva CL, Conly J. Aerosol generating procedures and risk of transmission of acute respiratory infections to healthcare workers: a systematic review. PloS One2012;7:e35797.

118 Centers for Disease Control and Prevention (CDC). Guidance on personal protective equipment to be used by healthcare workers during management of patients with Ebola virus disease in US hospitals, including procedures for putting on (donning) and removing (doffing) 2014. www.cdc.gov/vhf/ebola/hcp/procedures-for-ppe.html.

119 Chughtai AA, Seale H, Dung TC, Maher L, Nga PT, MacIntyre CR. Current practices and barriers to the use of facemasks and respirators among hospital based healthcare workers (HCW) in Vietnam. Am J Infect Control2015;43:72-7.

120 Beckman S, Materna B, Goldmacher S, Zipprich J, D'Alessandro M, Novak D, et al. Evaluation of respiratory protection programs and practices in California hospitals during the 2009-2010 H1N1 influenza pandemic. Am J Infect Control2013;41:1024-31.

121 Rebmann T, Wagner W. Infection preventionists' experience during the first months of the 2009 novel H1N1 influenza A pandemic. Am J Infect Control2009;37:e5-e16.

122 Occupational Safety and Health Administration (OSHA). US Department of Labor. Proposed guidance on workplace stockpiling of respirators and facemasks for pandemic influenza. www.osha.gov/dsg/guidance/ proposedGuidanceStockpilingRespirator.pdf.

123 Phin NF, Rylands AJ, Allan J, Edwards C, Enstone JE, Nguyen-Van-Tam JS. Personal protective equipment in an influenza pandemic: a UK simulation exercise. J Hosp Infect2009;71:15-21.

124 Swaminathan A, Martin R, Gamon S, Aboltins C, Athan E, Braitberg G, et al. Personal protective equipment and antiviral drug use during hospitalization for suspected avian or pandemic influenza. Emerg Infect Dis2007;13:1541-7.

125 Derrick JL, Gomersall CD. Protecting healthcare staff from severe acute respiratory syndrome: filtration capacity of multiple surgical masks. J Hosp Infect2005;59:365-8.

126 Albano L, Matuozzo A, Marinelli P, Di Giuseppe G. Knowledge, attitudes and behaviour of hospital health-care workers regarding influenza A/H1N1: a cross sectional survey. BMC Infect Dis2014;14:208.

127 Seale H, Corbett S, Dwyer DE, MacIntyre CR. Feasibility exercise to evaluate the use of particulate respirators by emergency department staff during the 2007 influenza season. Infect Control Hosp Epidemiol 2009;30:710-2.

128 Nickell LA, Crighton EJ, Tracy CS, Al-Enazy H, Bolaji Y, Hanjrah S, et al. Psychosocial effects of SARS on hospital staff: survey of a large tertiary care institution. CMAJ 2004;170:793-8.

129 Gammon J, Morgan-Samuel H, Gould D. A review of the evidence for suboptimal compliance of healthcare practitioners to standard/ universal infection control precautions. J Clin Nurs2008;17:157-67.

130 La Torre G, Mannocci A, Ursillo P, Bontempi C, Firenze A, Panico MG, et al. Prevalence of influenza vaccination among nurses and ancillary workers in Italy: systematic review and meta analysis. Hum Vaccines2011;7:728-33.

131 Pittet D. Improving adherence to hand hygiene practice: a multidisciplinary approach. Emerg Infect Dis2001;7:234-40.

132 Gershon RR, Vlahov D, Felknor SA, Vesley D, Johnson PC, Delclos GL, et al. Compliance with universal precautions among health care workers at three regional hospitals. Am J Infect Control1995;23:225-36.

133 Nichol K, McGeer A, Bigelow P, O'Brien-Pallas L, Scott J, Holness DL. Behind the mask: determinants of nurse's adherence to facial protective equipment. Am J Infect Control2013;41:8-13.

134 Moore D, Gamage B, Bryce E, Copes R, Yassi A. Protecting health care workers from SARS and other respiratory pathogens: organizational and individual factors that affect adherence to infection control guidelines. Am J Infect Control2005;33:88-96.

135 Caplan A, Shah NR. Managing the human toll caused by seasonal influenza: New York State's mandate to vaccinate or mask. JAMA 2013;310:1797-8.

136 Occupational Safety and Health Administration (OSHA). US Department of Labor. Respiratory Protection. OSHA 3079. 2002 (revised). www. osha.gov/Publications/osha3079.pdf.

137 National Institute for Occupational Safety and Health (NIOSH). NIOSH guide to the selection and use of particulate respirators. 1995. www. cdc.gov/niosh/docs/96-101/.

138 European Directive. Guidelines on the application of council directive 89/686/EEC of 21 December 1989 on the approximation of the laws of the member states relating to personal protective equipment. http://ec.europa.eu/enterprise/sectors/mechanical/files/ppe/ ppe_guidelines_en.pdf.

139 Standards Australia Limited/Standards New Zealand. Respiratory protective devices. Australian/New Zealand Standard. AS/NZS 1716. 2012. shop.standards.co.nz/catalog/1716:2012%28AS%7CNZS%29/ scope?.

140 Danyluk Q, Hon CY, Neudorf M, Yassi A, Bryce E, Janssen B, et al. Health care workers and respiratory protection: is the user seal check a surrogate for respirator fit-testing? J Occupat Environ Hyg2011;8:267-70.

141 Occupational Safety and Health Administration (OSHA). US Department of Labor. Respirator fit testing. 1994. www.osha.gov/pls/oshaweb/ owadisp.show_document?p_table=FEDERAL_REGISTER&p_id=13426.

142 Noti JD, Lindsley WG, Blachere FM, Cao G, Kashon ML, Thewlis RE, et al. Detection of infectious influenza virus in cough aerosols generated in a simulated patient examination room. Clin Infect Dis 2012;54:1569-77.

143 Wise ME, De Perio M, Halpin J, Jhung M, Magill S, Black SR, et al. Transmission of pandemic (H1N1) 2009 influenza to healthcare personnel in the United States. Clin Infect Dis2011;52(suppl 1):S198-204.

144 Bryce E, Forrester L, Scharf S, Eshghpour M. What do healthcare workers think? A survey of facial protection equipment user preferences. J Hosp Infect2008;68:241-7.

145 Gershon RR, Magda LA, Canton AN, Riley HE, Wiggins F, Young W, et al. Pandemic-related ability and willingness in home healthcare workers. Am J Disaster Med2010;5:15-26.

146 Lautenbach E, Saint S, Henderson DK, Harris AD. Initial response of health care institutions to emergence of H1N1 influenza: experiences, obstacles, and perceived future needs. Clin Infect Dis 2010;50:523-7.

147 Winter S, Thomas JH, Stephens DP, Davis JS. Particulate face masks for protection against airborne pathogens—one size does not fit all: an observational study. Crit Care Resusc2010;12:24-7.

148 Chughtai AA, Seale H, MacIntyre CR. Availability, consistency and evidence-base of policies and guidelines on the use of mask and respirator to protect hospital health care workers: a global analysis. BMC Res Notes2013;6:216.

149 WHO. WHO policy on TB infection control in health-care facilities, congregate settings and households. 2009. www.who.int/tb/ publications/2009/infection_control/en/

150 Centers for Disease Control and Prevention. Interim guidance on infection control measures for 2009 H1N1 influenza in healthcare settings, including protection of healthcare personnel. 2010. www.cdc. gov/h1n1flu/guidelines_infection_control.htm.

151 WHO. Infection prevention and control during health care for probable or confirmed cases of novel coronavirus (nCoV) infection. 2013. www.who.int/csr/disease/coronavirus_infections/ IPCnCoVguidance_06May13.pdf?ua=1.

152 WHO. Infection prevention and control guidance for care of patients in health-care settings, with focus on Ebola. 2014. www.who.int/csr/ resources/publications/ebola/filovirus_infection_control/en/.

153 Chughtai AA, MacIntyre CR, Peng Y, Wang Q, Toor ZI, Dung TC, et al. Examining the policies and guidelines around the use of masks and respirators by healthcare workers in China, Pakistan and Vietnam. J Infect Prevent2014; published online 10 Dec. doi:10.1177/1757177414560251.

154 Cohen J. When Ebola protection fails. Science2014;346:17-8.

155 WHO. Consensus document on the epidemiology of severe acute respiratory syndrome (SARS). 2003. www.who.int/csr/sars/en/ WHOconsensus.pdf.

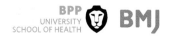

Communicating risk

Haroon Ahmed, general practice specialty academic trainee[1][2], Gurudutt Naik, associate academic fellow[3], Hannah Willoughby, general practice specialty academic trainee[2], Adrian G K Edwards, research professor in general practice[3]

[1]The Foundry Town Clinic, Aberdare, UK

[2]Department of Postgraduate General Practice Education, Cardiff University School of Medicine, Cardiff, UK

[3]Cochrane Institute of Primary Care and Public Health, Cardiff University School of Medicine, Cardiff CF14 4YS, UK

Correspondence to: A G K Edwards
edwardsag@cf.ac.uk

Cite this as: BMJ 2012;344:e3996

DOI: 10.1136/bmj.e3996

http://www.bmj.com/content/344/bmj.e3996

The communication of risk is an important and often difficult aspect of clinical practice. This clinical review aims to provide practising clinicians with a comprehensive and up to date overview of current evidence in this developing area.

What is risk communication?

Risk is the probability that a hazard will give rise to harm.[1] Risk communication is defined as the open two way exchange of information and opinion about harms and benefits, with the aim of improving the understanding of risk and of promoting better decisions about clinical management.[2] Risk communication should therefore cover the probability of the risk occurring, the importance of the adverse event being described, and the effect of the event on the patient.[3]

Risk messages are common. We hear that "there is a risk of flooding" or "the terrorism threat level is orange." In medicine, we may tell people that their "risk of a heart attack is 15%" or "stopping smoking will reduce their risk of lung cancer," but what do clinicians hope to achieve by providing this information? Box 1 outlines a clinical scenario that requires effective risk communication.

Communicating risk involves providing the patient with a balanced evidence based summary of the risks and harms associated with a service, test, or treatment.[3] In Ms Jones's case, it would be important to deal with her personal risk of breast cancer (based on her risk factors) and how this risk compares with the general population. To make an informed decision, she would also need to know whether screening would reduce the risk of an adverse outcome should she develop breast cancer and how this reduction in risk compares with no screening. She would also need to know the harms of screening. The clinician should present this information to her in the most transparent and understandable (rather than persuasive) way and accept that her informed decision on her own care may not necessarily be the one that reduces her risk. This highlights the complexities of risk communication. People perceive risk differently depending on their awareness and understanding of the risk in question and also depending on the way the risk information is presented to them.[1]

Therefore, effective risk communication should involve the sharing of information that improves risk perception and understanding and that allows shared decision making. Sometimes this may be at odds with apparent "public health" messages that may, for example, promote uptake of screening tests to achieve programme effectiveness at population levels. However, the clinician should accept that the final decision depends as much on the patient's own values as it does on the risk information presented.

The literature on risk communication is diverse and some areas of risk communication are still without strong evidence.[4] This review discusses the importance of effective risk communication and summarises the evidence behind the various methods of presenting risk information.

Why is risk communication important?

Where there is good evidence of the benefits of an intervention, risk communication should aim to go beyond simply sharing information and endeavour to change beliefs or promote behavioural change.[4] This is achievable, because theories of behavioural change highlight the association between risk perception (belief about the likelihood of personal harm from any given "risk") and health related behaviour.[5] For example, adults who think that they are at high risk of an illness (such as influenza) are more likely than others to take up vaccination.[6] However, many healthcare decisions have no single "best treatment" and require trade-offs between harms and benefits.[7] The provision of risk information in these scenarios should therefore promote patient involvement, informed decision making, and shared management plans.

How risk information is presented (for example, graphically, visually, verbally) is important and influences the degree to which perceived risk will affect behavioural change, such as with cardiovascular risk information.[8][9] Attention is needed not just on accurately predicting cardiovascular risk but also on how best to present that risk, stimulate changes in health behaviour, and reduce risk levels. Risk communication is important because it is something that most clinicians do every day. If done effectively it can trigger changes in beliefs or behaviour, but for this to occur the risk has to be communicated effectively.

How good (or bad) are clinicians at communicating risk?

Risk communication research has focused more on what we are doing rather than on how well we are doing it. An observational study of 70 consultations in primary care reported that cardiovascular risk was mainly communicated using verbal qualifiers (telling patients that their risk is "high," "medium," or "low"), but that patients' subjective understanding was significantly higher when visual formats were used.[10] Qualitative research reported that a sample of gynaecologists in Germany often did not correctly explain the benefits and harms of mammography screening to women.[11] Further work by Gigerenzer and colleagues highlights doctors' difficulties with explaining positive

SUMMARY POINTS

- Risk communication is the open two way exchange of information and opinion about harms and benefits; it aims to improve understanding of risk and promote better decisions about clinical management
- Strong evidence suggests that the format in which risk information is presented affects patients' understanding and perception of risk
- There is emerging evidence that effective risk communication can lead to more informed decision making in screening
- Decision aids can be an effective adjunct to risk communication and can improve knowledge, awareness, and decision making
- The presentation of data uncertainty is one of the most difficult aspects of risk communication

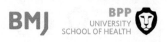

BOX 1 MS JONES'S DILEMMA

Ms Jones has just celebrated her 50th birthday. She is fit and well and takes no regular drugs. She comes to the surgery to discuss mammography screening. Ms Jones has no family history of cancer, had her first period aged 14 years, and her first child aged 26. Her sister has told her that a mammogram will detect a cancer before she feels a lump, so that any cancer will be diagnosed earlier, which "can only be a good thing." Ms Jones is more sceptical, having read stories in the press of women who had mammograms and biopsies and were then told it was a "false alarm." She wishes to know more about the benefits and harms of mammography screening before making a final decision.

predictive values of mammography, interpreting risks associated with the use of the contraceptive pill, and understanding survival rates for cancer.[12] [13]

Barriers to effective risk communication

Effective risk communication can be difficult to achieve for many reasons. The most commonly reported reason is the difficulty that patients and doctors have understanding numbers.[12] [13] [14] [15] Gigerenzer coined the term "collective statistical illiteracy" to describe how doctors, patients, journalists, politicians, and society at large have trouble understanding and interpreting health statistics.[12] Basic numeracy is also a problem—for example, only 21% of a sample of highly educated American adults could correctly identify one in 1000 as being equivalent to 0.1%.[14] Clinicians need to be adept at understanding numbers and explaining them in a way that patients can comprehend.

Methods available to communicate risk

Risk information can be communicated using several different methods and formats. Here we summarise these methods, provide examples, and discuss recent advances in the evidence base for their use.

Framing

"Framing manipulation" is the presentation of logically equivalent information in different ways.[16] It can be further subdivided into "attribute framing" and "goal framing."

Attribute framing is the positive versus negative description of a specific attribute of a single item or state. For example, Ms Jones could be told that there is an 82% chance that she will survive for five years after a diagnosis of breast cancer (positive attribute framing), or that she has an 18% chance of dying within five years of such a diagnosis (negative attribute framing). Akl and colleagues systematically reviewed 35 trials of positive versus negative attribute framing for their effects on cognitive and behavioural outcomes.[17] Interventions were perceived as more beneficial when presented using positive framing messages, but there was little evidence that framing affected patients' understanding or behaviour.

Goal framing describes the consequences of performing or not performing an act, presented as a gain versus a loss. For example, "screening will improve your chance of survival from cancer" versus "not participating in screening will reduce your chance of survival from cancer." Patients perceived screening as more effective when presented with a loss message, but again there was no evidence of an effect on patients' understanding or behaviour.[17]

Presenting risk reduction

Risk reduction can be presented using relative risk reduction (RRR), absolute risk reduction (ARR), or numbers needed to treat (NNT).

The RRR is the reduction of risk in the intervention group relative to the risk in the control group. For a risk of 20% in the control group and a risk of 10% in the intervention group, the RRR would be 50%. The ARR is the difference in risks between two groups, which for these same figures would be 10%. The NNT is the number of patients who need to be treated (or screened) to prevent one additional adverse outcome (NNT=10 for the above figures).

Ms Jones could be presented with the following statements[18] [19]:

- RRR: Early detection with mammography reduces the risk of dying from breast cancer by 15%
- ARR: Early detection with mammography reduces the risk of dying from breast cancer by 0.05%
- NNT: 2000 women need to have regular mammograms for more than 10 years to prolong one life.

A recent review of evidence suggested that using RRR makes treatment benefits and changes in risk seem larger than they are and recommended that information on risk reduction be consistently presented using ARR.[20] A Cochrane systematic review compared the use of ARR, RRR, and NNT in 35 trials.[21] No studies reported effects of using these risk reduction formats on patients' decision making or behaviour. The review did assess effects on patients' objective understanding, perception of benefit, and persuasiveness. It concluded that:

- RRR and ARR are equally well understood and both formats are better understood by patients and clinicians than is NNT
- RRR is perceived to be larger and is more persuasive than ARR and NNT
- ARR is perceived to indicate a larger effect than when the same information is expressed using NNT but is no more persuasive.

Personalising risk information

The risk of breast cancer can be presented as a general population based risk estimate (generalised risk information) or on the basis of the individual's own risk factors (personalised risk information). Personalised risk information can be presented as an absolute risk or as a numerical estimate of risk; it can categorise the individual as belonging to high, medium, or low risk groups; or it may simply list the individual's risk factors. Because personalised risk information is based on the individual's own characteristics, it is thought to provide a more accurate picture of risk and to improve decision making.[22] A risk tool (such as www.cancer.gov/bcrisktool; fig 1) could be used to provide Ms Jones with her personalised risk of developing invasive breast cancer. Several tools are also available for calculating cardiovascular risk, such as QRISK (http://qrisk.org).

A Cochrane review of 22 randomised controlled trials suggests that, compared with general risk information, personalised risk communication (whether written, spoken, or visually presented) in the context of screening tests can lead to more accurate risk perception, improved knowledge, and increased uptake of screening tests.[22] Since the

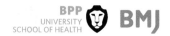

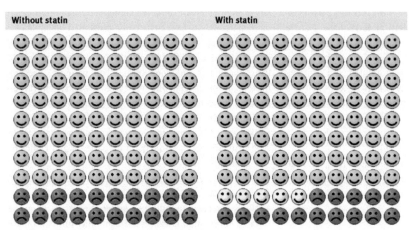

The breast cancer risk assessment tool (www.cancer.gov/bcrisktool)

Risk factors
Does the woman have a medical history of any breast cancer, ductal carcinoma in situ (DCIS), or lobular carcinoma in situ (LCIS)? NO
What is the woman's age? 50 years
What was the woman's age at the time of her first menstrual period? 14 years
What was the woman's age at the time of her first live birth of a child? 25-29 years
How many of the woman's first degree relatives (mother, sisters, or daughters) have had breast cancer? 0
Has the woman ever had a breast biopsy? NO
What is the woman's race/ethnicity? WHITE

Risk estimates
Five year risk
This woman (age 50): 1%
Average woman (age 50): 1.3%
Explanation
On the basis of the information provided, the woman's estimated risk for developing invasive breast cancer over the next 5 years is 1% compared with a risk of 1.3% for a woman of the same age and ethnicity from the general population. This calculation also means that the woman's risk of NOT getting breast cancer over the next 5 years is 99%
Lifetime risk
This woman (to age 90): 9.1%
Average woman (to age 90): 11.2%
Explanation
The woman's estimated risk for developing invasive breast cancer over her lifetime (to age 90) is 9.1% compared with a risk of 11.2% for a woman of the same age and ethnicity from the general population

Fig 1 Calculating Ms Jones's risk of invasive breast cancer using her personal risk factors

Without statin	With statin

If 100 people each take a statin (such as simvastatin) for 10 years:
• About 5 people will be "saved" from having a cardiovascular event by taking the statin (the yellow faces above)
• About 80 people will not have a cardiovascular event but would not have done so even if they had not taken a statin (the green faces above)
• About 15 people will still have a cardiovascular event (the red faces above), even though they take a statin

Fig 2 The NHS National Prescribing Centre provides pictographs to help explain the reduction in cardiovascular risk from taking statins in people with a moderate risk of a cardiovascular event (20% over 10 years). For more details see www.npc.nhs.uk

Here is a list of issues many women think about when choosing surgery
Click in the box next to the ones that are important to you. You do not have to click in every box

Avoid looking lop sided [info] ☐
Avoid mastectomy [info] ☐
Avoid more unexpected surgery [info] ☐
Remove the breast [info] ☐
Less chance of cancer returning [info] ☑
Avoid radiotherapy [info] ☐
Smaller scar and less change to breast size [info] ☐
Keep the breast [info] ☐

Unsure
Lumpectomy   Mastectomy

[Reset] [Next >]

Fig 3 Breast Cancer Decision Explorer (BresDex; www.bresdex.com). A decision aid to help women with breast cancer choose between mastectomy and breast conserving surgery

publication of that review, three randomised controlled trials have shown that providing personalised risk information leads to more informed decision making about participation in colorectal cancer and prenatal screening.[23] [24] [25]

Natural frequencies
A natural frequency is a joint frequency of two events, such as the number of women with breast cancer who have a positive mammogram.[26]

The use of natural frequencies, rather than percentages or probabilities, probably improves understanding of risks and benefits.[26] [27] Akl and colleagues showed that clinicians and patients find natural frequencies easier to understand than probabilities, suggesting that decisions based on frequencies are more informed than those based on probabilities.[21] There is also growing evidence to support the use of pictographs (fig 2) to present natural frequencies, with evidence suggesting that these are well understood and that they effectively support communication about individual statistics.[8] [20]

Decision aids
Decision aids aim to help patients participate in healthcare decisions by providing clear evidence based information on the choices available. They should communicate the benefit and harm of each option and promote informed decision making. A systematic review of 86 randomised controlled trials found that the use of decision aids improves patient knowledge and risk perception and increases patients' participation in decision making, promoting informed decision making that is consistent with patient values.[28] This review also suggested that although decision aids can improve patient-doctor communication, they have not been shown to improve actual health outcomes. Another systematic review of randomised controlled trials showed that decision aids can also increase the clinician's adoption of shared decision making.[29]

Although there is good evidence to support the cognitive benefits of decision aids, evidence for behavioural change is weaker. One systematic review suggested that decision aids have variable effects on patient behaviour.[28] For certain decisions, patients exposed to a decision aid behaved differently from those who did not use a decision aid. For example, patients exposed to a decision aid were less likely to opt for prostate specific antigen screening (risk ratio 0.85, 95% confidence interval 0.74 to 0.98). However, for other decisions (such as participating in colorectal screening), there was no evidence to suggest that patients exposed to the decision aid behaved any differently from those who were not.

BOX 2 HELPING MS JONES TO MAKE AN INFORMED DECISION

The NHS National Prescribing Centre (www.npc.nhs.uk) provides a breast screening decision aid. This explains that if 1000 women aged 50-70 years attend regular mammography screening for 10 years, 970 women will not have breast cancer, although 130 of these women will have undergone unnecessary extra investigations. Thirty women will have breast cancer diagnosed. Of these 30 women:

• In four, the breast cancers would have been clinically inconsequential

• In 23 of these women, the fact that the breast cancer was picked up by screening will have no effect on their outcome

• Three women will live longer because their breast cancer was detected early through screening

---

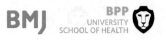

Intervention	Icon	Description
Beneficial		For which effectiveness has been demonstrated by clear evidence from systematic reviews, randomised controlled trials, or the best alternative source of information, and for which expectation of harms is small compared with the benefits
Likely to be beneficial		For which effectiveness is less well established than for those listed under "beneficial"
Trade-off between benefits and harms		For which clinicians and patients should weigh up the beneficial and harmful effects according to individual circumstances and priorities
Unknown effectiveness		For which there are currently insufficient data or data of inadequate quality
Unlikely to be beneficial		For which lack of effectiveness is less well established than for those listed under "likely to be ineffective or harmful"
Likely to be ineffective or harmful		For which ineffectiveness or associated harm has been demonstrated by clear evidence

Fig 4 Presenting data uncertainty. Categories of evidence: an approach used by the *BMJ Clinical Evidence* series[7]

SOURCES AND SELECTION CRITERIA

We are updating a Cochrane systematic review on risk communication in screening. Published studies and review papers identified during the search period for this review (2008-2011) were consulted for this article. We also searched PubMed and the Cochrane library for primary research articles, systematic reviews, and commentaries by authoritative authors in the field of risk communication published in the past 12 months.

QUESTIONS FOR FUTURE RESEARCH

- Can effective risk communication lead to behavioural change when the evidence supports specific outcomes?
- Are there methods of presenting data uncertainty that can improve understanding, knowledge, and decision making?

TIPS FOR NON-SPECIALISTS

- Become familiar with tools that provide decision support for common consultations and use them as adjuncts to normal consulting
- Consider using absolute risks when discussing risk reduction with patients
- Direct patients to decision aids for interventions where more than one option is available and informed decision making depends on patients' personal preferences and values

---

ADDITIONAL EDUCATIONAL RESOURCES

Resources for healthcare professionals
- NHS National Prescribing Centre (www.npc.nhs.uk/patient_decision_aids/)—Large number of freely available patient decision aids that can be downloaded, printed, and used during consultations

Resources for patients
- Option Grids (www.optiongrid.co.uk/)—"Option grids" are brief tools that describe options for several commonly encountered healthcare decisions
- Patient UK (www.patient.co.uk/search.asp?searchterm=brief+decision+aid&searchcoll=All&x=0&y=0)—Brief decision aids for a variety of conditions

An increasing number of online decision aids include risk communication elements, such as for decisions about screening (for example, prostate specific antigen testing; www.prosdex.com), surgical treatment (for example, choosing between breast conserving surgery or mastectomy for breast cancer; www.bresdex.com; fig 3), or medication (for example, choosing to take a statin; www.npc.nhs.uk). Clinicians' use of these aids during consultations could increase shared decision making and improve patients' knowledge and understanding. Furthermore, patients who use decision aids are consistently more ready to make a decision than those receiving usual care.[28] In the case of Ms Jones, she could be directed to the breast screening decision aid above to help her reach an informed decision about whether to participate in mammography screening (box 2).

Uncertainty

Other areas of risk communication remain inconclusive, including the quantity of information that should be presented, the order in which to present information, the use of summary tables, and best practice on presenting risk information when the evidence base is unclear. The presentation of uncertainty about data has been highlighted as one of the most difficult elements of risk communication,[30] and empirical research studies are still needed in this area. Politi and colleagues report the problems of communicating uncertainty in a narrative review.[30] They highlight the conceptual differences in the definition of uncertainty and in its measurement. The available research suggests that the response to uncertainty depends very much on the clinician's and patient's personal characteristics and values. Cross sectional surveys suggest that the communication of scientific uncertainty about medical tests and treatments depends on doctors' perceptions of their patients' reaction to uncertainty.[31] Further research also suggests that patients are unclear about the degree of uncertainty in medical decisions, with 39% of 2944 American adults believing that the Food and Drug Administration approves only "extremely effective" drugs.[32] Communicating uncertainty may also lead to lower decision satisfaction among patients.[33]

The degree of scientific uncertainty that complicates medical decision making can be highlighted using the example of Ms Jones. Is it appropriate to present Ms Jones with the risk of breast cancer in the UK using a prevalence estimate? Should we provide her with confidence limits for the prevalence estimate so that she can see the uncertainty associated with the estimate? When we informed Ms Jones that "mammography would reduce her risk of breast cancer by 15%," should we also have discussed the strength and validity of the research that the review was based on? For example, when the review looked only at adequately randomised trials, outcome did not differ between patients who underwent screening and controls.[18] Numerical literacy and understanding are even more important when communicating data uncertainty, and the clinician needs to balance information provision with the understanding and knowledge needed to make a decision. In an attempt to achieve this aim, several methods have been adopted, but there is little evidence for their effectiveness.[30] The most commonly used method is to summarise the quality of evidence pertaining to a given health intervention using a rating system and simple descriptive terms to describe the degree of uncertainty (fig 4).

In summary, evidence suggests that ARR is a more balanced and understandable representation of risk reduction for patients and clinicians than RRR or NNT. Natural frequencies are easier to understand and interpret than percentages or probabilities. Emerging evidence supports the use of personalised risk communication for promoting informed decision making in screening. There is also good evidence to support decision aids as a practical support to risk communication. Finally, it is difficult to communicate data uncertainty; there is little clear guidance on best practice approaches, and this area needs further empirical research.

Contributors: HA, GN, and AGKE conducted the searches and reviewed the papers that informed this article. HA and HW wrote the first draft.

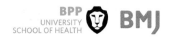

All authors helped critically revise the article and form the final draft. AGKE is guarantor.

Competing interests: All authors have completed the ICMJE uniform disclosure form at www.icmje.org/coi_disclosure.pdf (available on request from the corresponding author) and declare: no support from any organisation for the submitted work; no financial relationships with any organisations that might have an interest in the submitted work in the previous three years, AGKE has been involved in the development of the decision aids cited (Prosdex and Bresdex), which are hosted by Cardiff University on a not for profit basis and are publicly available.

Provenance and peer review: Commissioned; externally peer reviewed.

1 Edwards A, Elwyn G. Understanding risk and lessons for clinical risk communication about treatment preferences. *Qual Health Care* 2001;10(suppl 1):i9-13.
2 Ahl AS, Acree JA, Gipson PS, McDowell RM, Miller L, McElvaine MD. Standardization of nomenclature for animal health risk analysis. *Rev Sci Tech* 1993;12:1045-53.
3 Edwards A. Risk communication. In: Edwards A, Elwyn G, eds. Shared decision making in health care: achieving evidence-based patient choice. 2nd ed: Oxford University Press, 2009:135-42.
4 Brewer NT. Goals. In: Fischhoff B, Brewer NT, Downs JS, eds. Communicating risks and benefits: an evidence-based user's guide. US Department of Health and Human Services, Food and Drug Administration, 2011:3-10.
5 Weinstein ND, Klein WM. Resistance of personal risk perceptions to debiasing interventions. *Health Psychol* 1995;14:132-40.
6 Brewer NT, Chapman GB, Gibbons FX, Gerrard M, McCaul KD, Weinstein ND. Meta-analysis of the relationship between risk perception and health behavior: the example of vaccination. *Health Psychol* 2007;26:136-45.
7 How much do we know? *BMJ Clin Evidence* http://ncims.com/articles/HWClinical%20Evidence.pdf.
8 Lipkus IM. Numeric, verbal, and visual formats of conveying health risks: suggested best practices and future recommendations. *Med Decis Making* 2007;27:696-713.
9 Waldron C-A, van der Weijden T, Ludt S, Gallacher J, Elwyn G. What are effective strategies to communicate cardiovascular risk information to patients? A systematic review. *Patient Educ Couns* 2011;82:169-81.
10 Neuner-Jehle S, Senn O, Wegwarth O, Rosemann T, Steurer J. How do family physicians communicate about cardiovascular risk? Frequencies and determinants of different communication formats. *BMC Fam Pract* 2011;12:15.
11 Wegwarth O, Gigerenzer G. "There is nothing to worry about": gynecologists' counseling on mammography. *Patient Educ Couns* 2011;84:251-6.
12 Gigerenzer G, Gaissmaier W, Kurz-Milcke E, Schwartz LM, Woloshin S. Helping doctors and patients make sense of health statistics. *Psychol Sci Public Interest* 2007;8:53-96.
13 Gigerenzer G. How innumeracy can be exploited. In: Reckoning with risk—learning to live with uncertainty. 1st ed. Penguin Press, 2002:201-10.
14 Lipkus IM, Samsa G, Rimmer BK. General performance on a numeracy scale among highly educated samples. *Med Decis Making* 2001;21:37-44.
15 Moyer VA. What we don't know can hurt our patients: physician innumeracy and overuse of screening tests. *Ann Intern Med* 2012;156:392-3.
16 Edwards A, Elwyn G, Covey J, Matthews E, Pill R. Presenting risk information—a review of the effects of "framing" and other manipulations on patient outcomes. *J Health Commun* 2001;6:61-82.
17 Akl EA, Oxman AD, Herrin J, Vist GE, Terrenato I, Sperati F, et al. Framing of health information messages. *Cochrane Database Syst Rev* 2011;12:CD006777.
18 Gotzsche PC, Nielsen M. Screening for breast cancer with mammography. *Cochrane Database Syst Rev* 2011;1:CD001877.
19 Gotzsche PC, Hartling OJ, Nielsen M, Brodersen J. Screening for breast cancer with mammography. Nordic Cochrane Centre, 2012. http://www.cochrane.dk/screening/mammography-leaflet.pdf.
20 Fagerlin A, Zikmund-Fisher BJ, Ubel PA. Helping patients decide: ten steps to better risk communication. *J Natl Cancer Inst* 2011;103:1436-43.
21 Akl EA, Oxman AD, Herrin J, Vist GE, Terrenato I, Sperati F, et al. Using alternative statistical formats for presenting risks and risk reductions. *Cochrane Database Syst Rev* 2011;3:CD006776.
22 Edwards AG, Evans R, Dundon J, Haigh S, Hood K, Elwyn GJ. Personalised risk communication for informed decision making about taking screening tests. *Cochrane Database Syst Rev* 2006;4:CD001865.
23 Smith SK, Trevena L, Simpson JM, Barratt A, Nutbeam D, McCaffery KJ. A decision aid to support informed choices about bowel cancer screening among adults with low education: randomised controlled trial. *BMJ* 2010;341:c5370.
24 Steckelberg A, Hulfenhaus C, Haastert B, Muhlhauser I. Effect of evidence based risk information on "informed choice" in colorectal cancer screening: randomised controlled trial. *BMJ* 2011;342:d3193.
25 Nagle C, Gunn J, Bell R, Lewis S, Meiser B, Metcalfe S, et al. Use of a decision aid for prenatal testing of fetal abnormalities to improve women's informed decision making: a cluster randomised controlled trial (ISRCTN22532458). *BJOG* 2008;115:339-47.
26 Gigerenzer G. What are natural frequencies? *BMJ* 2011;343:d6386.
27 Gigerenzer G, Galesic M. Why do single event probabilities confuse patients? *BMJ* 2012;344:e245.
28 Stacey D, Bennett CL, Barry MJ, Col NF, Eden KB, Holmes-Rovner M, et al. Decision aids for people facing health treatment or screening decisions. *Cochrane Database Syst Rev* 2011;1:CD001431.
29 Legare F, Ratte S, Stacey D, Kryworuchko J, Gravel K, Graham ID, et al. Interventions for improving the adoption of shared decision making by healthcare professionals. *Cochrane Database Syst Rev* 2010;5:CD006732.
30 Politi MC, Han PK, Col NF. Communicating the uncertainty of harms and benefits of medical interventions. *Med Decis Making* 2007;27:681-95.
31 Portnoy DB, Han PK, Ferrer RA, Klein WM, Clauser SB. Physicians' attitudes about communicating and managing scientific uncertainty differ by perceived ambiguity aversion of their patients. *Health Expect* 2011; published online 12 August.
32 Schwartz LM, Woloshin S. Communicating uncertainties about prescription drugs to the public: a national randomized trial. *Arch Intern Med* 2011;171:1463-8.
33 Politi MC, Clark MA, Ombao H, Dizon D, Elwyn G. Communicating uncertainty can lead to less decision satisfaction: a necessary cost of involving patients in shared decision making? *Health Expect* 2011;14:84-91.

More titles in
The BMJ Series

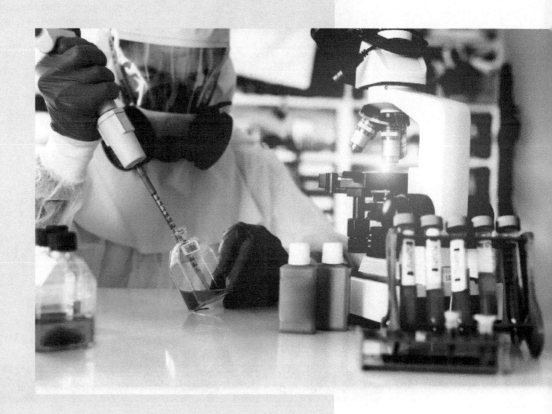

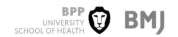
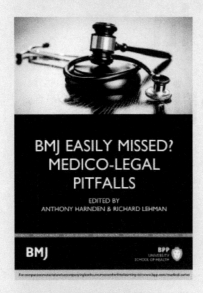
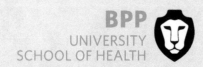

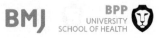
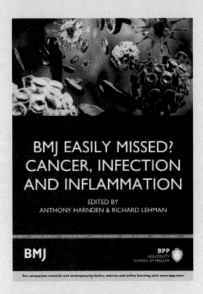
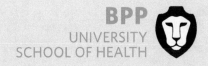

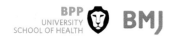

More titles in The BMJ Research Methods and Reporting Series

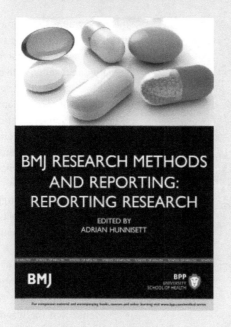

BMJ RESEARCH METHODS AND REPORTING: REPORTING RESEARCH

EDITED BY
ADRIAN HUNNISETT

This book is the third of three volumes drawing together a collection of articles previously published in the BMJ covering contemporary issues in research. In this volume, the articles give key messages about the 'nuts and bolts' of doing research, particularly with reference to how research findings should be reported. Each article also provides linked information and explicit evidence to support the statements made. The topics covered take a look at guidelines such as CONSORT, SPIRIT, GPP2, PRISMA and the IDEAL framework for surgical innovation. It also gives some guidance on economic evaluations, policy and service interventions and publication guidelines, as well as providing useful tips on preparing data for publication. Each article is written by an expert in the field and the volume brings together a masterclass in research reporting.

£29.99
February 2016
Paperback
978-1-472745-57-6

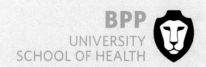

BPP
UNIVERSITY
SCHOOL OF HEALTH

www.bpp.com/medical-series

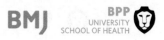
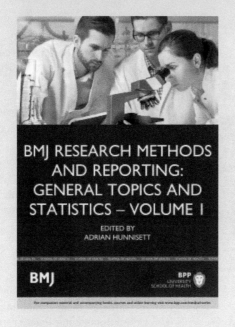
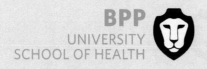

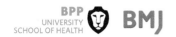
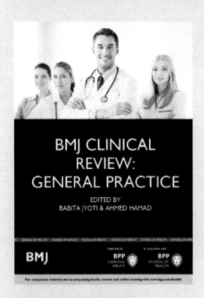
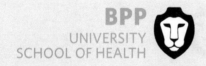

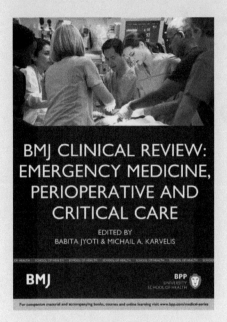
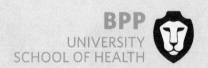

More titles from BPP School of Health

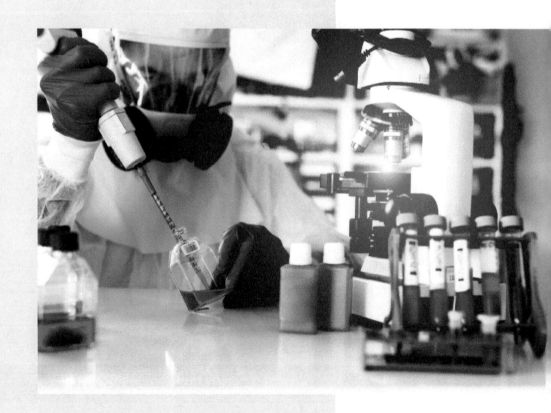

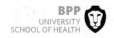

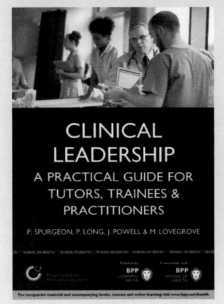
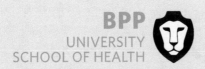

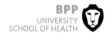

More titles in The Progressing Your Medical Career Series

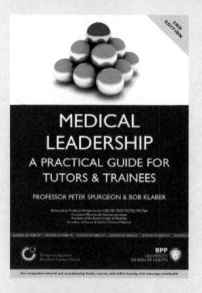

£19.99

April 2016

Paperback

9781-472745-59-0

Are you a doctor or medical student who wishes to acquire and develop your leadership and management skills? Do you recognise the role and influence of strong leadership and management in modern medicine?

Clinical leadership is something in which all doctors should have an important role in terms of driving forward high quality care for their patients. In this up-to-date guide Peter Spurgeon and Robert Klaber take you through the latest leadership and management thinking, and how this links in with the Medical Leadership Competency Framework. As well as influencing undergraduate curricula and some of the concepts underpinning revalidation, this framework forms the basis of the leadership component of the curricula for all medical specialties, so a practical knowledge of it is essential for all doctors in training.

Using case studies and practical exercises to provide a strong work-based emphasis, this practical guide will enable you to build on your existing experiences to develop your leadership and management skills, and to develop strategies and approaches to improving care for your patients.

This book addresses:

- Why strong leadership and management are crucial to delivering high quality care

- The theory and evidence behind the Medical Leadership Competency Framework

- The practical aspects of leadership learning in a wide range of clinical environments (eg handover, EM, ward etc)

- How Consultants and trainers can best facilitate leadership learning for their trainees and students within the clinical work-place

Whether you are a medical student just starting out on your career, or an established doctor wishing to develop yourself as a clinical leader, this practical, easy-to-use guide will give you the techniques and knowledge you require to excel.

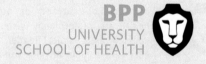

www.bpp.com/medical-series

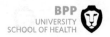
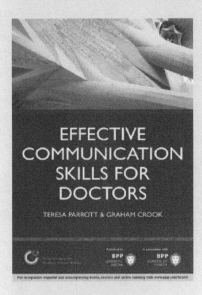
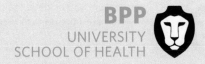

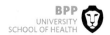
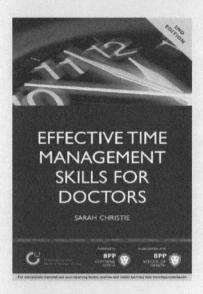
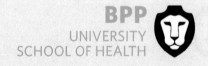

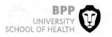
More titles in The Progressing Your Medical Career Series

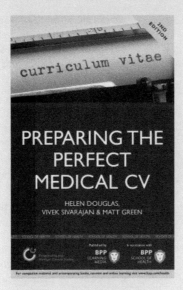

£19.99

October 2011

Paperback

978-1-445381-62-6

Are you unsure of how to structure your Medical CV? Would you like to know how to ensure you stand out from the crowd?

With competition for medical posts at an all time high it is vital that your Medical CV stands out over your fellow applicants. This comprehensive, unique and easy-to-read guide has been written with this in mind to help prospective medical students, current medical students and doctors of all grades prepare a Medical CV of the highest quality. Whether you are applying to medical school, currently completing your medical degree or a doctor progressing through your career (foundation doctor, specialty trainee in general practice, surgery or medicine, GP career grade or Consultant) this guide includes specific guidance for applicants at every level.

This time-saving and detailed guide:

- Explains what selection panels are looking for when reviewing applications at all levels.

- Discusses how to structure your Medical CV to ensure you stand out for the right reasons.

- Explores what information to include (and not to include) in your CV.

- Covers what to consider when maintaining a portfolio at every step of your career, including, for revalidation and relicensing purposes.

- Provides examples of high quality CVs to illustrate the above.

This unique guide will show you how to prepare your CV for every step of your medical career from pre-Medical School right through to Consultant level and should be a constant companion to ensure you secure your first choice post every time.

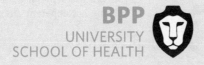

www.bpp.com/medical-series

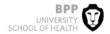
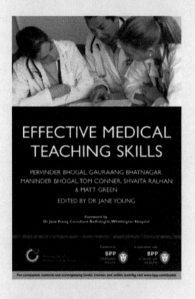
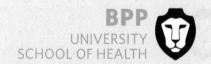

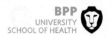
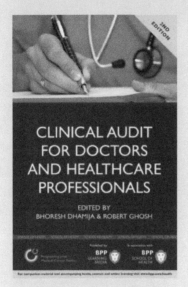
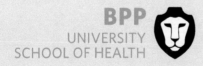

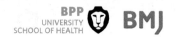